Olena Berezovska

Hormonal Intelligence:

How Hormones Shape Health and Well-being

International Academy of Healthy Life

2025

Hormonal Intelligence: How Hormones Shape Health and Well-being

Olena Berezovska

ISBN 978-1-0691603-8-6

p. 478

Published by the International Academy of Healthy Life

Hormonal Intelligence is a comprehensive guide to understanding how hormones influence every aspect of human health—physically, emotionally, and mentally. Drawing on decades of clinical experience and scientific research, Dr. Olena Berezovska walks readers through the intricate workings of the endocrine system, explaining how hormones are produced and regulated and how imbalances can affect everything from menstruation and pregnancy to mood, skin, and sexual health. She addresses common myths, misconceptions, and modern trends in hormone-related diagnostics and treatment with clarity and compassion, offering reliable, evidence-based insights for healthcare professionals and curious readers alike.

Beyond textbook definitions, this book explores how hormones interact with lifestyle, nutrition, stress, and aging. From childhood to menopause, from love and desire to depression and cancer risk, *Hormonal Intelligence* offers an accessible and nuanced understanding of the silent chemical messengers that govern well-being. Every chapter is firmly grounded in real-world relevance, helping readers understand the practical implications of their hormonal health.

Printed in Canada

CONTENTS

CONTENTS

Introduction

Dear Friends,

I am delighted to welcome you to the pages of my new book! Your interest in this topic is crucial, as understanding hormones is not just a personal journey, but a collective one. If the title caught your attention, you've already guessed that this work is dedicated to hormones — especially their profound impact on women's lives.

Why a book about hormones? Hasn't enough already been written and said on the topic? You're right! Hormones have been the subject of hundreds of articles, books, and films. However, amidst this wealth of information, there is a need for clarity. The topic of hormones remains not only relevant but also highly popular. However, this widespread attention has led to a flood of misinformation — rumors, myths, and even the misuse of hormones despite their potential side effects.

Hormones play a crucial role in human health, but their influence is even more pronounced for women. Hormonal fluctuations occur not only with age but also during pregnancy, breastfeeding, and the use of hormonal contraceptives, all of which can significantly impact a woman's well-being. This book focuses on the intricate relationship between hormones and women's health.

Are hormones our allies or adversaries? Which ones pose risks, and which are essential for balance? How many hormones does the human body produce? What does it mean when a hormone level is "high" or "low," and should it permanently be corrected? Can diet influence hormone levels? Should hormones be taken during pregnancy? Is there a link between hormones and cancer?

These are just a few pressing questions I will answer in the pages ahead. I am excited to embark on this journey with you, to separate fact from fiction and explore the fascinating world of hormones together.

Happy reading!

Chapter 1: Introduction to Hormones

Imagine the impact of a single word, spoken for the first time in 1905, that completely transformed our understanding of the human body. That word, as you might have guessed, is **'hormone '**.

On July 20, 1905, a group of brilliant minds, including English physiologist Ernest Starling, a professor at the University of London, came together to publicly introduce the term *'hormone '*. This word, derived from the Greek meaning *'to excite* or *to stimulate '*, emerged during a lunchtime discussion in Cambridge, where these pioneers debated how to describe certain mysterious substances already recognized by chemists and physicians.

This conversation sparked a new way of thinking about bodily functions, leading Starling to describe these chemical messengers in his landmark lecture, "Chemical Control of Body Functioning." He explained that these substances were produced by one organ, traveled through the bloodstream, and influenced target organs elsewhere in the body. Though he wasn't referring to any specific hormone then, his definition paved the way for groundbreaking research.

The first hormone had been discovered a decade earlier. In 1894, English researchers George Oliver and Edward Schäfer, along with Polish physiologist Napoleon Cybulski, independently identified a substance now known as **epinephrine** (adrenaline). This hormone, originally described as *'the primary substance of the adrenal glands that increases blood pressure,' plays a crucial role in the*

12

body's fight-or-flight response. Jokichi Takamine, an American scientist of Japanese origin, later determined its chemical structure. This marked the true beginning of hormone research and the rise of endocrinology.

Following adrenaline, other hormones were identified, including **secretin, thyroxine**, and **insulin**. By 1923, four hormones had been formally recognized, laying the foundation for the expanding study of hormonal science.

Even today, over a century of research later, we are still uncovering new complexities about these powerful chemical messengers. While we have unraveled much about their functions, hormones remain one of the most intricate and fascinating aspects of biology, challenging scientists with new discoveries and mysteries yet to be solved.

1.1. What Hormones Are

Over a century ago, even without knowing the names of hormones or understanding their origins, quantities, or forms, scientists recognized their role as *messengers* — chemical signals that travel from one part of the body to another, regulating vital functions.

The concept of chemical messengers was not new in the early 20th century. As early as the 19th century, scientists had hypothesized the existence of substances that facilitated communication between cells and tissues in humans and animals. These ideas stemmed from experiments in which extracts from the thyroid, adrenal glands, testes, and pancreas of animals were introduced into humans, primarily as treatments for various illnesses. These extracts were often called "*elixirs of life*" or "*youth tonics.*" When these treatments proved effective, researchers inferred that they contained substances missing in the patient's body — a concept that later formed the basis of **hormonal deficiency disorders.**

Historical observations of hormonal imbalance have been striking, though often made in vastly different contexts. One such example, deeply rooted in the past, comes from the 16th to 18th centuries when castrati singers gained widespread fame in European theaters. These were young boys, primarily from low-income families or orphans, who were sold into the possession of theaters and castrated before puberty to preserve their exceptionally high-pitched voices, often described as "angelic." The weight of this historical context is palpable, inviting us to explore the implications of this practice.

The absence of male sex hormones profoundly altered their development, resulting in elongated limbs, unusually developed ribcages, and a lack of typical male characteristics. This profound alteration, exemplified by the singers, underscores the significant impact of hormonal imbalance on human development. It provides early — albeit crude — evidence that specific organs produce substances capable of shaping physiology. One of the most renowned castrati, Farinelli, famously sang lullabies for the King of Spain. His portrait now hangs in Handel's house, a lasting reminder of this unusual historical practice.

Today, we know that the human body produces approximately 50 hormones. The list would be two to three times longer if we included

their metabolites—compounds that retain some hormonal activity.

Based on their chemical structure, hormones are categorized into four main groups:

- Amines

- Proteins and Peptides (amino acid derivatives)

- Steroids (cholesterol derivatives)

- Fatty acid derivatives

In addition to natural hormones produced by the body, scientists have developed hundreds, if not thousands, of synthetic hormones that mimic natural hormonal activity. These artificial hormones, such as birth control pills, hormone replacement therapy drugs, and corticosteroids, are widely used in hormonal contraception, hormone replacement therapy, and treatments for various diseases, significantly expanding how hormones can be harnessed for medical purposes.

1.2.   What Role Do Hormones Play?

There is virtually no organ, system, or essential biological process in the human body that functions independently of hormones. From metabolism, puberty, and reproduction to aging, adaptation, and survival, hormones govern nearly every aspect of life.

Since hormones have numerous and diverse effects, compiling a complete list of their influence on different organs and tissues would be extensive. Instead, we will examine each hormone individually to provide a clear understanding of its role in the body.

More precisely, hormones act through a complex network of direct and feedback communication between the endocrine glands, which produce them, and the nervous system, which regulates their release and function. Hormonal feedback is a crucial mechanism that helps maintain hormonal balance. The same hormone can have different effects depending on a person's age, physiological state, or health condition.

For example, prolactin:

- In pregnant women, it stimulates the mammary glands to produce milk.

- In non-pregnant women, high prolactin levels can inhibit the maturation of reproductive cells, affecting fertility.

Interestingly, the structure and function of hormones are nearly identical across most animals, though some variations exist. This underscores their fundamental role in the biological world, shaping human health and the development and survival of countless species.

1.3. Where Are Hormones Produced?

Hormones are primarily produced in endocrine glands. However, the term' endocrine gland' is somewhat conditional. For instance, if we look at the sequence of processes in the ovary, the first phase of the menstrual cycle is entirely focused on the maturation of the reproductive cell. During this period, most of the hormones produced by the ovary are used within the ovary itself, demonstrating its *paracrine function*. This means that the hormones produced by the ovary act locally, influencing the function of nearby cells or tissues, rather than being released into the bloodstream to act on distant cells.

In the second phase, the ovary's function shifts to *endocrine activity*, producing hormones necessary for the implantation of a fertilized egg and the development of pregnancy. At this stage, most of the hormones produced by the ovary enter the bloodstream and circulate throughout the body, primarily to support the uterus and mammary glands.

Thus, some organs that produce hormones utilize them both internally and systemically.

The most important endocrine glands include:

- **The hypothalamic-pituitary system**
- **The thyroid gland**
- **The parathyroid glands**
- **The pancreas**
- **The adrenal glands**
- **The gonads (ovaries and testes)**

The synthesis of any human hormone follows a specific natural sequence. First, signals are sent to the brain, indicating a deficiency of a particular hormone, typically from the tissues that rely on it. As the control center, the brain sends a signal to the pituitary gland, a small gland located at the base of the brain. This signal may pass through various structural units of the central nervous system before reaching the pituitary. The pituitary gland, often referred to as the **'master gland**,' then produces hormones that stimulate other endocrine glands located on the periphery, far from the brain. Once they receive the command, these glands utilize raw materials delivered via the bloodstream to produce the required hormone. The hormone is then transported through the blood and other bodily fluids to the tissues that initially signaled the demand.

In other words, hormone production regulation resembles a consumer-producer relationship, managed by centralized control, with specific methods of transmitting information and transporting the "product." However, some systems exhibit a degree of autonomy from the hypothalamic-pituitary system.

1.4. How Are Hormones Absorbed?

The production and absorption of hormones occur in several stages. The glands that produce hormones always maintain a reserve supply, acting as storage units. This means that **as long as an endocrine gland or tissue exists, the body will always have a certain level of hormones**. Moreover, **the production of the same hormone can occur in multiple parts of the body, not just in a single gland.** This serves as a compensatory mechanism in case an endocrine gland is damaged, showcasing the body's remarkable adaptability. However, internal mechanisms cannot compensate for all gland functions.

The next stage is the transportation of hormones to **target cells** (target tissues or organs). Most hormones bind to proteins, traveling through the bloodstream in a bound form. This binding neutralizes their effects, preventing hormones from acting too aggressively or negatively on organs. We will delve deeper into this aspect when we cover steroid hormones, as hormone-binding proteins play a crucial role in regulating hormone effects.

Target cells have special receptors on their surface — essentially lock-and-key mechanisms — that recognize the hormone molecule as a "key." When a hormone binds to its receptor, it triggers a cellular response, prompting the cell to produce the necessary substances or reactions.

The amount of hormones produced in the human body is small, as are the ranges of their normal levels. However, the reference values laboratories use to assess hormone levels are based on statistical averages, representing most people in a specific region. When interpreting these values, it is also important to consider age, pregnancy, and individual health conditions. This emphasis on individual health conditions empowers individuals to take control of their health, as hormonal norms vary significantly among individuals.

1.5.   Should Hormone Levels Be Tested?

I often hear women talk about "hormonal imbalances" frequently as an explanation for menstrual cycle irregularities. Remember that neither "*hormonal imbalance*" nor "*menstrual cycle irregularity*" is a diagnosis! A menstrual cycle irregularity is merely a symptom (a sign) and does not indicate a specific illness. We'll discuss the menstrual cycle in a separate chapter.

The concept of a "hormonal imbalance" is medically absurd. Which hormone, exactly, is out of balance? The human body produces around 50 different hormones, so they can't be out of balance simultaneously. Yet, women are often sent for extensive hormone panels, many of which are unrelated to their specific problems and frequently show results within normal ranges.

We do not treat hormone levels. We treat diseases! For instance, we treat conditions like diabetes, thyroid disorders, and adrenal insufficiency. **A diagnosis cannot be made based on the level of a single hormone.**

Endocrine diseases, which are caused by dysfunctions of the endocrine glands, present a complex puzzle for diagnosis. Achieving an accurate diagnosis can be a time-consuming process, often requiring months of testing and observation.

Key points to understand about interpreting hormone tests:

- Reference values (normal ranges) are relative and depend on the test, region, and country.

- Sex and age must be considered.

- Pregnancy status must also be considered.

- Hormone levels may be reported in different units of measurement, which can vary even within the same country or city and may not align with international standards.

Testing hormone levels has become a trend in commercial medicine. The once-popular saying, "Nerves cause all diseases," has now been replaced with "*Hormones cause all diseases.*" Add to this the myths about "poor immunity" and various genetic mutations, and suddenly, it seems like healthy people don't exist.

But this is not true! While the health industry claims to focus on human well-being, it has increasingly transformed into an industry of illness. Walking out of a doctor's office with a diagnosis of "healthy" has somehow become awkward and unacceptable — for both doctors and patients.

When assessing any health complaints or symptoms, it is crucial not to exaggerate minor issues while overlooking more significant ones. Endocrinology, the study of hormones and related disorders, has long been treated as secondary in medical education, receiving far fewer teaching hours than other specialties. Until recently, endocrinology was one of the least popular fields, and even among obstetricians-gynecologists, only a few specialize in female endocrinology. Even fewer endocrinologists deeply understand women's hormonal health, let alone the hormonal changes that occur during pregnancy.

Over the past two decades, the medical landscape has evolved significantly. The once-prevailing belief that 'All diseases are caused by nerves' has fallen out of favor, particularly as nerve-related conditions are notoriously difficult to treat. The hyper-marketing of antidepressants in developed countries has become the de facto 'treatment' for all nerve-related diseases.

At the same time, life expectancy has increased dramatically. In some countries, a third of the population is now of retirement age. Modern retirees often lead active lives, travel, and pay closer attention to their health. Slowing the aging process has become fashionable, with many aiming to live 100 years or more.

Hormones have been used not only as experimental treatments but also in quackery for centuries, even when their nature and role were utterly unknown. Think of the age-old "*elixirs of youth*" and "*elixirs of life.*" Today, in the internet era, where even the most deceptive advertising can spread instantly, a renewed interest in hormones has surged. Catchphrases like "All diseases are caused by hormones" and "Hormones cure all diseases" have become tools for manipulation, playing on people's desire to be forever young, healthy, and yet, paradoxically, constantly "sick."

This creates a vicious cycle:

- Feeling well? Don't trust it! Poor ecology, stress, and other modern horrors make proper health impossible. Check your hormones!

- Hormones are normal? Please don't believe it. Problems often lurk undetected. Dig deeper. Even if everything seems fine, start preventive treatment against future deficiencies, aging, or countless diseases.

- Feeling unwell? It must be due to hormonal imbalances. After all, every single process in the body depends on hormones.

Hormones play a crucial role in regulating metabolism, growth, and development and maintaining the balance of other bodily functions. However, it's important to remember that not every health issue is due to a hormonal imbalance. Fear of illness and aging are closely linked but also provide

fertile ground for the rapid rise of excessive testing and unjustified treatments for false diagnoses.

This book is not designed to instill fear. Instead, it aims to provide you with the unvarnished truth about what modern, evidence-based medicine knows regarding hormones and endocrine diseases.

Understand this: it's not all bad!

Many women try to address their health issues independently, which is not inherently wrong. Most of us want answers to questions like:

- "What's happening to me?"

- "Is this dangerous for my health?"

- "Should I see a doctor?"

With medical services becoming increasingly expensive and often not covered by insurance (or unaffordable for those without insurance), many women prefer to undergo testing on their own before consulting a doctor. However, it's important to remember that self-diagnosis and treatment can be risky. **If you're experiencing persistent or severe symptoms, it's best to consult a healthcare professional for a proper diagnosis and treatment plan.**

You can waste a great deal of time and money on unnecessary tests for diseases you do not have and likely never will. Globally, it is standard practice for a doctor to determine which tests are necessary based on your complaints, symptoms, and medical history. The doctor's role is to suspect a disease, make a preliminary diagnosis, and explain the rationale for specific tests. If your doctor suggests monitoring the situation for a few weeks or months, it does not mean they are wrong. On the contrary, it may be the most reasonable course of action. Trusting your doctor's judgment can give you confidence and security in your medical journey.

Rushing to find problems or ordering tests based on trends can lead to false conclusions, unnecessary treatments, and even harm. **Every test must have a clear medical justification, and every diagnostic method must be validated.** There should be no 'just in case' checks. It's crucial to be cautious and aware of the potential harm that unnecessary tests can bring.

Serious diseases exist, but not everyone is at the same risk of developing them. One woman may have a higher likelihood of a specific condition, while another may have a much lower risk — everything is individual. **Understanding individual health risks should reassure you that your unique situation is being considered. No one can suffer from every possible disease, even the most dangerous ones.** Likewise, no one develops all the 'trendy' conditions that seem to be diagnosed everywhere today.

The rise of "*commercial diagnoses*" imposed for profit does not reflect the actual prevalence of diseases. That is why it is essential to carefully assess whether hormone testing is necessary, especially without clear clinical indications.

There is no "*within normal limits, but still abnormal.*" This misleading claim is often used to scare patients into spending money. Statements like, "Your hormone level is within the lower (or upper) range of normal, but that's bad and needs to be corrected," come from non-professionals. **Normal is normal, and it should not be manipulated.**

What if a test result slightly deviates from the reference range? For example, if a hormone level is measured at 3.3 in specific units, but the laboratory defines anything above 3.2 as abnormal — is this a real problem? No. It might be entirely normal for that individual. It could be a laboratory error. It could be a random fluctuation — after all, **the substances in our bodies are dynamic, constantly changing from day to day, month to month, and year to year, even in the same person. Isolated lab results hold no practical significance without evaluating symptoms and clinical complaints.**

Testing should be necessary, reasonable, and not excessive. There is no benefit in checking every possible hormone level or undergoing a battery of unnecessary analyses. **If you take 1,000 tests, at least 10% of the results will show minor deviations from the reference range simply because every individual is unique, and physiological norms vary.** Understanding this will help you approach hormone testing rationally and avoid unnecessary medical interventions.

Chapter 2. Endocrine Glands

This chapter will discuss the most important **endocrine glands** and their significance for the human body.

2.1. The Hypothalamus

The hypothalamus is one of the oldest (and smallest) brain parts and plays a vital role in human life. This part of the brain weighs only 4 grams compared to the 1,400 grams of the entire brain. Its structure is unique, with many nerve fibers as well as cells that produce several types of hormones.

The hypothalamus is responsible for the most essential life functions:

- Energy metabolism
- Metabolic exchange and control
- Nutrition and gastrointestinal function
- Water-salt balance and electrolyte regulation
- Body temperature regulation
- Energy and nutrient storage
- Regulation of sleep and wake cycles
- Reproductive function (maturation of sex cells, pregnancy, lactation)
- Breastfeeding
- Stress response

These points could be further detailed, but one conclusion is clear — this is an essential endocrine gland.

The hypothalamus is conventionally divided into three parts, each with different functions. Based on the structure of the cells, there are three systems of endocrine or hormonal action. Some neurons produce hormones, such as oxytocin and vasopressin, which travel through blood vessels to the posterior part of another crucial gland — the pituitary gland, where they are distributed to the entire body when needed.

Other *neuroendocrine cells* have direct contact with the pituitary and stimulate or suppress the production of pituitary hormones. *Gonadotropin-releasing hormones* are an example of this.

The third group of cells is involved in the independent (autonomous) control of hormone production in other organs, such as insulin production by the pancreas.

The hypothalamus, a key player in the brain's limbic system, is not just a regulator of bodily functions. It also plays a significant role in the formation of emotions, working in tandem with the **amygdala**. This link to our emotional experiences makes the study of the hypothalamus even more intriguing.

Let's now take a closer look at the main hormones produced by the hypothalamus:

HORMONE NAME	ROLE	DEFICIENCY	EXCESS
Thyrotropin-releasing hormone	Stimulates production of thyroid-stimulating	Thyroid dysfunction	No known cases of excess

(TRH)	hormone (thyrotropin) and partially influences prolactin production		
Gonadotropin-releasing hormone (GnRH)	Initiates puberty and stimulates gonadotropin production by the pituitary	Intense physical exertion, starvation (anorexia)	Rare hypothalamic-pituitary tumors causing excess testosterone and estrogen production
Growth hormone-releasing hormone (GHRH)	Controls the production of growth hormone	Growth delay, stunted physical development, reduced muscle mass, increased fat accumulation	Hypothalamic tumors may cause pituitary enlargement, acromegaly, diabetes, high blood pressure, gigantism
Corticotropin-releasing hormone (CRH)	Controls production of adrenocorticotropic hormone; also produced by the placenta, influencing pregnancy duration	Alzheimer's disease, chronic fatigue syndrome, placental deficiency leading to pregnancy loss	Depression, anorexia, insomnia, exacerbation of autoimmune diseases
Somatostatin	Inhibits production of thyroid-stimulating hormone and growth hormone;	Insufficient data	Somatostatinoma tumor, diabetes, gallstone formation

	also produced by the pancreas		
Dopamine (Prolactin-inhibiting hormone)	Inhibits prolactin production, regulates motor function centers	Parkinson's disease	Conflicting data
Vasopressin (Antidiuretic hormone, ADH)	Regulates kidney function and urine production	Excessive urine output, leading to diabetes insipidus	Water retention, low sodium levels (hyponatremia)
Oxytocin	Stimulates uterine contractions during labor, promotes milk production in response to nursing, strengthens maternal-infant bonding	Unknown	Benign prostatic hyperplasia

Releasing hormones are also often referred to as releasing factors or *liberins*. All of them are protein-based substances. In the animal kingdom, three types of *gonadotropin-releasing hormones* (GnRH) have been identified, and human GnRH is 85% identical to those found in many mammals.

The examination of the hypothalamus and its hormone production, though rarely performed, holds immense significance. These hormones are not just involved in numerous physiological processes, but they also play multiple crucial roles in regulating bodily functions simultaneously.

It is crucial to note that synthetic analogs of these hormones play a pivotal role in treating various medical conditions. Most commonly, gonadotropin-releasing hormone agonists are employed in the treatment of infertility, prostate cancer, and both congenital and acquired hormone deficiencies. Oxytocin is widely used during and after childbirth to enhance uterine contractions, while vasopressin is utilized in the treatment of diabetes insipidus. Dopamine has proven effective in managing different types of shock; however, due to its numerous side effects, its dosage must be carefully controlled.

2.1.1. Does Hypothalamic Disease Exist?

Given the hypothalamus's crucial role in regulating numerous bodily functions, could there be a distinct condition known as hypothalamic disease?

In medical practice, hypothalamic disease is typically discussed in the context of physical trauma that damages specific areas of the hypothalamus. Since this part of the brain regulates multiple physiological processes, hormone production deficiencies can manifest in many symptoms. These symptoms, numbering over a hundred, can include insomnia, fatigue, infertility, menstrual irregularities, and thyroid dysfunction, among others. Many of these symptoms overlap with disorders of the endocrine organs under hypothalamic control, making diagnosis a complex and intricate process that requires thoroughness and attention to detail.

Because the pituitary gland is closely linked to the hypothalamus, hormonal dysfunctions often affect both structures. Assessing the extent of hypothalamic damage can be particularly challenging, underscoring the importance of a detailed medical history, including past head injuries or brain surgeries. This comprehensive patient assessment is crucial in diagnosing conditions that are frequently classified as **hypothalamic-pituitary disorders** rather than isolated hypothalamic diseases.

Thus, while hypothalamic dysfunction does exist, it is a rare and often overlooked diagnosis in clinical practice. This underscores the need for vigilance and a high level of suspicion when dealing with complex cases that may involve the hypothalamus.

2.1.2. Oxytocin — The Hormone of Love?

In recent years, medical conferences on endocrinology have increasingly focused on menopause, diabetes, and thyroid disorders — conditions that have become remarkably prevalent. However, oxytocin, a hormone widely used in obstetrics worldwide, has also attracted significant scientific interest.

Biologist Sue Carter, director of the Kinsey Institute at Indiana University, has devoted extensive research to the effects of oxytocin administered during labor on child development. Her work has made her one of the most sought-after speakers in recent years. Dr. Carter is not the first scientist to express concerns about the potential behavioral effects of oxytocin in animals and humans or question its widespread use in obstetrics. She has demonstrated with her colleagues that oxytocin, often called the "hormone of maternal love", is crucial in forming long-term monogamous bonds, fostering maternal instincts, and regulating aggressive behavior.

Recent studies have explored oxytocin's influence on child development, particularly its role in shaping human behavior from the prenatal period onward (epigenetic effects of oxytocin). While early research suggested that oxytocin does not cross the blood-brain barrier, newer findings indicate otherwise, showing that it directly affects the brain. However, the precise mechanisms of this influence remain poorly understood.

Scientists have identified that the gene responsible for oxytocin receptor function (the **oxytocin receptor gene**) in children is activated by three key factors: the process of childbirth itself, maternal behavior, and externally administered oxytocin (as a medication). Naturally elevated oxytocin levels during labor do not negatively impact the child. However, the administration of high doses of oxytocin to induce or accelerate labor, often without sufficient medical justification, can have long-term effects on the *social brain* of the child, the brain regions responsible for social behavior and interpersonal relationships. This underscores the need for a more cautious approach to oxytocin use in obstetrics.

Neuroendocrine research on oxytocin's effects on the human brain remains a relatively new but rapidly evolving field in evidence-based medicine. However, emerging data already compel forward-thinking physicians to reassess medical interventions during childbirth. Are these interventions excessive? Is the modern approach to labor too aggressive toward women? Could the increasing prevalence of behavioral disorders, including autism and anorexia (as proposed by Michel Odent, a French obstetrician and childbirth specialist), be linked to the overuse of medications, particularly steroid hormones and oxytocin?

These and many other pressing questions require an urgent and critical reassessment of long-standing beliefs about pregnancy and childbirth. The time to act is now, as we need to reassess our practices and make necessary changes to ensure the safety and well-being of our patients.

2.2. The Pituitary Gland

For centuries, the pituitary gland remained a mystery, yet its significance was noted as early as 1365 BCE when an Egyptian pharaoh described acromegaly — a condition caused by excessive growth hormone. The Greek physician and philosopher Galen, who also discovered pulmonary circulation, was the first to describe the structure of the pituitary gland in 150 CE. His belief that the gland pumped fluid (phlegm) from the brain to the nasopharynx marked a significant step in our understanding of this vital organ.

By the early 18th century, physicians had identified conditions such as **amenorrhea** (absence of menstrual cycles), **acromegaly** (widening and thickening of facial bones), and **diabetes insipidus**. Efforts to understand these disorders led to surgical attempts to remove the pituitary gland. The first transsphenoidal surgery, accessing the gland through the sphenoid bone of the skull, was performed in 1907 by Austrian neurosurgeon Hermann Schloffer. Later, between 1910 and 1925, American physician Harvey Cushing performed over 200 similar procedures, further advancing pituitary surgery.

The pituitary gland, a marvel of nature, is located at the base of the brain within a bony cavity called the **sella turcica** (Latin for "*Turkish saddle*"). This unique name is derived from the distinctive shape of traditional Turkish saddles, which resemble this anatomical structure. The use of such descriptive names by anatomists in the past adds an intriguing layer to the study of human anatomy.

The pituitary gland measures 5–15 mm and weighs approximately 0.5 g. It consists of two main parts: the anterior and posterior lobes.

The **anterior pituitary** houses six distinct types of glandular cells, each responsible for producing a single hormone. Let's take a closer look at one of these hormones.

2.2.1. Thyroid-stimulating hormone (TSH)

Thyroid-stimulating hormone (TSH, also known as thyrotropin), plays a pivotal role in regulating the function of the thyroid gland, an important component of the endocrine system.

Measuring TSH levels has become a standard recommendation for all women planning pregnancy and during the initial trimester, underscoring its importance in reproductive health.

TSH is composed of two amino acid chains:

- The *alpha chain* is identical in **TSH, FSH, LH,** and **hCG**.

- The *beta chain* is unique to each hormone and determines its specific function.

TSH production is regulated by both - the hypothalamus and the thyroid gland. The hypothalamus secretes **thyrotropin-releasing hormone (TRH)**, which stimulates TSH production. A deficiency of thyroid hormones in the blood signals the need to "activate" TSH production.

It's worth noting that TSH not only regulates thyroid function but also has a significant impact on prolactin production. This dual role can lead to elevated prolactin levels and associated breast discomfort in women with thyroid dysfunction. Conversely, somatostatin suppresses TSH production.

Thyroid cells have receptors on their surface (G-protein-coupled receptors, or GPCRs) that bind TSH, activating the cells to produce thyroxine (T4), the primary hormone of the thyroid gland.

Antibodies Against TSH

Unfortunately, TSH can trigger the production of *autoantibodies*, which the body mistakenly creates against its cells. These antibodies were first identified in 1956 in patients with *Graves' disease* (also known as diffuse toxic goiter), confirming the condition's autoimmune nature.

These antibodies belong to the IgG class and bind to TSH molecules, interfering with hormone uptake and its effect on thyroid cells. The exact mechanism behind their production remains unknown, as do effective methods for reducing their levels.

What Should the TSH Levels Be?

Measuring TSH levels has become a pivotal indicator of thyroid function and a primary tool in diagnosing thyroid disorders. This knowledge empowers healthcare professionals and individuals alike to understand and manage thyroid dysfunction, whether hyperthyroidism (overactivity) or hypothyroidism (underactivity), which can occur at various life stages, including pregnancy and postpartum. This will be discussed in more detail in another chapter.

Thyroid issues are more common in women, affecting approximately 15% of women and 4% of men at least once in their lives. This understanding of the prevalence of thyroid dysfunction in women helps to validate their experiences. However, how can thyroid dysfunction be suspected when symptoms are mild or unclear?

Because TSH directly regulates thyroid function, a low but within-normal-range TSH level generally suggests that the thyroid functions well. Extremely low TSH levels indicate hyperthyroidism, while insufficient thyroxine production (hypothyroidism) triggers the hypothalamic-pituitary system to increase TSH production, leading to high TSH levels.

TSH is secreted by the pituitary gland in a pulsatile manner, causing daily fluctuations. In healthy individuals, TSH levels can vary by up to 50% due to individual differences. Importantly, TSH production has a significant genetic component (involving the PDE8B and CAPZB genes), which is a fascinating area of study. This genetic influence means twins tend to have nearly identical TSH patterns and levels if living under similar conditions. This suggests some individuals may have TSH levels outside the standard reference range while maintaining normal thyroid function.

Is It Essential to Have TSH < 2.5 µIU/mL During Pregnancy?

Family doctors and obstetricians-gynecologists, with their increasing focus on thyroid function, play a crucial role in advising women planning an early pregnancy to measure TSH levels.

A TSH level of 2.5 µIU/mL or lower has become the international standard for the first trimester of pregnancy.

But on what basis did the American Thyroid Association propose this maximum TSH level for the first trimester in 2011? The exact reasoning remains unclear. These recommendations did not fully account for pregnancy outcomes. However, concerns about the overdiagnosis of thyroid diseases led many physician groups to investigate further. Their diligent studies confirmed that lower TSH levels are associated with better pregnancy outcomes and improved newborn health, providing reassurance and confidence in physicians' care.

Deciding to prescribe thyroid medication should always be individualized, considering your unique risk factors. This approach empowers you to participate actively in healthcare decisions, ensuring your needs and circumstances are considered.

Iodine and TSH

In recent years, the global concern about **iodine deficiency** has sparked frequent discussions. Simultaneously, iodine has been added to many foods and dietary supplements. Physicians frequently recommend iodine supplementation, emphasizing its benefits and the *'global deficiency.'*

But can iodine intake become excessive, and how does this affect TSH levels?

Iodine plays a critical role in normal thyroid function and hormone production. A severe iodine deficiency can impair thyroid function, but mild deficiencies rarely cause significant hormonal disruptions.

When iodine intake is sufficient or excessive, a paradoxical relationship with TSH levels emerges. Contrary to what might seem logical, increased iodine intake tends to lead to higher TSH levels. This paradox can be confusing, but it's a crucial aspect to understand for both doctors and patients.

This response is believed to be a protective reaction of the thyroid gland to high doses of iodine. Such effects are carefully considered when interpreting test results to avoid misdiagnosis, ensuring your confidence in the healthcare system.

Weight and TSH

The intricate relationship between thyroid function and weight is of paramount importance. Understanding how a normally functioning thyroid influences weight, and vice versa, can provide crucial insights into the management of thyroid dysfunction and weight fluctuations.

Research has revealed a fascinating connection between TSH levels and body weight. Thyroid hormones, under the influence of TSH, play a pivotal role in energy metabolism and can even influence appetite. This indirect control over food intake is a key factor in weight management. Moreover, TSH's involvement in fat metabolism and storage in adipose tissue adds another layer of intrigue to the complex relationship between thyroid function and weight.

One of the most intriguing aspects of the thyroid-weight relationship is the uncertainty about the cause-effect relationship. For instance, it's unclear whether thyroid changes cause weight gain or vice versa. This uncertainty piques our curiosity and keeps us engaged in the ongoing research in this field.

In smokers, no clear relationship between TSH and weight has been identified. However, smoking is known to hurt thyroid function.

As you continue reading this book, you will learn more about the thyroid gland.

2.2.1. Follicle-Stimulating Hormone (FSH)

The name *"follicle-stimulating hormone"* suggests that this substance influences certain follicles. It is an essential hormone in the lives of both women and men.

We will discuss the menstrual cycle in another chapter. Still, it is important to mention that the female gonads, reproductive organs or ovaries, contain many fluid-filled sacs (**follicles**) that house germ cells. The ovaries naturally have a multi-follicular structure, and without a functioning follicular system, egg cells would not mature, and hormone production would not occur. FSH, along with other hormones, plays a crucial role in the menstrual cycle by stimulating the growth and development of these follicles. It directly influences follicle development and the maturation of eggs within them.

In men, FSH, together with testosterone, is involved in the maturation of sperm cells and sperm production. In the testes, *granulosa cells* and *Sertoli cells* contain FSH receptors, which respond to FSH. However, the exact mechanism that triggers germ cell maturation remains unknown, making artificial regulation of this process impossible.

The condition and activation of FSH receptors are genetically controlled. Reproductive medicine and genetics aim to determine which genes and mutations influence germ cell maturation and the ability to reproduce. This is a highly complex and multifactorial issue; research has just begun.

FSH also plays a significant role in bone health. In postmenopausal women, as menopause sets in, the risk of bone fractures increases due to bone loss, a condition known as osteoporosis. FSH, along with other hormones, regulates bone density and remodeling. Studies have shown that women with mutations in the gene responsible for FSH receptor function not only experience difficulties with egg maturation and conception but also have a higher risk of osteoporosis due to the decreased bone density caused by FSH deficiency.

FSH receptors in other tissues and organs suggest these tissues may also respond to FSH. FSH receptors have been identified in the following ways:

- The inner lining of blood vessels,

- The cervix,

- The endometrium,

- The glands of the cervical canal,

- The muscle tissue of the uterus.

In pregnant women, FSH receptors has been found in the umbilical cord vessels, placenta, and fetal membranes. However, FSH production by the maternal pituitary gland is suppressed during pregnancy.

FSH receptors have also been found in the blood vessels of certain tumors, suggesting that FSH may play a role in tumor blood supply. This has led researchers to explore the potential use of *FSH antagonists*, which are substances that block the action of FSH, in cancer treatment. By blocking FSH, these antagonists could potentially disrupt the blood supply to tumors, thereby inhibiting their growth. However, more research is needed to fully understand the potential of FSH antagonists in cancer treatment.

When Is It Important to Check FSH Levels?

FSH is not directly involved in any disease but is an excellent indicator of ovarian function. FSH levels are most measured when diagnosing the following conditions:

- Disorders of puberty, whether premature or delayed

- Menstrual irregularities, such as oligomenorrhea or amenorrhea

- Infertility, including male infertility

- Perimenopause and menopause

In many cases, FSH testing is included in a standard hormonal panel alongside *luteinizing hormone* and *estradiol.*

FSH levels fluctuate throughout the menstrual cycle in the absence of hormonal contraceptives. If menstrual cycles are regular, measuring FSH usually has little practical value. However, when testing is necessary, it is crucial to check FSH levels on the third day of the menstrual cycle, with the first day counted from the onset of menstrual bleeding.

When menstrual cycles are absent or irregular, FSH can be measured on any day. In some cases, menstrual bleeding is artificially induced first, and the test is performed after withdrawal bleeding occurs.

FSH is a reliable marker for confirming menopause, but for a secure diagnosis, two independent tests within one month are necessary.

High FSH Levels

High FSH levels are most observed in women entering the menopausal transition. This hormone can start rising one to two years before menopause, but persistently high FSH is a key marker of *ovarian failure*, signaling the cessation of egg maturation. This can occur due to early menopause (before age 40), ovarian surgery, ovarian insufficiency, or premature depletion of the ovarian reserve. High FSH is also seen in cases of underdeveloped gonads (ovaries), *Turner syndrome, Klinefelter syndrome*, and certain forms of *congenital adrenal hyperplasia*.

In men, elevated FSH levels indicate *testicular insufficiency*. In women with systemic lupus erythematosus, high FSH levels are also frequently observed. This can be due to the disease's impact on the ovaries, leading to premature ovarian failure and high FSH levels.

Now, let's address some common myths about high FSH. As mentioned, single lab results without considering symptoms and clinical presentation have little practical value. Therefore, detecting high FSH is not always a bad sign.

It's crucial to understand that FSH production and secretion occur in a pulsatile manner, meaning its levels naturally fluctuate throughout the day. This variability is a normal part of the body's hormonal balance, not a cause for immediate concern. **Rising FSH levels indicate that the body attempts to stimulate egg maturation and ovarian function**. In other words, the body recognizes a dysfunction at some level, though doctors may not always be clear about what has gone wrong. This is a natural response of the body to maintain reproductive health.

Although FSH plays a role in stimulating egg maturation, it does not directly measure the process itself. Instead, it indicates ovarian reserve, which refers to the estimated number of eggs remaining in the ovaries. When the ovarian reserve is low, FSH levels rise as the body attempts to stimulate the maturation of the remaining eggs. However, this does not necessarily mean that a woman is in menopause. It simply means that the ovaries are not responding to the FSH as they should, possibly due to various reasons such as age or certain medical conditions.

Many women in their 20s and 30s may have elevated FSH levels for various reasons while still experiencing regular menstrual cycles. This is not always due to ovarian dysfunction. For example, pituitary tumors can be associated with high FSH levels and may also disrupt ovarian function.

Of course, high FSH levels can make conception more complicated, and women in this situation often require assisted reproductive technologies to achieve pregnancy. The availability of these technologies offers hope and potential solutions for those facing fertility challenges.

The higher the FSH level, the more challenging it becomes to conceive, as it is typically associated with a diminished ovarian reserve. It is essential to understand that there is currently no medication capable of lowering FSH levels or restoring them to normal level. This knowledge can help manage expectations and guide decisions about fertility treatments. Understanding the implications of high FSH levels on fertility treatments can help manage expectations and guide decisions about the most appropriate course of action.

Ultimately, FSH is simply an indicator of ovarian function and egg maturation. It's important to remember that it is not the cause of impaired egg development but rather a marker that can help identify potential issues with ovarian health. Understanding this can empower you to have informed discussions with your healthcare provider about your reproductive health, ensuring that you are an active participant in your own care.

Low FSH Levels

For some reason, doctors and patients tend to focus more on high FSH levels, while low FSH is also not normal. FSH, or follicle-stimulating hormone, is a key hormone in the reproductive system. It plays a crucial role in stimulating the growth of ovarian follicles in women and the production of sperm in men. Low levels of this hormone are most observed in *gonadal insufficiency (hypogonadism)*, which can be either congenital or acquired. In men, this leads to a cessation of sperm production, while in women, menstrual cycles stop.

Since the pituitary gland produces FSH, disorders affecting it can lead to decreased FSH levels. These include *hypothalamic suppression, hypopituitarism,* and *Kallmann syndrome.* Certain medications that suppress ovarian and testicular function, such as GnRH antagonists and agonists, can also lower FSH levels.

Low FSH is also observed in polycystic ovary syndrome (PCOS), particularly in combination with obesity, excessive hair growth, and infertility. Elevated prolactin levels and the use or excessive production of estrogens can also suppress FSH secretion.

In rare instances, genetic mutations affecting FSH production can disrupt ovulation in women and spermatogenesis in men, leading to infertility in both sexes. In essence, FSH is a crucial indicator of testicular and ovarian dysfunction, providing valuable diagnostic information.

Regardless of the low FSH levels, it is crucial to consider a patient's symptoms and evaluate each case individually. This personalized approach is key to providing comprehensive care and addressing each patient's unique needs.

Synthetic FSH Analogues

In the 1960s, physicians began using hormonal medications derived from the urine of postmenopausal women. These included *menotropin,* or *human menopausal gonadotropin* (hMG), which contained both FSH and LH.

Urine from postmenopausal women was used because women in this stage of life have incredibly high levels of FSH and LH in their blood and urine. In 1949, a simple method was developed to extract gonadotropins from urine. Early medications contained equal amounts of FSH and LH, but as the importance of FSH in egg maturation, a process crucial for fertility, became evident, the proportion of FSH increased.

Later, technological advancements, such as improved extraction and purification methods, enabled the production of *urofollitropin* from urine, with minimal amounts of other biological substances previously present in urinary-derived medications. Some formulations included trace amounts of hCG.

Today, several medications, including those containing FSH either in pure form or in combination with

LH, hCG, and other substances, are widely used in reproductive medicine. These drugs play a crucial role in stimulating follicular growth, a practice that has become a cornerstone of modern reproductive medicine.

Egg cells are essential for both natural conception and assisted reproduction (IVF). The type and dosage of medication used for *ovulation stimulation* depend on the specific goal of the treatment. In some cases, the aim is to obtain only a few eggs, while in others, such as IVF, more than 10 eggs may be required. The doctor's expertise and approach also play a crucial role. Their understanding of how different medications work, their distinctions, advantages, and limitations influences the choice of treatment strategy.

2.2.3. Luteotropic Hormone (LH)

Luteotropic hormone, or luteinizing hormone (LH, lutropin, lutrophin, luteotropin), is a important player in the reproductive process and is equally important as FSH. These two hormones often work in tandem, and their specific ratio is crucial for the normal functioning of both the female and male bodies. LH, as a gonadotropin, significantly influences the activity of the ovaries and testes.

The term 'luteotropic' signifies this pituitary hormone's role in the ovary's *corpus luteum*. However, LH's function in the female body extends beyond supporting the corpus luteum. It plays a crucial role in stimulating the production of female sex hormones by the granulosa cells of ovarian follicles, directly impacting reproductive health and highlighting its significant role in the female reproductive system.

LH levels peak before ovulation, followed by a brief progesterone surge. These two hormones rise, depending on each other, triggers the release of a mature egg from the follicle, a process known as **ovulation**. Without LH, egg maturation cannot occur.

After ovulation, LH gradually rises, influencing the transformation of the ruptured follicle — first into a *hemorrhagic body* (filled with blood) and then into a corpus luteum, which produces progesterone. Thus, LH regulates ovarian hormonal activity.

LH production, which regulates testosterone, estrogen, and progesterone synthesis, depends on *hypothalamic-pituitary activity*. Throughout the day and menstrual cycle, LH pulsation occurs in different modes:

- High-amplitude pulsation (large LH surges without precise time intervals)

- Minimal pulsation (low LH production)

- Sleep-state pulsation (chaotic frequency and amplitude of LH secretion)

- Regular 90-minute pulsation

All these modes are normal and can alternate in a healthy woman. However, LH pulsation determines the secretion of other hormones, including progesterone. **The 90-minute uniform pulsation, commonly described in textbooks, is not a constant feature but is more frequently observed during peak progesterone production.**

Additionally, the pulsatile release of LH is influenced by age, stress levels, fatigue, intense physical activity, and various endocrine disorders. LH secretion patterns vary, and pulsation frequency shifts may occur unexpectedly due to internal and external factors. Therefore, a single hormone test rarely provides an accurate picture of a woman's hormonal state and can lead to misdiagnosis.

Another important hormone, *human chorionic gonadotropin* (hCG), which appears during pregnancy, has a similar structure to LH, allowing both hormones to interact with the same cell receptors. It is believed that their coordinated action supports successful embryo implantation. As pregnancy progresses, LH levels decrease due to hCG activity, which takes over the role of LH in maintaining the corpus luteum and supporting the early stages of pregnancy. **This shift in hormonal activity is a key factor in the changes that occur in the female body during pregnancy**.

In men, LH stimulates the production and release of male sex hormones in the testes, often called *interstitial cell-stimulating hormone* (ICSH). This process is crucial for the development and maintenance of male reproductive organs and secondary sexual characteristics. LH also plays a role in the regulation of sperm production, further underlining its importance in male reproductive health.

LH testing is a vital and indispensable component of fertility assessments for women with infertility issues. It is also a key measurement when irregular menstrual cycles occur. Complaints of fatigue, unexplained weight loss, and decreased appetite may also indicate the need for LH testing, underlining its crucial role in reproductive health and the urgency of its inclusion in fertility assessments.

LH levels are often tested in men when testosterone levels are low, libido is reduced, or muscle mass decreases.

Interestingly, the production of both FSH and LH is regulated by the same hypothalamic hormone — GnRH. However, the precise mechanism by which GnRH controls the secretion of these two distinct hormones remains unknown.

Excess LH and FSH are metabolized in the liver and excreted via the kidneys in urine.

Since LH interacts with multiple hormones, a single LH measurement has little practical significance.

High and Low LH

The two most common conditions associated with elevated LH levels are *menopause* and *polycystic ovary syndrome* (PCOS). If LH levels are extremely high, a pituitary tumor should be ruled out.

The clinical significance of low LH levels is not yet fully understood. The hormone may be low in cases of pituitary disorders, stress, anorexia, and starvation. A genetic defect can also lead to low LH levels, often manifesting as hypogonadism.

Isolated *luteinizing hormone deficiency* is extremely rare and usually occurs with FSH deficiency.

Despite LH playing a crucial role in the human body, greater attention has been given to the LH-to-FSH ratio as these hormones interact, something we will discuss further.

The LH-to-FSH Ratio and Vice Versa

Many women diagnosed with polycystic ovary syndrome (PCOS) have likely heard about the **LH-to-FSH ratio**. For years, an elevated ratio was considered one of the diagnostic criteria for PCOS. However, the assumption that a high **LH/FSH ratio** (above 3) is characteristic of this condition lacked scientific evidence. New research has shown that the LH-to-FSH ratio is the same in healthy women and those with PCOS. Only a small subgroup of women with PCOS (those who do not ovulate) may exhibit a slight increase in this ratio, but it remains below 3 in most cases. This complexity in understanding LH levels in PCOS is an intriguing area of research.

Why, then, does the LH-to-FSH ratio increase in some women? As I mentioned earlier, the secretion of these two hormones occurs in a pulsatile manner, reflecting the release of gonadotropin-releasing hormone (GnRH) from the hypothalamus. **In healthy women, the pulsatile release of FSH and LH is synchronized**, with FSH stimulating the growth of ovarian follicles and LH triggering ovulation. However, in women with PCOS, the frequency of LH pulses increases while FSH secretion remains the same or slightly decreases. This leads to higher LH levels relative to FSH.

Luteinizing hormone stimulates the production of male sex hormones in the ovaries. When LH levels are elevated, this can lead to hyperandrogenism, a key clinical and laboratory marker of PCOS. This excess of male sex hormones can lead to symptoms such as acne, hirsutism, and irregular menstrual cycles in women with PCOS.

Studying the mechanism of LH and FSH secretion in women with PCOS has led researchers to discover that the

frequency of hypothalamic GnRH pulsations determines LH production, while slower pulsations drive FSH secretion. This may explain how a single hypothalamic hormone controls the secretion of two different pituitary hormones. However, this remains a theoretical assumption requiring further research. The urgency and importance of understanding what regulates and stimulates these pulsations in healthy women and those with endocrine disorders cannot be overstated.

In girls, the pulsatile secretion of gonadotropins does not establish a clear pattern until the menstrual cycles become regular, typically by the later stages of puberty (around 19–22 years of age).

Interestingly, in over 80% of women with PCOS, the LH-to-FSH ratio does not exceed 2.5 (in nearly 30% of cases, it is less than 1). In comparison, approximately 13% have a ratio between 2.5 and 3.5, and the remaining women have a ratio above 3.5. Thus, for most women with PCOS, this ratio remains within the normal range. This is why it is no longer considered a diagnostic criterion for PCOS (which we will discuss in a separate chapter).

The **FSH/LH ratio,** a key measure in medicine, is a complex entity with distinct clinical significance. It undergoes fluctuations throughout the menstrual cycle as the cycle phases change. This complexity prompts the question: Can it be used to assess menstrual cycle quality?

A low FSH-to-LH ratio (below 1.4) in the early days of the cycle is associated with longer menstrual cycles, an extended follicular phase, lower ovulation rates, and reduced conception frequency. However, the luteal phase and progesterone production remain unchanged. Overall, when combined with a low FSH level on days 3–5 of the cycle, this ratio is linked to a prolonged follicular phase but does not hold prognostic value for the luteal phase.

The FSH/LH ratio is a crucial factor in reproductive medicine and is used to determine the optimal medication and dosage for ovulation induction. It's important to understand that the response to treatment is highly individualized. Some women produce many *oocytes* (eggs) after receiving a small dose of gonadotropins or other medications, while others exhibit ovarian resistance even when treated with high doses. This variability in response underscores the need for an optimal prognostic test to improve infertility treatment success.

Even when FSH and LH levels are within the normal range, their ratio may be either low or high. Studies have shown that if the FSH/LH ratio exceeds three on day 3 of the cycle, the response to ovulation stimulation may weaken, and IVF success rates lower. Additionally, these women may experience elevated FSH levels for several months after stimulation. Conversely, a low FSH/LH ratio (below 2) is linked to a lower ovulation rate and is often observed in women with diminished ovarian reserve. However, with the development of new medications and stimulation protocols, the prognostic value of the FSH-to-LH ratio has been reduced.

The FSH/LH ratio changes with age, making it an unreliable parameter in women over 40. Therefore, its measurement is not recommended in this age group.

Moreover, the optimal FSH/LH ratio for predicting ovulation and conception remains unknown.

Synthetic LH Forms and Their Application

LH is a pharmaceutical component in *menotropins*, combined with FSH and several other reproductive medicine drugs. Recombinant LH is also available, though its production is costly. Interestingly, human chorionic gonadotropin (hCG), which can be easily extracted from the urine of pregnant women, has been found to exert effects like those of LH.

2.2.4. Prolactin

One could write an entire book about prolactin — **it influences more cells, tissues, and organs than all other hormones combined.** This is not an exaggeration; it is a fact.

Due to an apparent error in medical terminology dictionaries, prolactin — a pituitary hormone responsible for breast development and milk production, was mistakenly referred to as "luteotropic hormone" in certain publications. However, prolactin has its proper synonyms: lactotropin and lactotrophic hormone (LTH). It is rarely called a lactostimulating hormone. The prefix *"lacto"* connects it to the mammary glands, and referring to prolactin as a luteotropic hormone, as some dictionaries do, is incorrect.

On one hand, prolactin has been the subject of intense study, mainly because of its role in milk production, which has fascinated researchers since its discovery. On the other hand, it remains a mystery how a single hormone can exert such a diverse range of effects on the body.

Most prolactin is produced by specialized pituitary cells called lactotroph cells, but it can also be synthesized outside the pituitary gland—in the mammary glands, uterus, T-lymphocytes, and placenta.

Prolactin regulation is unique among pituitary hormones. Typically, the hypothalamus stimulates pituitary hormone production by releasing hormones. However, prolactin is an exception — it is actively suppressed by the hypothalamus, and its levels rise when this suppression is lifted. While dopamine is widely recognized as the primary inhibitor of prolactin secretion, no distinct *prolactin-inhibiting factor* has ever been isolated.

Another unique aspect of prolactin is that, unlike other pituitary hormones, it lacks a feedback loop with the organs that utilize it. Most pituitary hormones regulate endocrine glands that, in turn, produce their hormones — for example, TSH controls thyroid function, while gonadotropins regulate sex hormones and progesterone production. **Prolactin, however, does not stimulate the secretion of other hormones because the mammary glands do not produce hormones.** This means elevated prolactin levels remain unchecked, even by the pituitary. **Prolactin molecules may act directly on the hypothalamus, triggering dopamine release and inhibiting its production — a remarkable self-regulation mechanism.**

Structurally, prolactin closely resembles *growth hormone* and *placental lactogen*, all encoded by a single gene on chromosome 6. It is believed that this hormone family emerged approximately 400 million years ago in early rodents.

Several variants of prolactin exist, though their significance remains poorly understood. Prolactin binds to the same cell receptors as growth hormone, but the interaction mechanisms are highly complex and still under investigation. Interestingly, the first prolactin receptors were isolated from rat liver cells.

The most well-studied functions of prolactin include:

- Regulation of mammary gland development
- Initiation and maintenance of milk production (lactation)
- Influence on reproductive function
- Role in immune system activity
- Regulation of metabolic processes (osmoregulation)
- Impact on human behavior

However, prolactin's influence extends far beyond these functions — it is attributed to over 300 roles in the human body, and researchers continue to uncover more. The field of prolactin research is dynamic and ever evolving, with new discoveries being made regularly, keeping scientists engaged and excited about the potential of this hormone.

We understand its crucial role in pregnancy and breastfeeding. We also know that excessive prolactin can disrupt egg maturation. But when it comes to its significance in non-pregnant, non-lactating women or in men — there is still much to learn.

The highest prolactin levels are observed in late pregnancy, during the third trimester. These levels surpass those seen postpartum and even during lactation. The fetus is exposed to exceptionally high levels of prolactin, leading researchers to believe that this hormone plays a crucial role in fetal maturation and may also be involved in triggering labor.

During pregnancy, the placenta produces a specific type of prolactin, sometimes considered prolactin and sometimes a prolactin-like substance. **Placental lactogen** shares structural similarities with growth hormone and pituitary prolactin, making it difficult to determine which is more closely related. Additionally, a specialized layer of endometrial tissue, the *decidua*, produces its prolactin. This production begins in the luteal phase of the menstrual cycle under the influence of progesterone and continues throughout pregnancy, increasing significantly after embryo implantation.

Amniotic fluid also exhibits hormonal activity, partly due to several forms of prolactin.

The muscular layer of the uterus (*myometrium*) can also synthesize prolactin, though the specific cells responsible remain unknown. This intriguing mystery adds to the complexity of understanding prolactin. Interestingly, the regulation of prolactin production in the myometrium and endometrium differs entirely. The function of myometrial prolactin, a puzzle yet to be solved, adds to the enigma of this hormone.

One of the most intriguing aspects of prolactin is that it can be synthesized by brain cells.

Another mysterious characteristic of prolactin is its genetic stability. Unlike other hormones, no genetic mutations (polymorphisms) have been identified in prolactin or its receptors. Yet lactotrophic (prolactin-producing) cells occupy between 20% and 50% of the anterior pituitary's volume. Remarkably, no known genetic disorder is associated with a defect in the gene responsible for prolactin synthesis. As a result, **no known condition is characterized by isolated prolactin deficiency.**

Since no humans exist without prolactin, we cannot fully understand the consequences of its complete absence or its full biological significance.

The only prolactin-related condition that receives medical attention is **hyperprolactinemia** (elevated prolactin levels). This condition can lead to a range of symptoms, including irregular menstrual periods, infertility, and, in some cases, milk production in men or non-pregnant women.

To this day, the minimum prolactin levels required for normal human function remain unknown. Even when prolactin-producing sections of the pituitary are absent, such as after pituitary tumor removal, prolactin does not entirely disappear from the body. This is due to extra pituitary prolactin production sources, including the immune system, skin, and breast tissue.

In cases of acute prolactin deficiency, growth hormone can bind to prolactin receptors and perform their function, essentially acting as a substitute.

There is growing evidence that prolactin is not just a hormone but also a unique molecule known as a **cytokine**. This multifunctionality of prolactin, acting as a hormone and a cytokine, adds to its intrigue. Cytokines are small protein molecules communicating signals between cells by binding to specific receptors. Some forms of prolactin are tiny and may act as signal carriers.

Although milk production occurs in all mammals, no animal model perfectly mirrors human prolactin regulation, production, and function. This makes studying prolactin in humans particularly challenging. The lack of a perfect animal model underscores the complexity and importance of this research.

Characteristics of Prolactin Secretion

The secretion of prolactin by the pituitary gland has distinct features. The first and most well-studied mechanism of prolactin release is triggered by suckling, particularly during lactation and breastfeeding. This is considered an *acute type of prolactin secretion* or a **classic neuroendocrine reflex**, which occurs over a short period — just a few hours. **The longer the act of suckling, the more prolactin is released.** The quality of suckling, particularly its active nature, also plays a significant role. For optimal prolactin (and milk) production, the baby must be starving and suckle with a strong appetite.

Estradiol stimulates another type of prolactin secretion — *chronic secretion*, which follows a *circadian rhythm*. In many animals, rising estrogen levels in the afternoon lead to increased prolactin secretion, which continues to rise daily. This hormonal interaction is a key factor in the regulation of prolactin levels.

Prolactin secretion has yet another unique aspect — it is closely linked to sleep. Hormone levels begin to rise with the onset of sleep (specifically nighttime sleep), starting from the first stage of slow-wave sleep (non-REM), which lasts 5–10 minutes. Throughout the day, prolactin levels peak approximately 13–14 times every 90 minutes. This

59

underscores the importance of sleep-in regulating prolactin levels. Food intake, especially protein consumption, also affects prolactin production. This means prolactin levels fluctuate significantly within 24 hours, with up to 25% variations.

Prolactin secretion also follows a day-night cycle during pregnancy. This rhythmic secretion supports the corpus luteum and its progesterone production in early pregnancy. The day-night cycle of prolactin secretion during pregnancy is crucial for maintaining the corpus luteum, which produces progesterone. Progesterone is essential for maintaining the uterine lining and supporting the early stages of pregnancy.

Some studies suggest that prolactin levels increase near ovulation and remain elevated throughout the second half of the cycle. Others refute these fluctuations. In practice, the specific day of the menstrual cycle is not a determining factor when testing for prolactin levels. The conflicting data on prolactin levels near ovulation may indicate that individual variations and other factors could influence these levels, which should be considered when interpreting test results.

With the onset of menopause, prolactin levels remain within the normal range in nearly half of all women. In others, levels may slightly increase or decrease, but these changes are minimal and do not significantly impact health.

Measuring Prolactin Levels

A single blood test is typically sufficient to determine prolactin excess. Blood does not need to be drawn in the morning after waking up or after a meal — the test can be performed at any time. Any prolactin measurement above the upper reference limit is considered **hyperprolactinemia**, but it is crucial to account for factors that may temporarily elevate prolactin levels.

In approximately 30% of cases, mild prolactin elevation is due to stress, including anxiety and fear — commonly referred to as *white coat syndrome*. A prolonged or traumatic venipuncture attempt (such as struggling to find a vein) can also lead to a temporary prolactin surge.

In cases where prolactin results appear questionable, a repeat blood draw 20–30 minutes later may be recommended to account for the hormone's pulsatile secretion. However, most women leave the lab after the test and return only when results are available. For this reason, a repeat measurement is typically only conducted if the physician, based on the patient's medical history and symptoms, has concerns about the accuracy of the initial results.

Prolactin and the Brain

As previously discussed, prolactin plays an important role in shaping human behavior. This is a significant function, as it is the brain cells themselves that can synthesize their own prolactin.

When prolactin receptors were discovered in various brain regions, it was initially assumed that these receptors were absorbing pituitary prolactin, which circulates in the bloodstream. However, studies on individuals who had undergone pituitary removal revealed a surprising fact-prolactin was still present in the brain. This unexpected discovery challenged the initial assumption and led to the conclusion that brain tissue is an independent source of prolactin. Further research confirmed that the brain can produce prolactin, often associated with other hormones or their metabolic byproducts. For instance, through estrogen receptors, prolactin influences the production of steroid hormones in the testes and ovaries.

If oxytocin is often referred to as the 'hormone of love,' particularly maternal love, then prolactin could be seen as the 'hormone of maternal care.' During lactation and breastfeeding, oxytocin and prolactin work in harmony, each supporting the other to foster maternal behaviors.

Animal studies have shown that prolactin is essential for developing maternal instincts, particularly in fostering care for offspring. These instincts may begin forming during pregnancy and may be influenced by placental lactogens. However, maternal behaviors intensify as prolactin levels rise.

Prolactin, in addition to its role in maternal care, is also believed to stimulate appetite. This is a key factor in understanding why pregnant and breastfeeding women often experience an increased appetite, consume more food, and gain extra weight. Even in non-lactating women, elevated prolactin levels (hyperprolactinemia) can lead to weight gain due to increased appetite.

During stress, prolactin levels rise in brain tissue. It is thought that prolactin can reduce stress responses and calm the nervous system. This connection between stress, prolactin levels, and appetite is a key factor in understanding why people often reach for the refrigerator under stress, mindlessly snacking to self-soothe.

Elevated Prolactin Levels – Hyperprolactinemia

Elevated prolactin levels in the blood, known as *hyperprolactinemia*, can indicate an underlying condition or appear as an isolated symptom affecting bodily functions, particularly in women. In some cases, it may also be a physiological norm, which means it's within the normal range for a healthy individual and not necessarily a cause for concern.

When analyzing prolactin levels, it is crucial to exercise caution and consider the units of measurement to avoid misinterpretation. Normal prolactin levels are generally considered to be up to 30 ng/mL, although different organizations may have slightly varying standards. Levels exceeding 50 ng/mL are often indicative of a pituitary tumor (*prolactinoma*).

When can elevated prolactin be considered normal?

- During adolescence (only in girls).
- During pregnancy.
- Up to three months postpartum.
- During lactation and breastfeeding.
- After nipple stimulation (including after sexual activity).

Conditions associated with elevated prolactin levels:

- Acute and chronic stress.

- Intense physical exertion.

- Insomnia.

- Fasting and hypoglycemia (low blood sugar).

- Thyroid disorders.

- Surgical procedures.

- Use of certain medications.

Drug-induced hyperprolactinemia is one of the most common causes of elevated prolactin levels, particularly in women. The list of medications that can trigger prolactin elevation is extensive and includes *dopamine antagonists, estrogens, antidepressants*, certain *painkillers, antihistamines, antiepileptics,* and *hormonal contraceptives*. **Always read the package insert for possible side effects!**

Prolactin levels can increase not only while taking hormonal contraceptives but also after discontinuing them. This post-discontinuation increase, known as the *withdrawal effect*, is typical. About 30% of women using combined oral contraceptives (*COCs*), especially high-dose formulations, experience mild to moderate prolactin elevation. Estrogen therapy for medical purposes can also contribute to increased prolactin levels.

To confirm whether a medication is the cause of hyperprolactinemia, it is recommended to discontinue the drug for **three days** (if the treatment plan allows) and then remeasure prolactin levels. A level decrease would indicate a medication-related cause, though not necessarily typical.

If a woman suffers from a chronic illness, her prolactin levels may initially rise. However, prolactin levels may eventually decrease due to prolonged stress and disruption of the hormone's pulsatile secretion.

In 20–40% of cases, high prolactin levels are linked to pituitary tumors, including isolated *prolactinomas* and mixed adenomas. Tumors smaller than 10 mm in diameter are classified as *microadenomas*, while those more significant than 10 mm are *macroadenomas*. *Microadenomas* are more commonly found in women of reproductive age, whereas *macroadenomas* are more frequent in postmenopausal women. Adenomas may be *functional* (actively producing prolactin) or *non-functional* (inactive).

Hyperprolactinemia can also occur due to *pituitary or hypothalamic disorders,* such as *hypophysitis*, after radiation therapy or following a pituitary injury. Other brain tumors (*gliomas, craniopharyngiomas*) can also affect prolactin production. Additionally, ovarian *dermoid cysts* and renal tumors (*hypernephroma*), as well as lung cancer, are sometimes associated with high prolactin levels. *Chronic kidney failure*, particularly in combination with hemodialysis, is another known cause of hyperprolactinemia.

In 10–20% of cases, *idiopathic hyperprolactinemia* occurs, meaning the underlying cause is unknown. However, the complexity of diagnosing hyperprolactinemia is evident, as standard lab tests do not always differentiate *macroprolactin* (a large prolactin variant, which we will discuss later).

Hyperprolactinemia is more straightforward to detect in women than in men, as women more frequently report symptoms. The most common complaints include:

- Irregular menstrual cycles (*oligomenorrhea*).

- Absence of menstruation (*amenorrhea*).

- Nipple discharge (*galactorrhea*).

- Decreased libido.

- Infertility.

- Decreased bone mass (*osteoporosis*).

However, these symptoms do not always manifest. Likewise, they are not always specific to hyperprolactinemia. For instance, nipple discharge can persist for years after breastfeeding has ended. Infertility can have numerous other causes. Osteoporosis is common in menopausal women. Therefore, each case requires an individualized approach.

Mildly elevated prolactin levels can be associated with various symptoms, while even significantly high levels may not cause any noticeable complaints. This variability in symptom manifestation underscores the need for careful observation and individualized care.

There is evidence suggesting a connection between hyperprolactinemia and breast cancer in premenopausal and menopausal women, as well as prostate cancer in men. However, the exact mechanism remains unclear. While prolactin stimulates breast tissue growth (proliferation, which refers to rapid increase or growth), its direct role in classic breast cancer development is not well established.

Macroprolactin

The large variety of prolactin variants complicates the assessment of the actual levels of the biologically active form — the one capable of interacting with different cells and tissues. Depending on molecular size, prolactin exists in the following forms:

- Monomeric (14–23 kDa)

- Dimeric (48–56 kDa)

- Polymeric (macroprolactin) (100–150 kDa)

Monomeric prolactin is biologically active and circulates most frequently in human blood. Polymeric forms, known as macroprolactin, represent a complex of monomeric prolactin bound to IgG antibodies. Due to its large molecular size, macroprolactin has minimal interaction with cell receptors and, in most cases, cannot pass through blood vessel walls, remaining in circulation.

Macroprolactinemia is quite common — 10% to 40% of hyperprolactinemia cases are caused by this form of prolactin in both adults and children. On average, 15% of circulating prolactin is macroprolactin. Elevated macroprolactin levels do not cause symptoms. However, if complaints arise, it may indicate an increase in different forms of prolactin, such as in pituitary prolactinomas, in which case further investigation is required. There are also anti-prolactin antibodies that can bind to prolactin molecules.

Macroprolactinemia is sometimes called *"analytical hyperprolactinemia?"* because it can lead to inconsistencies in lab test interpretations. It is crucial to consider the method used to measure prolactin in serum. Most laboratories do not differentiate macroprolactin separately.

Treatment of Hyperprolactinemia

Now that you are aware of the many causes of elevated prolactin levels and understand that prolactin exists in different forms, including macroprolactin, which is harmless to the body, the decision to treat hyperprolactinemia depends on answering the following questions:

1. Which form of prolactin is elevated?

2. Can prolactin levels be lowered by addressing the underlying cause?

3. What symptoms are present, and how severe are they?

When evaluating symptoms, it is crucial to distinguish primary issues from those secondary to hyperprolactinemia. Elevated prolactin levels may be merely an indirect or incidental finding unrelated to the patient's complaints. In most cases, macroprolactinemia does not require any intervention, but a careful evaluation of symptoms is always necessary.

If the underlying cause is known, it should be eliminated or its impact minimized. Otherwise, attempts to lower prolactin will be unsuccessful, or any improvement will be short-lived. **In 30% of cases, hyperprolactinemia resolves on its own without any treatment, with prolactin levels returning to normal.** This is most common in cases of *idiopathic hyperprolactinemia*, where no definitive cause is identified.

If a prolactinoma causes hyperprolactinemia, the treatment depends on the tumor's size and associated symptoms, which can include *menstrual irregularities, infertility, and visual disturbances*. The standard treatment involves medications such as cabergoline (Dostinex) or bromocriptine. These medications are effective in reducing tumor size in over 60% of cases, normalizing menstrual cycles in 80% of cases, and improving reproductive function. About 50% of women conceive after treatment, and in nearly 90% of cases, nipple discharge (galactorrhea) stops. Prolactin levels return to normal in almost 70% of cases.

The dosage and duration of treatment for hyperprolactinemia depend on how quickly the woman's concerns are resolved. Prolactin levels are monitored one month after starting treatment to assess its effectiveness. Follow-up MRI scans are performed annually for microadenomas and every 3 months for macroadenomas to monitor tumor size and any potential recurrence.

Treatment must be discontinued upon pregnancy confirmation, as prolactin levels naturally rise from the early weeks of gestation. Only in rare cases of large prolactinomas may bromocriptine treatment be continued during pregnancy. **There is no conclusive evidence linking high prolactin levels to early pregnancy loss**. If treatment is ineffective or if the prolactinoma is large, surgical removal of the tumor is considered.

If prolactin levels are high and symptoms are present, medical treatment is necessary. However, it's crucial to understand the source of the excess prolactin. It's important to note that dopamine receptor agonists (bromocriptine and Dostinex) do not lower prolactin levels unless the pituitary gland is the source of excess production. **If prolactin**

comes from an extrapituitary source, prescribing these medications is incorrect.

Mildly elevated prolactin levels do not cause menstrual irregularities or infertility, meaning treatment is unnecessary. For moderate to severe hyperprolactinemia (excluding macroprolactinemia), medical therapy can be considered with prolactin levels monitored after a month.

We will return to prolactin later in this book, but let's move on to other equally essential hormones of the human body.

2.2.5. Growth Hormone

As I mentioned earlier, prolactin has a close relative, one could even call it a sibling, capable of performing similar functions: growth hormone, which is also produced by the pituitary gland. Somatotropin is an "ancient" hormone, one of the earliest to appear in the animal kingdom. Growth hormone, prolactin, and insulin (its precursor, proinsulin) originate from the same protein substance, regulated by the same gene.

Describing growth hormone (somatotropin) as the *'king of energy'* is not an exaggeration. It holds a pivotal role in energy storage during times of plenty and regulates the use of carbohydrates, fats, and proteins when food is scarce. Even in well-nourished individuals, energy levels follow a daily cycle (fasting at night, eating during the day), a process controlled by growth hormone. This intricate regulation of energy by growth hormone is a fascinating and unique aspect of its function.

But what about growth itself? If it is called the "growth hormone," does that mean it is solely responsible for growth? The answer is not that simple. This hormone is crucial for newborns' development and the transition from childhood to adulthood. However, growth is a complex process involving many other hormones and substances. An excess of growth hormone leads to gigantism, while a deficiency results in dwarfism. Yet, today, numerous growth-related syndromes have been identified that are independent of growth hormone. The exact role of this hormone in human growth is a complex puzzle that remains unclear and requires further study, adding to the intrigue of its function.

The human body produces several **growth factors** in addition to growth hormone. Some of these interact with growth hormone, such as **insulin-like growth factor (IGF-1)**, which plays a role in skeletal and muscle development. Others function independently of growth hormone.

On one hand, growth hormone is produced by the pituitary gland, making it an endocrine hormone. On the other hand, even after the pituitary gland's removal, some growth hormone circulates in the blood, suggesting that alternative sources exist. Growth hormone receptors are found in almost every organ and tissue of the human body. The nervous, immune, reproductive, musculoskeletal, cardiovascular, gastrointestinal, and respiratory systems utilize growth hormone locally as a *paracrine* hormone to regulate the growth of cells and tissues. Some of these tissues can also produce growth hormone for their own needs.

There are several *isoforms* of growth hormone, each performing a specific function, though their roles are not yet fully understood.

71

Interest in growth hormone among scientists and physicians has grown significantly compared to the previous century for several reasons. From conception onward, the human body is in constant growth, first at the fetal stage, then through infancy, childhood, and adolescence. There are alternating periods of rapid and slow growth throughout childhood, though the mechanisms that trigger these fluctuations remain unknown. However, growth hormone is undoubtedly involved. Ongoing research sheds light on these mechanisms, offering hope for a better understanding of growth regulation. Continually exploring growth hormone and its functions provides optimism for future discoveries. Eventually, every individual reaches a stage where growth ceases, typically around age 25, known as **somatopause**.

What happens to growth hormone when the body stops growing? Its levels begin to decline by approximately 15% every decade starting at age 30. Gradually but steadily, muscle and bone mass decrease, fat accumulates, memory and cognitive function deteriorate, and various physiological processes slow down. It would seem logical that supplementing growth hormone could slow down aging — an idea widely promoted in the anti-aging industry. However, such therapy has proven to be completely ineffective.

Recent studies on the gene set of centenarians, in search of a 'longevity gene,' revealed an intriguing finding. Most people who reach the age of 100 tend to be shorter in stature, suggesting a possible link between longevity and a gene that regulates growth hormone production. This discovery and ongoing research challenge the notion that high growth hormone levels guarantee a longer life. It's fascinating as scientists continue identifying other 'longevity genes' that may contribute to human health and lifespan.

Women have higher growth hormone levels than men, primarily because estrogen levels influence its production — these hormones are closely interconnected. The more estrogen present, the more growth hormone is produced. This physiological phenomenon presents a paradox: growth hormone plays a key role in bone growth, muscle development, and fat reduction (by promoting fat breakdown). Logically, women should be larger and more muscular than men! Could this be an error? No, it is not.

When menopause occurs and estrogen levels drop, growth hormone levels decrease as well, leading to bone loss (osteoporosis), muscle atrophy, and fat accumulation. However, obesity due to reduced growth hormone is not exclusive to women; it occurs in all individuals when growth hormone levels decline. The female body remains full of mysteries requiring further study and understanding.

Growth hormone's multifaceted functions make them a prime target for speculation, particularly regarding their role in aging. The commercial market for growth hormone-based products promises everything - from rejuvenation and weight loss to improved skin quality and memory enhancement.

One of the most debated topics surrounding growth hormone is whether it contributes to cancer, particularly breast cancer. It is well known that many hormones are associated with the development of various malignancies. For instance, steroid hormones (which will be discussed in later chapters) are classified as carcinogens, meaning they have the potential to promote cancer.

Natural growth hormone, as it circulates in the human body, has not been linked to cancer — at

least, no such connection has been found. However, the external administration of growth hormone may have a different impact, mainly through IGF-1, a breakdown product of growth hormone in the liver. Elevated IGF-1 levels have been detected in prostate cancer patients and women in the premenopausal stage with breast cancer. However, individuals with naturally high growth hormone production do not show an increased cancer risk. Furthermore, those with growth hormone deficiency have a nearly 50% lower incidence of cancer compared to the general population. Thus, the relationship between growth hormone and cancer remains unproven and poorly understood, underscoring the urgent need for further research in this area.

Like other pituitary hormones, growth hormone is secreted in a pulsatile manner. For healthy individuals, routine testing of growth hormone levels is unnecessary. In clinical practice, such tests are mainly performed on children. Growth hormone abnormalities are rare; a single blood test is often insufficient due to the hormone's daily fluctuations. Therefore, stimulation or suppression tests are commonly used for more accurate assessment.

Growth hormone testing is conducted in children with growth delay, accelerated growth, or puberty disorders. In adults, testing may be performed when there is rapid muscle loss, sudden obesity, or conditions such as acromegaly.

Growth hormone naturally declines with age, and while this decline is a physiological process, there are no official medical recommendations for administering growth hormone to counteract age-related decreases.

2.2.6. Adrenocorticotropic Hormone

The adrenocorticotropic hormone (ACTH, adrenocorticotropin, corticotropin) is a vital hormone the anterior pituitary gland produces. Despite not being trendy, its role in regulating the production of adrenal hormones and the body's response to stress is of the utmost importance. It is the key player in managing stress in the body, a function that directly impacts our daily lives and well-being.

The name **adrenocorticotropin** indicates that this hormone plays a significant role in controlling the production of adrenal cortex hormones — primarily **cortisol**. Its influence on producing other adrenal hormones is minimal, but its power and influence over cortisol production are immense. In the fetus, this hormone stimulates the production of the male hormone **DHEA-S**, which serves as a precursor for estrogen.

The precursor of ACTH is **pro-opiomelanocortin** (POMC) — a complex name, but an essential substance that acts as the "parent" for several other hormone-like compounds: *lipotropin* (a precursor of endorphins), *β-endorphin* and *met-enkephalin* (proteins involved in pain response), and *melanocyte-stimulating hormone* (MSH) (which controls melanin production and skin pigmentation).

From previous chapters, you have learned about pituitary hormones such as gonadotropins, which regulate the human reproductive system (gonads). The connection between the hypothalamus, pituitary gland, and ovaries is called the **hypothalamic-pituitary-ovarian axis**. This axis is crucial for the normal functioning of the reproductive system. However, since the pituitary gland produces corticotropin, which is essential for the body's stress

response and survival, it can block the production of gonadotropin-releasing hormone (GnRH), effectively suppressing the hypothalamic-pituitary-ovarian axis and shutting down reproductive function. This means **the body prioritizes survival over reproduction under stress, leading to a slowdown or cessation of reproductive function.**

How does this manifest in the body? Egg maturation is disrupted or ceases entirely, and menstrual cycles disappear. We will discuss menstrual cycle disorders in another chapter. Still, the most common issue is hypothalamic anovulation/amenorrhea, which accounts for up to 70% of ovulation and menstrual cycle disorders. "Hypothalamic" means that reproduction is inhibited at the hypothalamus level by suppressing GnRH production. As a result, FSH and LH are not produced sufficiently, leaving the ovaries inactive and ovulation absent.

Stress is the body's response to numerous stimuli. It can manifest at any level — psycho-emotional, physical, or metabolic — but its effect on the brain, including the hypothalamus and pituitary gland, remains the same. As ACTH levels rise, the adrenal glands increase cortisol production. Cortisol is the stress hormone — the king of stress!

Acute short-term stress most often stimulates egg maturation, meaning it does not immediately suppress a woman's reproductive function. Chronic prolonged stress, on the other hand, suppresses gonadotropin production, leading to anovulation.

The measurement of ACTH levels has not found widespread application in medicine. However, it is a crucial component of laboratory panels for suspected endocrine disorders, primarily *Addison's disease* (adrenal insufficiency), *Cushing's syndrome,* and *adrenal cortex hyperplasia.* In these conditions, abnormal ACTH levels can provide important diagnostic information, aiding in identifying and managing these disorders.

A synthetic ACTH analog is widely used in the treatment of many diseases, even those not directly related to pituitary function, such as multiple sclerosis, certain autoimmune conditions, severe allergic reactions, and rheumatoid arthritis. ACTH itself does not cure these diseases, meaning it does not eliminate the underlying condition, but it can alleviate many of the symptoms.

2.2.7. Melanocyte-Stimulating Hormone

MSH, a unique hormone due to its specific action on *melanocytes,* the skin cells responsible for pigment, plays a crucial role in determining skin color and forming pigmented formations. These include birthmarks, moles, and even malignant tumors like melanomas.

There are two forms of MSH. *Alpha-MSH*, responsible for tanning under the influence of ultraviolet radiation, is a key player in the skin's defense against UV light. It triggers the production of melanin, which protects the cell, particularly its nucleus, from the damaging effects of UV light.

Beta-MSH is a hormone that helps regulate body weight, energy homeostasis, and metabolism.

ACTH increases glucocorticoid levels, reducing the skin's inflammatory response to sun exposure, especially prolonged exposure, which enhances the effect of alpha-MSH. Additionally, beta-endorphins, produced simultaneously with these two hormones, help suppress pain perception following a skin burn.

It's fascinating to note that synthetic forms of MSH can achieve an artificial tan without ultraviolet exposure. Even more intriguing, some synthetic MSH variants have been found to aid in treating erectile dysfunction in men, showcasing the diverse potential of this hormone.

MSH is also produced by other brain cells, where it plays a role in appetite suppression. Individuals with genetic mutations affecting MSH receptors tend to develop obesity.

2.2.8. Pituitary Disorders

From the previous chapters, you already understand the pituitary gland's intricate role. As an endocrine gland, it is also vulnerable to diseases. Moreover, it can be assailed by autoimmune antibodies, known as *anti-pituitary antibodies* (APA). These antibodies can damage pituitary tissue and instigate inflammation, culminating in lymphocytic hypophysitis.

It's worth noting that pituitary antibodies, the culprits behind these disorders, have been discovered in individuals grappling with type 1 diabetes and thyroiditis, further underscoring the intricate interplay within the endocrine system.

Regrettably, the role of these antibodies is still shrouded in mystery, making the diagnostic and treatment methods for this rare condition elusive. However, in most cases, pituitary cell destruction occurs in specific areas, leading to a deficiency in producing only one or two hormones. For instance, if the cells that produce TSH (thyroid-stimulating hormone) are destroyed, thyroid dysfunction may develop. If FSH (follicle-stimulating hormone) production is blocked, both men and women may have infertility. This complexity makes the diagnosis of *lymphocytic hypophysitis* particularly daunting.

Another condition known as *empty sella syndrome* can occur either due to a tumor that grows and compresses the surrounding pituitary tissue or because the *soft meninges* (brain lining) enter the pituitary cavity, displacing glandular tissue. This leads to disruptions in pituitary hormone production and may also trigger the development of autoimmune antibodies against specific hormones. Such a condition is often observed after pituitary surgery or radiation therapy. Some women with obesity and increased intracranial pressure may show signs of empty sella syndrome.

Whether the syndrome is congenital (primary) or manifests in childhood, it can be associated with disruptions in sexual development and other endocrine disorders. Treatment in these cases focuses on rectifying hormonal imbalances, underscoring the importance of early intervention and comprehensive care.

Other pituitary disorders with a chromosomal-genetic origin are exceedingly rare, underscoring the need for heightened awareness and vigilance in the medical community.

2.3. Thymus Gland

The **thymus**, or **thymus gland**, is an organ involved in the body's defense mechanisms and the formation of immunity. It is located behind the sternum. It gradually decreases in size from birth, and in adults, it measures only about 1 cm in diameter.

While not an endocrine gland, the thymus has historically been misclassified as such in almost all medical textbooks and popular medical literature. This misclassification sparked debates among doctors years ago, but scientific and medical progress eventually prevailed, leading to a more accurate understanding of the thymus's function.

Despite not being an endocrine organ, the thymus plays a crucial role in immune function. In the 1960s, **thymosin** was discovered in the thymus and mistakenly identified as a hormone. Later, the substance, initially called thymosin, was found to consist of about forty different compounds. These compounds in the thymus play a significant role in *hematopoiesis* (blood cell formation) and immune function, primarily in T-lymphocyte production and maturation.

Traces of certain hormones can be found in thymus tissue, but these enter through the bloodstream rather than being produced by the thymus itself.

Thus, the term "thymus gland" is misleading, as this organ is neither structurally nor functionally a gland.

2.4. Pancreas

The pancreas is a marvel of nature, uniquely performing both an endocrine function—producing hormones, and a crucial role in digestion. It secretes pancreatic juice, a special fluid that contains numerous substances essential for breaking down food, processing fats, proteins, and carbohydrates, and absorbing nutrients.

The pancreas contains several hundred thousand clusters of cells, forming the *islets of Langerhans*, named after their discoverer, the German pathologist Paul Langerhans. These clusters function as endocrine glands and consist of five types of cells:

- Alpha cells produce glucagon.

- Beta cells produce insulin and amylin.

- Delta cells produce somatostatin.

- PP cells produce pancreatic polypeptides.

- Epsilon cells produce ghrelin.

2.4.1. Glucagon

While insulin is a familiar hormone for most adults, the importance of **glucagon** is often overlooked. Glucagon, as insulin's antagonist, is vital in increasing blood sugar and fatty acid levels, particularly during fasting periods, such as overnight or between long meal intervals, to maintain normal blood glucose levels.

People with type 1 diabetes often experience low blood sugar (*hypoglycemia*) due to a lack of glucagon. In contrast, type 2 diabetes is frequently associated with *hyperglycemia* (high blood sugar levels). **Glucagon is the primary hormone that regulates glucose levels and suppresses insulin activity**. It works by binding to glucagon receptors, which are present in various tissues and organs throughout the body. The highest levels of glucagon are observed between 6 and 12 AM.

Glucagon affects multiple organs:

- In the liver, it increases fat breakdown, stimulates glucose production, and enhances liver cell survival (hepatocytes).

- In the brain, it creates a feeling of satiety.

- It increases heart rate, although heart cells may experience energy depletion.

- It stimulates intestinal motility.

- It raises body temperature.

- It breaks down white body fat.

- The kidneys filter and retain more fluids.

- It helps regulate body weight.

These are just some of glucagon's many functions. Additionally, glucagon is widely used as a pharmaceutical drug.

Given the widespread concern about weight control, maintaining normal glucagon levels is crucial for weight loss and maintenance. This practical advice can benefit adult women, who often face this constant dilemma.

2.4.2. Insulin

There is no need to introduce insulin — it is frequently mentioned today due to the rising number of people worldwide suffering from obesity, which is often accompanied by type 2 diabetes. This form of diabetes, also known as *alimentary diabetes*, develops due to excessive carbohydrate consumption (sugar, flour-based foods, etc.). Insulin and glucose metabolism are also discussed during pregnancy, as some women develop *gestational diabetes*. Additionally, insulin levels are evaluated when assessing the menstrual cycle and suspected *polycystic ovary syndrome* (PCOS) cases.

Insulin has an effect opposite to glucagon — it lowers blood sugar levels. As soon as blood glucose rises, insulin production is triggered, prompting skeletal muscles to utilize more glucose and store it as *glycogen*.

When discussing diabetes and blood sugar control, the focus is often placed on diet and antidiabetic medications. However, it's crucial to remember that **physical activity should be the primary factor in regulating blood sugar**. This knowledge empowers individuals to take an active role in managing their health.

Skeletal muscles are the number one consumer of sugar. The more they contract, the more glucose they use, as they require more energy. Conversely, a sedentary lifestyle leads to excess sugar, which, through a series of mechanisms, is eventually stored as body fat.

Insulin is crucial in protein synthesis, using amino acids circulating in the blood. It affects liver cells (*hepatocytes*), which synthesize glycogen while simultaneously inhibiting the enzymes responsible for its

83

breakdown. Insulin also affects brain cells, particularly the hypothalamus, helping to suppress appetite. This comprehensive understanding of insulin's functions provides a more profound knowledge of its role in the body.

Glucose Tolerance Test

Various diabetes diagnostic tests assess glucose absorption by the body. The most common is the *screening test* (Glucose Challenge Test) and the *diagnostic test* (Glucose Tolerance Test, or GTT). GTT is gaining popularity due to its diagnostic significance.

Who should take this test? It is used not only for diagnosing diabetes but also in many other cases. Excess weight and obesity are often associated with *metabolic syndrome*, a condition in which metabolic processes throughout the body are disrupted. While it may remain compensated and cause no immediate symptoms, it significantly increases the risk of cardiovascular disease. Therefore, GTT is recommended in the following cases:

- Body Mass Index (BMI) over 25

- Blood pressure ≥ 130/85 mmHg

- Fasting blood glucose level ≥ 5.5 mmol/L

- Triglyceride level ≥ 1.7 mmol/L

Although GTT measures blood sugar levels two hours after consuming 75 or 100 g of glucose solution, some researchers believe the one-hour post-glucose level better predicts diabetes risk and metabolic syndrome.

A significant drawback of the glucose tolerance test is the lack of universal standards for evaluating blood sugar levels. Reference values vary between health organizations, such as the WHO, endocrine societies, and professional associations.

Blood Insulin Testing

Measuring insulin levels in the blood would provide a clear picture of its production. However, studies have shown that **insulin concentration in the blood does not reflect its absorption by tissues, meaning it does not accurately indicate insulin resistance**. As a result, this measurement has limited practical significance in medicine. High insulin levels may be observed in the early stages of metabolic syndrome, but they can also signal excessive insulin production, which occurs in conditions such as *insulinomas*.

Measuring insulin levels is a complex task due to the vast array of laboratory tests available, each with its unique approach. This lack of a universal standard for insulin measurement poses a significant challenge, as there are no internationally accepted guidelines for determining insulin levels.

The question of insulin resistance most commonly arises when evaluating women suspected of having polycystic ovary syndrome (PCOS). However, the low sensitivity of current tests has sparked considerable debate among doctors, highlighting the complex nature of insulin resistance. A comparative analysis of several insulin resistance tests showed that results varied widely depending on the method used. Additionally, insulin resistance fluctuates constantly within an individual and may even normalize periodically, adding to the challenge of understanding this condition.

Insulin resistance is a complex condition that involves more than just tissue absorption of insulin. However, researchers actively investigate additional biomarkers to clarify the relationship between insulin and cells. This ongoing research provides hope for a better understanding of insulin resistance and the development of predictive tools for assessing the risk of diabetes and cardiovascular diseases.

Other Pancreatic Hormones

Amylin, a hormone produced alongside insulin, plays a crucial role in stabilizing blood glucose levels and inducing a feeling of fullness by slowing gastric emptying. While its significance was previously overlooked, it is now recognized as important as insulin. It has been increasingly used in diabetes treatment, often with insulin.

Somatostatin is a growth hormone inhibitor that suppresses insulin and glucagon production. When released into the stomach, it inhibits the secretion of gastric juice and hydrochloric acid. It also affects the production of various other substances in the body.

Pancreatic polypeptide, in contrast, reduces pancreatic juice secretion but stimulates gastric juice production. However, little is known about its role.

Ghrelin is considered the *hunger hormone*. It is released when blood sugar levels are low, triggering hunger sensations.

Cells in the gastrointestinal tract produce a range of other hormone-like substances that act locally, primarily in digestion and nutrient absorption. However, some compounds also affect the nervous system and other tissues.

2.5. Ovaries

Where does a woman's unique journey begin? With her ovaries. These remarkable organs are the cornerstone of the female body and play a pivotal role in the miracle of life.

A woman receives her **primary reproductive cells** in the first weeks after conception — before the ovaries even exist. As the fetal gonads develop in utero, these cells settle in the ovaries. Many women are unaware that the entire supply of reproductive cells (follicles), initially numbering in the millions, of which only 300–400 will mature into eggs, declines rapidly, never regenerates, and cannot be replaced. This is the so-called **ovarian reserve**, a crucial factor in a woman's fertility. Doctors assess this reserve in adulthood when a woman has difficulty conceiving or symptoms of ovarian insufficiency, as a low ovarian reserve can indicate a reduced chance of conception.

The ovaries are complex and endowed with two inseparable functions: egg maturation and hormone production. As follicles mature, they produce male and female sex hormones and progesterone, a delicate dance that influences the entire body's function.

Follicle maturation is crucial for conception and maintaining normal estrogen, testosterone, and progesterone levels, which in turn influence the entire body's function.

The ovaries are paired organs, and nature has ensured that even if one ovary is lost, a woman can still conceive thanks to the function of the remaining ovary. The right ovary is always larger than the left, as it has a better blood supply, so ovulation occurs more frequently in the right ovary. This asymmetry in ovulation can be significant in cases where one ovary is compromised, as it ensures that the woman still has a good chance of conceiving from the remaining ovary.

It is a myth that eggs mature in the ovaries alternately. In reality, no one knows what determines the order of egg maturation. However, in nearly 70% of cases, ovulation occurs in the right ovary. It is usual for ovulation to occur in the same ovary for several consecutive cycles. We will discuss the menstrual cycle in detail in a later chapter.

Hormone production and egg maturation are not independent processes. They are intricately interconnected, forming a delicate balance for the female reproductive system. *Ovarian insufficiency*, therefore, is not just a hormonal imbalance but also a disruption in egg development.

It's important to note that a follicular ovarian structure is a standard characteristic of all mammals and not a cause for concern. Some doctors mistakenly diagnose polycystic ovary syndrome (PCOS) based solely on the presence of multiple follicles, which are often referred to as 'small cysts.' This misconception can lead to unnecessary worry, but it's important to remember that **a follicular ovarian structure is a normal and essential part of the female reproductive system.**

Oocytes (eggs) are surrounded by granulosa cells (somatic or granular cells) and embedded in the ovarian stroma, a soft structural framework containing connective tissue, muscle tissue, and blood vessels. The entire ovary is enclosed in a connective tissue capsule.

A follicle containing a primary oocyte is also called a *germinal vesicle*. It is surrounded by granulosa cells, which play a crucial role in hormone production. Around this granulosa cell layer is a thin basal membrane; externally, *theca cells*, appearing only in nearly mature follicles. Theca cells are responsible for producing androgens, which are then converted into estrogen by the granulosa cells, thereby contributing to the maturation of the follicle.

2.5.1. The Role of Gonadotropins in Egg Maturation

For a long time, gynecology was guided by the "**two-cell, two-gonadotropin**" theory, which described the process of egg maturation (**folliculogenesis**) and hormone production by theca and granulosa cells under the influence of follicle-stimulating hormone (FSH) and luteinizing hormone (LH). This theory has been widely published in medical literature and textbooks.

According to this theory, granulosa cells are the primary source of estradiol, which is formed by the conversion of androgens (produced by theca cells) into female sex hormones through a process known as *aromatization*. Aromatization depends on FSH levels, which bind to and activate granulosa cell receptors.

The intricate dance of hormonal changes observed throughout the menstrual cycle, including fluctuations in gonadotropins, estradiol, and progesterone, has long supported the 'two-cell, two-gonadotropin' theory. However, it's worth noting that many medical textbooks have described these hormonal shifts inaccurately, adding a layer of complexity to our understanding.

The commonly accepted explanation has been as follows:

- In the first phase of the cycle, rising FSH stimulates follicular growth and estrogen production.

- After ovulation, increasing LH stimulates progesterone production by the corpus luteum.

- Thus, FSH and estrogen dominate the follicular phase, while LH and progesterone dominate the luteal phase.

Most doctors still follow this model when ordering FSH, LH, and estrogen tests on days 3–8 of the cycle and progesterone and LH (again) on days 9–21.

However, the reality is that FSH and LH levels remain relatively stable throughout the menstrual cycle, except for the pre-ovulatory surge. This surge, which occurs around the middle of the menstrual cycle, is a sudden increase in FSH and LH levels that triggers ovulation. Estradiol levels are also low at the beginning of the follicular phase, but in the luteal phase, they are slightly higher than in the first half of the cycle.

Estrogen production indeed requires the interaction of two types of cells — theca and granulosa. However, some researchers have found that theca cells can produce both androgens and estrogens. Others argue that theca cells primarily produce progesterone due to the lack of aromatase, an enzyme necessary for converting androgens into estrogens.

Considering these stages of sex hormone synthesis, it becomes clear that the "two-cell, two-gonadotropin" theory is not entirely accurate. This theory portrays progesterone as a secondary hormone produced by the corpus luteum only after ovulation. Progesterone plays a far more significant role — it is the primary, foundational hormone intricately woven into every function of ovarian cells, influencing their activity. The inaccuracies in this theory could lead to misinterpretation of test results and mismanagement of reproductive health conditions, underscoring the need for a reevaluation of current understanding and practices.

Progesterone inhibits granulosa cell growth in the ovaries, effectively suppressing follicular development. This explains why, during pregnancy, when progesterone levels are high, follicular growth and ovulation do not occur.

Of course, egg maturation and ovulation require specific hormone levels and proportions in the blood. However, if we analyze the sequence of processes in the ovary, the first phase of the cycle is entirely focused on egg maturation. The hormones produced during this period are primarily used within the ovary itself, which is why the ovary is said to have a paracrine function during this phase. This means that the hormones produced by the ovary act locally, influencing the growth and development of the follicles and the maturation of the egg.

In the second phase, the ovary's primary function shifts to endocrine activity, producing hormones necessary for implantation and pregnancy maintenance. During this phase, most hormones the ovary produces enter the bloodstream and are distributed throughout the body, particularly to the uterus and mammary glands.

The removal of the ovaries results in a deficiency of estrogen and progesterone, affecting the function of multiple organs, including other endocrine glands. This underscores the importance of *hormone replacement therapy* (HRT), which includes not only estrogen but also progesterone, ensuring a comprehensive approach to maintaining hormonal balance.

The ovaries can rightfully be called the kingdom of progesterone — this hormone, often overshadowed by estrogen, regulates the entire function of the ovary, a fact that deserves our full appreciation.

2.5.2. Steroid Hormones

It is time to talk about a special group of hormones known as **steroids**. Many people are familiar with steroids as medications.

All steroid compounds share a common structural feature — four carbon rings, often called the *steroid nucleus* or *gonane*. These rings are labeled with Latin letters (A, B, C, and D) from left to right.

Several hundred steroid compounds exist in nature, including plants, fungi, and animals. Modern pharmacology includes hundreds of synthetic steroids, such as corticosteroids and anabolic steroids. These are used not only in medicine to treat conditions like asthma and autoimmune diseases but also in various industrial fields, for instance, in the production of plastics and hormones for livestock.

It is believed that the appearance of steroids in nature is linked to the increase in atmospheric oxygen levels. Most biochemical processes in living organisms occur through the addition (*oxidation*) or removal of oxygen atoms.

Traditionally, steroid hormones are divided into **five** classes:

- Estrogens

- Progestogens (progesterone)

- Androgens

- Glucocorticoids

- Mineralocorticoids

All steroid hormones produced by the ovaries, testes, and adrenal glands are interconnected, and their function depends on three key factors at the cellular level:

1. The quality and quantity of receptors capable of binding to hormones

2. The presence of sufficient enzymes involved in steroid hormone metabolism

3. The site of hormone binding (cell surface, intracellular cytoplasm, nucleus, mitochondria)

Target Cells

Hormones, with their specific receptors, are like keys that fit only one kind of lock. This precision allows hormones to act only on target cells with specific receptors that can bind to hormone molecules or another mechanism for their absorption. This specificity is a testament to the intricate design of the endocrine system.

Under certain conditions, different hormones and chemical substances may interact with some receptors (receptor-blocking drugs, for example, are widely used to treat various diseases).

Understanding the relationship between endocrine glands, receptors, and hormones is crucial. To illustrate this, one can compare it to radio broadcasting. A radio station (endocrine gland) continuously transmits signals (hormones) over long distances (throughout the body). However, a radio receiver (organ) must be switched on and tuned to a specific frequency (hormone receptors) to receive and hear the broadcast. This analogy underscores the importance of understanding the endocrine system for maintaining health and treating diseases.

Steroid hormones act on specific target tissues. Target organs or target tissues are those hormones from the ovaries that directly influence and help them perform their function. In the female body, these include the uterus (but not all layers — only the endometrium and partially the myometrium) and the mammary glands, which require hormones for milk production.

Synthesis of Steroid Hormones

Steroid hormones, crucial for various bodily functions, are derivatives of **cholesterol**. These hormones include cortisol, which regulates metabolism and the body's response to stress, and testosterone, which is responsible for the development of male reproductive tissues. Despite the myths and misconceptions surrounding cholesterol, modern research at the molecular and atomic levels has enlightened us about its vital role in the normal functioning of the human body.

The term "cholesterol" originates from two Greek words: "chole" (bile) and "stereos" (solid, as in the word "steroids"). The French physician and chemist Poulletier de la Salle first isolated cholesterol in solid form from gallstones in 1769. The suffix "-ol" indicates that cholesterol belongs to the class of alcohols.

Cholesterol is a key player in the body's functions. It serves as the foundation for steroid hormones and bile acids. It is also a crucial structural component of cell membranes, ensuring their strength and water resistance. While every human cell can produce cholesterol, the liver, intestines, reproductive organs, and adrenal glands are the primary sites of its synthesis.

Fats obtained from food are essential for cholesterol production. Additionally, a significant amount of cholesterol is directly absorbed from dietary sources, mainly animal products. A deficiency of dietary fats can impair the production of not only cholesterol but also steroid hormones, especially sex hormones, potentially leading to reproductive dysfunction or even a complete shutdown of reproductive processes.

All biochemical processes in nature follow a staged or gradual pattern. This stage-by-stage nature may seem like a complex, multi-step mechanism, but it is also a system of interconnected simple processes. A failure at one level can be efficiently compensated for by alternative pathways involving different molecules, reassuring us of the body's resilience and ability to adapt.

The more essential a substance is for life, the simpler its synthesis mechanisms. Progesterone, one of the most critical steroid hormones, serves as the precursor for many other hormones. Its production and regulation are ensured through multiple independent mechanisms. An intermediate steroid compound called *pregnenolone* is synthesized from cholesterol and forms various steroid hormones, highlighting the body's efficient and straightforward approach to producing essential substances.

Organs that produce steroid hormones contain specific progesterone receptors. These hormone receptors, which are mostly lipid or protein structures, act like locks that can only be opened by the specific hormone molecule, the 'key '. **Each hormone has its unique receptors, and without this 'lock-and-key' interaction, the hormone cannot exert its biological effect on target cells or the organ. When the hormone binds to its receptor, it triggers a series of biochemical reactions within the cell, leading to the hormone's specific physiological effect.**

Transport of Steroid Hormones

There are several ways in which hormonal substances are transported throughout the human body. Most hormones travel in a protein-bound form. Hormones and other substances bound to proteins are referred to as **conjugated**. If hormone molecules and other compounds are not bound to proteins, they are in a non-conjugated state. Only up to 2% of steroid hormones in human blood exist in a free form. When a hormone is bound to a protein, it remains inactive, meaning it does not affect cells and tissues.

Human blood contains a vast array of organic substances and cellular structures. Proteins comprise 6–8% of blood volume, with the most common types being *albumins, globulins,* and *fibrinogen.* Albumins and globulins are also known as serum globulins or globular proteins, as their molecules have a compact, spherical shape.

Blood, Serum, and Plasma – What's the Difference?

Understanding the nuanced differences between blood, serum, and plasma is not just a matter of semantics. It's a crucial aspect of laboratory tests, as they often analyze different components. Certain substances may be measured in **whole blood, serum,** or **plasma** depending on the lab, yielding different results. Failing to consider these distinctions can lead to misinterpretation of lab findings. Armed with this knowledge, you can navigate the complexities of blood analysis with confidence and precision.

When blood is drawn from a vein (venous blood sampling is preferred over finger-prick sampling), the collected sample consists of whole blood, containing all its components. If an anticoagulant is added to prevent coagulation (clotting) and the sample is then centrifuged, the cellular components (red blood cells, white blood cells, platelets) settle at the bottom of the test tube. The remaining fluid, free of blood cells, is called plasma.

If coagulation factors, mainly fibrinogen, are removed from plasma, the resulting fluid is called serum. The remaining proteins in serum can be further separated using electrophoresis. Under the influence of an electric current, proteins migrate toward electrodes at different speeds, allowing for the isolation of various protein fractions in the blood.

Albumins

Albumins, making up approximately 50% of all blood proteins, are true multitaskers. Produced in the liver, they transport numerous small-molecule substances throughout the body. But their role doesn't stop there. They also play a crucial role in maintaining *osmotic pressure*, essential for regulating fluid balance in the blood. This multifunctionality is a testament to the intricate design of our biological systems.

Albumins, the unsung heroes of our blood, can bind to a wide array of substances. They can bind to water molecules, various ions (sodium, potassium, calcium), certain hormones, bilirubin, vitamins, lipids, and multiple medications. During pregnancy, the developing fetus produces *alpha-fetoprotein* (AFP), which albumins transport within the fetal bloodstream and across the placenta. This versatility is a testament to the adaptability of albumins in our bodies.

Albumin's Role in the Transport of Progesterone and Sex Hormones

Since the 1970s, the role of albumin in transporting progesterone and other sex hormones has been studied in animal models and humans. Research has been conducted across various age groups, medical conditions, and pregnant women. Since progesterone is one of the primary ovarian hormones, understanding its transport and metabolism provides deeper insight into the absorption and regulation of steroid hormones.

Under normal progesterone levels and outside of pregnancy, up to 80% of progesterone is bound to albumin. When progesterone concentrations increase, such as during pregnancy or after exogenous progesterone administration, the albumin-bound progesterone fraction decreases, even though total albumin levels may increase. However, the rise in protein levels does not always correlate with the increase in hormone levels (as observed during pregnancy). In such cases, some hormone molecules may bind to other proteins, such as globulins in red blood cells, or remain free.

Globulins

Serum globulins, a significant component of the body's transport system, are crucial in transporting various substances. There are three types: **alpha, beta, and gamma globulins**, each with its unique functions and contributions to the body's overall health.

- **Alpha-globulins** transport many vitamins and hormones, including estrogen, testosterone, and progesterone. However, only 20% of progesterone in the bloodstream is bound to globulins.

- **Beta-globulins** transport various substances, such as iron, which is carried in the form of transferrin.

- **Gamma-globulins**, a key immune system component, function as antibodies (often called immunoglobulins). They are produced in response to foreign agents entering the body or against the body's own damaged or abnormal cells (such as cancerous cells). The level of antibodies usually increases in response to infections, highlighting the body's remarkable defense mechanisms.

There are **five classes of antibodies** (Ig), which are produced either sequentially or simultaneously, depending on the type of foreign agent. Gamma-globulins are used for treating specific conditions and preventive purposes, as they are included in many vaccines. **Autoimmune antibodies**, which can target endocrine glands and affect hormone production, most commonly belong to class G (IgG).

Specific globulins that bind steroid hormones include several proteins capable of binding to sex hormones. One is **sex hormone-binding globulin** (SHBG), which belongs to the globulin family. Unlike sex hormones, progesterone binds to this protein infrequently, while androgens and estrogens are the primary steroid hormones associated with SHBG.

Another type of globulin is **corticosteroid-binding globulin** (CBG or transcortin), which primarily binds to cortisol. This large protein consists of 135 amino acids and is closely related to proteins that transport thyroid hormones.

While CBG binds 80–90% of cortisol in human blood plasma, it can also bind to progesterone.

Another important globulin is an **α1-acid glycoprotein** (AAG) or *orosomucoid*. CBG and AAG contain a high proportion of sugars found in all mammals. In pregnant females of certain animal species, the level of progesterone-bound protein increases several times faster than the level of corticosteroid-binding protein. In pregnant women, the concentration of α1-globulin increases significantly, binding primarily to progesterone and, to a lesser extent, to other steroids, including testosterone.

Understanding the transport mechanisms of steroid hormones, particularly sex hormones and progesterone, helps clarify the reasons behind fluctuations in hormone levels. Simply measuring an increase in hormone levels is insufficient — it is essential to determine whether the hormone is in its bound or free form. Additionally, in protein deficiency (such as malnutrition or fasting), the proportion of free hormones in the blood may increase.

Why is most progesterone bound to albumin rather than globulins? The degree of hormone binding depends on the type of protein and body temperature. Although globulins have a binding capacity 500 times greater than albumin, the concentration in the blood is significantly higher — for every molecule of CBG, there are 800 molecules of albumin. As a result, most of the progesterone (as well as other hormones) in the bloodstream is bound to albumin, with more than 50% of progesterone being albumin-bound during pregnancy.

Protein binding, a crucial aspect of steroid hormone metabolism, plays a protective role. Since steroid hormones are virtually insoluble in body fluids, produced naturally or introduced externally, protein binding facilitates their transport and protects them from enzymatic degradation, ensuring their stability and effectiveness.

2.5.3. Progesterone

Progesterone, as well as male and female sex hormones produced by the ovaries, has been mentioned multiple times throughout this book. We will continue exploring these remarkable substances, giving progesterone the leading role due to its evolutionary significance, biochemical perfection, and vital importance.

Progesterone, a truly unique compound, is synthesized by living organisms, including humans. Its essential role in the survival of many animal species and its diverse effects on humans, which can be both beneficial and harmful, depending on various factors, conditions, and external biochemical interventions, make it a fascinating subject of study.

Progesterone is known by several names: corpus luteum hormone, lutein hormone, progestational hormone, luteal hormone, luteohormone, lutein, the pregnancy hormone, pregnandione, and progesteronum. Some countries have their specific terminology for this hormone.

While it's not necessary to memorize the exact chemical structure of progesterone or have an in-depth understanding of metabolic pathways in the human body, it's important to remember specific key facts about its structure and function. These insights are valuable as they help us better understand how the human body works, what processes take place, and how they affect specific organs and the body.

First and foremost, progesterone is a steroid compound, as previously mentioned. This fact should prompt critical thinkers to recognize that steroids are interconnected like members of the same extended family — parents, siblings, grandchildren, great-grandchildren, etc. Progesterone also shares a "familial" connection with other steroid hormones, a topic we will explore further.

Progesterone, a hormone familiar to most women, has often been mistakenly labeled as a sex hormone in many sources, including medical literature. This misconception can be traced back to the early 20th century when male sex hormones were first identified. The discovery of male sex hormones led to the assumption that women must have female sex hormones, and since ovarian extracts contained progesterone, this false assumption took root and persisted for decades.

However, male and female sex hormones are present in all individuals, regardless of gender, albeit in different amounts and proportions. **Male sex hormones are androgens, while female sex hormones are estrogens.**

While progesterone does influence the female reproductive system and regulate the menstrual cycle, it is important to note that it is not a sex hormone. Understanding this distinction is crucial for a comprehensive grasp of human biology.

The placenta, a remarkable organ, takes charge of progesterone production during pregnancy, producing almost 15 times more than the ovaries in the first few weeks of gestation. **This independence in progesterone production is a fascinating aspect of pregnancy, as it is not reliant on the woman's ovaries or the corpus luteum of pregnancy**. Instead, it occurs independently and automatically through biochemical processes in the placenta, which is derived from the fertilized egg, not the mother.

It's reassuring to know that regardless of whether the fetus is male or female, the placenta (and partially the fetus itself) produces the same amount of progesterone. This natural balance ensures that **neither the baby's sex nor the mother's female biology influences progesterone production during pregnancy**. Additionally, the progesterone synthesized by the placenta is not absorbed by the mother's body — instead, it is utilized by the fetus to synthesize essential hormones and other biochemical compounds.

It's time to debunk a common misconception about hormonal balance. The key factor in a woman's hormonal balance is often believed to be the ratio of estrogen to progesterone. But if this were true, what would be the key factor in the hormonal regulation of the male body? The usual answer is testosterone levels, but is that the case? **When we consider biochemical pathways and the production of all sex hormones, it becomes clear that both men and women rely on a physiologically balanced proportion of three hormones — progesterone, testosterone, and estrogen — the actual 'holy trinity' of steroid hormones.**

It is essential to recognize that in the process of *gamete* (sex cell) maturation, the dominant ratio is not estrogen/progesterone but rather testosterone/estrogen, regulated through the *matrix hormone* — progesterone. **Progesterone plays a key role in this process, influencing the balance of testosterone and estrogen, which are crucial for the maturation of sex cells.** The exact proportion of these hormones is influenced not only by the menstrual cycle phase but also by age, diet, work-rest balance, stress levels, and other individual factors, often leading to natural fluctuations.

The ovaries, testes, and adrenal glands produce progesterone. In some cases, it is used locally, for example, by the ovaries for sex hormone synthesis or by the adrenal glands for steroid hormone production. Progesterone plays a crucial role in these processes, influencing the synthesis of sex hormones in the ovaries and steroid hormones in the adrenal glands. It is also transported to target tissues where its consumption is highest, primarily the uterus and mammary glands.

Hormone Levels in the Blood

Though present in small quantities, endogenous progesterone circulates freely in the body. The extent to which cells and tissues utilize this active progesterone instead of breaking it down and excreting it remains a mystery. When free progesterone levels rise, enzymes in the blood and other tissues swiftly target it to mitigate its potential adverse effects.

The bound form of progesterone (98–99% of total progesterone) is transported to various organs, tissues, and cells. This form moves more slowly through the body and partially degrades during transport despite being bound to proteins, especially in the liver. However, bound progesterone is inactive and does not influence target cells. The exact percentage of bound progesterone utilized by tissues also remains unclear.

The progesterone level measured in a woman's blood reflects the bound, inactive form, which does not accurately represent how much progesterone is absorbed by cells and how effectively it functions in the body.

This issue of hormone measurement is not limited to progesterone. For many years, physicians measuring hormone levels in blood failed to recognize the significant differences between bound, free, and total hormone levels. A hormone's biological impact is primarily determined by its free form, yet most laboratories still measure only total hormone levels (the sum of free and bound hormones). This complexity underscores the need for further research and understanding in this field.

In many cases, bound hormone levels may be elevated, such as during pregnancy, while free hormone levels remain normal. There may be multiple reasons for this if the conjugated (bound) hormone levels are high. Still, in most cases, it is a protective compensatory response: when excess hormone appears in circulation, the body neutralizes its activity by binding it to proteins and facilitating rapid elimination. This is why hormone metabolites (breakdown products) are often found in increased concentrations in bodily fluids such as blood, urine, or stool.

As medical science advances, hormone measurement methods are improving. For example, thyroid function is no longer diagnosed based solely on total T4 and T3 levels — modern testing considers free thyroid hormones as well as

TSH (thyroid-stimulating hormone) from the pituitary gland, which regulates thyroid function (thyroid disorders will be discussed in another chapter).

The same applies to male sex hormones — the free androgen index is far more relevant than total or bound testosterone. Similarly, prolactin levels should be evaluated by distinguishing between free and protein-bound forms.

Despite advancements in medical science, female endocrinology still grapples with the need for accurate hormone measurements. Many reproductive disorders are diagnosed based on incorrect hormone measurements and metabolites without considering their binding status. For instance, the biologically active forms of hormones, such as free estradiol and free progesterone, are often overlooked in favor of conclusions drawn from conjugated hormone levels. This oversight hampers accurately determining the percentage of a hormone absorbed by the body and how much is excreted in urine or stool.

Additionally, hormone levels fluctuate constantly. **Each day of the menstrual cycle and different times of the day have unique hormonal proportions**. Current knowledge of these fluctuations is limited. This underscores the urgent need for further research to understand these fluctuations and their implications.

While hormone fluctuation graphs exist, they are based on data from experimental studies and reflect individual cases rather than universal patterns. The highly variable nature of hormonal rhythms means these charts cannot be universally applied to all women.

Thus, modern female endocrinology faces serious dilemmas, not only in diagnosing endocrine disorders but also in choosing treatment strategies. An even more significant challenge arises when prescribing hormone therapy in perimenopausal and menopausal women.

Two Forms of Progesterone

Most women are unaware that progesterone exists in two distinct forms, produced by different sources and serving completely different roles.

The corpus luteum (luteal body) produces the most significant amount of progesterone in non-pregnant women, which is why it is often referred to as *luteal progesterone*. Its peak production occurs on the 7th day after ovulation, coinciding with the onset of implantation of the fertilized egg.

It was once believed that progesterone levels were uniform in all women of reproductive age. However, research has shown significant variations across different ethnic groups. In some populations, progesterone levels are up to 70% lower, yet fertility rates remain unchanged, challenging previous assumptions about "normal" hormonal ranges.

Luteal Progesterone

After ovulation, luteal progesterone performs the following functions:

- Stimulates further production of progesterone by the ovary.

- Suppresses endometrial proliferation (prevents excessive growth of the uterine lining).

- Stimulates proliferation of mammary glands (peaking around day 24 of the cycle).

- Reduces inflammatory processes in the ovaries and uterus.

- Triggers the differentiation program of the endometrium.

- Stimulates the growth of spiral arteries in the myometrium.

- Activates endometrial glands, enhancing their secretion of a specialized fluid.

- Attracts immune system cells to the uterus, which plays a role in establishing a healthy connection between the fertilized egg and the uterus.

- Creates the "implantation window" by forming *pinopodes* (specialized endometrial structures).

- Regulates the production of pituitary and hypothalamic hormones.

- Participates in female sexual behavior (suppressing sexual desire).

- Influences psycho-emotional state (often suppressing mood).

- Reduces intestinal and gallbladder motility.

  After conception, luteal progesterone also:

- Reduces uterine contractions, preventing early embryo expulsion during implantation.

- Stimulates decidual tissue formation, a crucial section of the endometrium where the embryo attaches.

Luteal progesterone has many other functions, as progesterone receptors are present in various organs throughout the human body.

A young, healthy woman with a 28-day menstrual cycle produces approximately 210 mg of progesterone per cycle, totaling about 2,500 mg per year.

Placental Progesterone

From weeks 7–8 of pregnancy, the developing placenta begins producing *placental progesterone*, reaching very high levels as pregnancy progresses. Although this progesterone crosses the placental barrier into the maternal bloodstream, most remains within placental tissue, amniotic fluid, and the fetal body.

As soon as placental progesterone production begins, ovarian progesterone production significantly decreases. Maternal blood progesterone levels gradually increase, peaking just before labor — this entire process is driven by placental progesterone.

Despite its high levels, the mother's body does not efficiently absorb placental progesterone. This is evident from the lack of a significant increase in other steroid hormones derived from progesterone and the absence of an increase in progesterone metabolites in blood and urine.

Placental progesterone exhibits a remarkable level of autonomy — not only from the mother's body but also from the fetus. While this independence is a mystery to scientists and physicians, it has significant implications for our understanding of pregnancy and fetal development.

By the end of pregnancy, the placenta produces the highest progesterone levels, with total hormone production reaching 300 mg daily — many times more than the ovaries produce.

What role does placental progesterone play for the mother? Traditionally, it is believed to perform the following functions:

- Suppresses the inflammatory response of the myometrium to the placenta.

- Prepares the mammary glands for lactation.

- Maintains a balance between uterine contractions and relaxation.

- Inhibits the production of prostaglandins in the uterus.

- Stimulates uterine contractions in full-term pregnancy.

In other words, the portion of placental progesterone that enters the maternal bloodstream primarily affects the uterus and mammary glands. At the same time, the fetus benefits from it much more than the mother.

The exact role of progesterone in fetal development remains unclear, as no correlation has been found between progesterone levels in the umbilical arteries, umbilical veins, and fetal circulation.

Once in the fetal liver, placental progesterone is converted into pregnanediol, which is used for steroid hormone synthesis. Progesterone also plays a role in cortisol production by the fetal adrenal glands. However, excessive cortisol levels, which can indicate fetal distress, lead to an increase in progesterone levels in the umbilical vein. Some studies have observed higher progesterone levels in cases of breech presentation and after Cesarean section, though other researchers dispute these findings.

While the regulation and metabolism of luteal progesterone in women are well understood, the mechanism behind placental progesterone production remains unknown. This presents an exciting area for future research. It is still unclear how the fetus signals the placenta to produce progesterone or how the placenta determines the required amount of this hormone. Further studies in these areas could significantly enhance our understanding of placental progesterone's role in pregnancy and fetal development.

Numerous clinical studies have confirmed that retroplacental progesterone does not correlate with maternal blood progesterone levels or umbilical cord progesterone levels. This underscores the extraordinary and unique independence of placental progesterone. It suggests that the placenta and the fetus operate independently in their respective programs for progesterone production and utilization.

Most progesterone remains in placental tissue, increasing as pregnancy progresses. The concentration of progesterone in *retroplacental blood* (between the placenta and endometrium) ranges from 380 to 4,650 nmol/L, while in maternal plasma, levels range from 100 to 620 nmol/L — almost 15 times higher than before pregnancy. In the umbilical cord vessels (fetal circulation), progesterone levels range from 90 to 1,800 nmol/L.

The fetus uses approximately 30% of placental progesterone for synthesizing various essential substances. Some progesterone enters the maternal bloodstream, but most remain in the placenta.

It's worth noting that no correlation has been found between fetal sex and progesterone levels in the umbilical cord, which adds to our understanding of placental progesterone dynamics.

Research has shown that **administering exogenous progesterone to the mother does not alter placental or fetal blood progesterone levels**. This further confirms the unique autonomy of placental progesterone production.

The Significance of Accurate Progesterone Level Measurement

The question of determining progesterone levels in a woman's body arises in various situations: diagnosing conditions, selecting hormone therapy, and monitoring treatment effectiveness. In each case, doctors aim to use the most accurate method for measuring progesterone levels. Once results are obtained, the next concern is whether they fall within the expected range. This approach seems straightforward, yet many diagnostic and treatment errors occur, not only due to incorrect hormone measurements but also because of misinterpretation of test results.

As mentioned earlier in this book, progesterone exists in the blood in free and protein-bound forms. It can also bind to red blood cells. This means progesterone levels in whole blood, serum, and plasma will differ.

It is assumed that serum progesterone levels should be at least 5 ng/mL to suppress endometrial growth. However, many studies have shown that administering progesterone in different forms often results in only a slight increase in blood levels. Despite this, clinical effects are still observed. How can this be explained? The key reason is that **progesterone levels in the blood do not reflect its concentration in tissues and cells that actively utilize it, including progesterone metabolites**. Specific organs rapidly absorb progesterone, including the endometrium, salivary glands, lungs, brain, kidneys, liver, skin (through the bloodstream), and fat deposits.

A completely outdated and uninformative method is the so-called *"hormonal mirror,"* determined through cytological smears or colposcopy, which many older-generation doctors still use, especially during pregnancy. Diagnosing progesterone deficiency or predicting pregnancy outcomes based on such methods is absurd.

Additionally, laboratories use different units of measurement for progesterone levels, including ng/mL, μg/L, and nmol/L. Comparing numerical values without considering the unit of measurement can lead to false conclusions.

Every laboratory establishes reference values, representing the minimum and maximum thresholds considered normal. However, these ranges apply only to the specific method used in that lab and do not necessarily reflect actual progesterone levels for a given population of women.

For example, if laboratory reagents are purchased from another country, the reference values may reflect the normal ranges for that country or region, not the population being tested.

Reference values for progesterone levels often fail to account for critical factors such as pregnancy status, ethnicity, nationality, and age, essential for accurately interpreting hormone test results.

Characteristics of Progesterone Levels in the Female Body

In addition to variations in progesterone levels across different blood fractions and bodily fluids, it is essential to remember that progesterone breaks down rapidly. As a result, its levels fluctuate throughout the menstrual cycle and within a single day. Due to the pulsatile secretion of gonadotropins, progesterone production also follows a pulsatile pattern. A single progesterone measurement does not accurately reflect a woman's hormonal status.

It's crucial to recognize that every woman is unique, and her progesterone levels may not fit the 'ideal' 28-day menstrual cycle often depicted in textbooks. Women with normal reproductive function can have cycles with both low and high progesterone levels. **Measuring progesterone levels on day 21 of the menstrual cycle is not a rational approach to assessing a woman's hormonal status.** A diagnosis should never be made based on a single progesterone measurement.

Progesterone levels fluctuate based on diet, alcohol consumption, smoking, physical activity, lifestyle, and other factors. The use of medications, including other steroid hormones prescribed by therapists, family doctors, surgeons, and other specialists, also significantly affects progesterone levels in women. This underscores the need for caution and awareness when considering these factors in hormonal health.

There is very little data on how progesterone levels differ among women of various ethnic groups worldwide. However, laboratory reference values often fail to account for these ethnic variations, applying standardized ranges that may not reflect the physiological norms of women in each population. What one laboratory considers an abnormal deviation from the norm may be a woman's natural physiological state.

Pregnancy is unique, as luteal progesterone levels decrease after 5 weeks while placental progesterone levels rise. However, only a tiny portion of placental progesterone enters the maternal bloodstream. Interestingly, progesterone levels in early pregnancy are higher during a woman's first pregnancy than in subsequent ones. Fetal sex, maternal weight, and age do not influence progesterone levels.

Another distinctive feature of pregnancy is the increase in free progesterone levels, which rises faster than total progesterone. Between weeks 24 and 40, the free progesterone fraction increases from 6% to 13% of total progesterone. Notably, just two hours after childbirth, free and bound progesterone levels drop sharply, but the proportion of free progesterone increases to 19% of total progesterone and may remain elevated for a prolonged period. Since laboratories do not measure free progesterone during pregnancy, incorrect conclusions about "progesterone deficiency" are often made.

Administering exogenous progesterone in medications temporarily increases free progesterone levels in the blood, but only briefly, as progesterone rapidly breaks down. Also, free and bound progesterone levels depend on the dosage, administration route, and other factors.

Numerous nuances regarding progesterone synthesis, absorption, and metabolism are discussed in other chapters of this book. Doctors must have a comprehensive understanding of these factors to ensure accurate diagnosis and treatment.

Myths About Minimum Progesterone Levels, Nutrition, and Lifestyle

Women often ask what minimum level of luteal progesterone is necessary for conception and a healthy pregnancy. Many doctors also seek to establish a link between pre-pregnancy progesterone levels and the likelihood of successful implantation and pregnancy progression.

Numerous international studies have been conducted on this topic, but scientists disagree. Some researchers suggest that a progesterone level of 5 ng/mL (16 nmol/L) is sufficient for early pregnancy development. Many reproductive clinics set their minimum threshold for luteal progesterone at 10–13 ng/mL (32–41 nmol/L). In most women, luteal progesterone levels range from 7 to 57 nmol/L.

However, reference values and progesterone measurement units vary across different laboratories, which can lead to significant confusion in the interpretation of test results. For instance, a woman might be told she has a 'low' progesterone level in one lab but a 'normal' level in another. Additionally, even with low progesterone levels, a woman may still carry a pregnancy to term. These discrepancies have given rise to numerous myths, fears, and misconceptions about the 'minimum progesterone levels' needed for pregnancy.

It's well-established that nutrition plays a crucial role in conception rates and fertility. This is evident from the lowest birth rates observed among white populations, especially in developed countries. The number of childless couples is rising, and most families have only one child, rarely two or three. However, when we examine pregnancy and birth rates in developing countries, they remain the highest globally, underscoring the importance of a healthy diet in fertility.

It's a testament to the resilience of women that they can conceive and give birth even in conditions of extreme poverty, war, malnutrition, and water shortages. Despite these harsh conditions, women in developing regions may experience up to 12 pregnancies in their lifetime, with an average of 7–8 children. Many children die due to hunger and life-threatening infections, yet women continue to bear children, inspiring us with their strength.

Nutrition only slightly influences fertility, although menstrual cycle regularity and ovulation are linked to body mass index (BMI) and fat tissue levels. Studies show that ovarian function depends on energy metabolism and can be disrupted by low and high energy availability. The most common cause of ovulation disorders among women in developed countries is stress, including energy stress. Any stress — physical, emotional, or nutritional (since nutrients are also a form of energy) — can disrupt ovulation.

The question of why stress primarily manifests as ovarian dysfunction in societies with abundant food supplies remains a topic of debate among experts and lacks a clear explanation. One hypothesis suggested that these reproductive issues are linked to progesterone deficiency, which affects conception and pregnancy maintenance. However, pre-ovulatory progesterone levels are naturally low, and progesterone deficiency is more commonly associated with infertility rather than pregnancy loss. The topic of stress will be further explored in other chapters of this book.

A study of American women from rural (non-industrialized) areas found that their progesterone levels were lower than those of urban women despite their higher conception and pregnancy rates. Since American women generally follow similar diets, nutrient deficiencies are unlikely to explain these differences, except in rare cases.

Scientists conducted an international study on Bolivian Aymara women living in high-altitude regions to investigate further. This group was chosen because their villages are isolated from urban areas and in mountainous regions. Their lifestyle involves hard physical labor and frequent food shortages. Additionally, contraceptive use among both men and women in this population was virtually nonexistent.

Previous studies have already shown that women in high-altitude Indigenous communities tend to have lower progesterone levels than women from cities and industrialized regions. The highest progesterone levels were typically observed in pregnant and lactating women.

The American and Bolivian study participants were matched for age to ensure accurate data. The average age of first-time mothers in Chicago was 31 years (compared to 30 years in Canada, 27–29 years in Europe, and 29 years in the U.S.). Although progesterone levels in reproductive-age women do not significantly change with age until menopause, Bolivian women were selected to match the age range of the American participants (27–28 years on average). However, most Bolivian women had already given birth at least four times by that age. After each childbirth, they breastfed for at least 1–2 years, and their *postpartum amenorrhea* (absence of menstruation) lasted at least one year.

The study found that progesterone levels in Bolivian women were significantly lower than in their American counterparts: 77% of American women's progesterone levels during the follicular phase, 67% during the luteal phase and 71% at the luteal peak

These measurements were taken during conception cycles. While differences in progesterone levels between American and Bolivian women during the follicular phase were not statistically significant, post-ovulatory and menstrual phase differences were substantial.

The rise in progesterone after ovulation was faster and higher in American women, especially near the progesterone peak. During implantation (8–10 days after ovulation), Bolivian women's progesterone levels were half those of American women. Regardless of whether conception occurred or not, progesterone levels were consistently lower in all Bolivian women's cycles compared to their American counterparts.

This led researchers to conclude that **low progesterone levels do not necessarily indicate infertility and may be a physiological characteristic of many healthy women**. This conclusion opens new avenues for understanding and interpreting progesterone levels in women.

Low progesterone levels are not exclusive to rural populations but are also observed in certain ethnic groups worldwide. For example, Japanese women naturally have lower progesterone levels than American and European women. Similarly, low progesterone levels have been documented in rural women from Poland, Nepal, and the Democratic Republic of Congo, with values comparable to Bolivian women living at 4,000 meters above sea level.

This finding suggests that geographic location does not directly influence progesterone fluctuations. However, a notable seasonal trend was observed — **progesterone levels decreased during food scarcity periods** (often in winter and early spring) among women across various populations.

Thus, progesterone levels in women's blood may depend on factors doctors often overlook. In cases of low progesterone, it is always crucial to consider symptoms and clinical signs of progesterone deficiency, which are discussed in the chapter on luteal phase insufficiency. This underscores the need for a comprehensive approach to evaluating progesterone levels.

The Concept of "Progesterone Action"

We have already discussed the role of progesterone in the female body, including during pregnancy (a separate chapter is dedicated to hormones and pregnancy). We have also examined the topic of progesterone level measurement. However, there is another subject surrounded by numerous myths — the so-called "*progesterone property*," "*progesterone action*," or "*progesterone activity*," often mentioned in literature when describing the characteristics of progesterone and its synthetic forms. What exactly do these properties mean, and how were they determined?

All progestogens, including natural and synthetic progesterone, share a common effect — their progestogenic action. **This term refers to their ability to act on an estrogen-prepared rabbit endometrium, inhibiting its growth and triggering secretory changes.** This effect on the rabbit endometrium was established as the gold standard of 'progestogenic activity.' However, beyond this progestogenic property, natural progesterone and synthetic progestins exhibit a fascinating array of biological effects on cells and tissues in animals and humans, adding a layer of complexity to our understanding of their actions.

Since progesterone synthesizes all steroid hormones, an important question arises: what additional properties does it have? Does its biochemical relationship with other steroids grant it some of their characteristics? Research has shown that progesterone can exhibit properties similar to or opposite to those of androgens, estrogens, glucocorticoids, and mineralocorticoids. These effects depend on several factors:

- Which receptors progesterone interacts with

- Which tissues are involved

- How progesterone is metabolized

- Its concentration in blood and tissues.

Structurally, progesterone is closest to male sex hormones, which is why it often has *androgenic properties*. This means that it can stimulate the development of male characteristics. Most medical progestins also exhibit androgenic activity. This effect is observed at high doses of progesterone. Lower doses, on the other hand, exert *anti-androgenic effects*. Depending on the dose, progesterone can also act as an anti-estrogen, an anti-glucocorticoid, or an anti-mineralocorticoid. Additionally, the impact of progestogens varies depending on the route of administration of the medication.

Beyond progestogens, the human body produces many other substances with effects similar to progesterone. For instance, the ovaries produce estrogen, the adrenal glands produce cortisol, and the placenta produces human chorionic gonadotropin (hCG). Several other organs also synthesize these substances.

Now, we will step away from progesterone to examine the role of other ovarian hormones. However, it's important to note that progesterone plays a key role in the body's hormonal system, and we will return to it multiple times throughout this book, underscoring its significance.

2.5.4. Male Sex Hormones

Dispelling the myths about male sex hormones is crucial for understanding their significant impact on women's health. The term 'male' can be misleading, but it's essential to realize that women have more male sex hormones (androgens) in their bodies than female sex hormones (estrogens). Furthermore, **female sex hormones are derived from male sex hormones — without androgens, estrogens would not exist.** This knowledge empowers us to understand better and manage women's health.

There are five primary androgens:

- Dehydroepiandrosterone sulfate (DHEA-S)

- Dehydroepiandrosterone (DHEA)

- Androstenedione (A)

- Testosterone (T)

- Dihydrotestosterone (DHT)

The first three are often referred to as prohormones — precursors to active hormones, because they can be converted into testosterone, thereby indirectly exhibiting androgenic activity. DHT is considered a testosterone metabolite or breakdown product, yet it possesses the highest hormonal activity alongside testosterone itself. Among all androgens, DHEA-S has the highest concentration in blood serum, but its biological activity is one of the lowest.

The ovaries produce 25% of androgens, mainly testosterone, while the adrenal glands produce 75%. In men, androgens are produced in the testes and adrenal glands.

Testosterone production by the ovaries and adrenal glands fluctuates depending on the menstrual cycle phase. As ovulation approaches, ovarian testosterone production increases (up to 65–75%) while adrenal production decreases. The ovaries also produce 50% of androstenedione and 20% of DHEA, whereas the adrenal glands synthesize nearly all DHEA-S and 80% of DHEA. Significantly elevated levels of these hormones may indicate adrenal dysfunction and warrant further evaluation.

Beyond the gonads and adrenal glands, the liver, fat tissue, and skin also serve as sources of androgens. Androstenedione and small amounts of DHEA are converted into testosterone in the skin. Fat tissue also stores steroid hormones, which can be converted into androgens when present in excess.

A woman produces 0.1 to 0.4 mg of testosterone daily, but serum testosterone levels fluctuate throughout the menstrual cycle. The highest testosterone levels occur mid-cycle, approximately 20% higher than at the beginning or end of the cycle. However, when testing testosterone levels in women, the specific day of the menstrual cycle is generally not a determining factor. During pregnancy, additional sources of testosterone emerge.

It is important to note that about 80% of testosterone binds to sex hormone-binding globulin (SHBG), a protein synthesized by the liver. Liver function is crucial in regulating active (free) and inactive (bound) testosterone levels in a woman's body.

Androgens, like all steroid hormones, are a fascinating area of study for medical researchers. Their effects go beyond the reproductive system, influencing various organs, including the brain, and even shaping human behavior. This intriguing aspect of androgens sparks curiosity and encourages further exploration in endocrinology.

As mentioned earlier, female sex hormones are synthesized from male sex hormones. This process, known as the *androgen-estrogen conversion pathway*, is one of the most fundamental aspects of female biological development. It involves the conversion of androgens, such as DHEA and androstenedione, into estrogens, primarily estradiol, in various tissues, including the ovaries, adrenal glands, and fat tissue.

It's a fascinating fact that puberty, a significant milestone in human development, begins with a rise in hormone levels, including male sex hormones, for both girls and boys. This underscores the intricate and shared biological processes that shape us all. For a more detailed discussion of puberty and the role of androgens in menstrual cycle development, I invite you to explore my book "Growing Up Strong: A Guide to Girls' Health and Well-Being."

The Androgen Effect: More Than Just Male Development

When discussing androgenic effects, the focus is typically on their role in male puberty and physical development. Androgens were first described in the 18th century, although their hormonal nature was not yet understood. In 1771, John Hunter performed a groundbreaking experiment in which he transplanted rooster testes into a hen, an important moment in the history of endocrinology. This caused the hen to develop a rooster's comb and wattle. Later, in 1849, the German scientist Arnold Berthold conducted a similarly significant experiment. He transplanted testes from a healthy rooster into a castrated one and observed the same effect — the regrowth of the comb and wattle and the restoration of typical rooster behavior. These experiments laid the foundation for our understanding of androgens. However, it was not until 1935 that Leopold Ruzicka identified the chemical structure of a substance extracted from testes, naming it testosterone.

The impact of testosterone and other androgens on human behavior is now a subject of extensive research. Scientists have discovered that brain cells contain androgen receptors of two subtypes — AR-A and AR-B. The primary influence of androgens on the brain is linked to the formation of aggressive behavior, both in men and women. An excess of male sex hormones further reinforces this connection, demonstrating how androgens shape human behavior. On the other hand, low androgen levels are associated with an increased risk of depression and irritability, especially in postmenopausal women.

Sudden fluctuations in testosterone levels, particularly sharp declines in androgens, have been observed in individuals with mood disorders and psychoses. Androgens are also believed to have a neuroprotective function, supporting the survival of nerve cells.

Thus, beyond serving as precursors to estrogens, playing a critical role in puberty, and regulating the menstrual cycle, androgens are also essential for the maturation of gametes (sex cells) in both men and women.

This underscores the crucial role of androgens in the reproductive process. Sex hormones are intricately interconnected and rely on a delicate hormonal balance.

But what happens when male sex hormone levels rise? Why do these levels increase? We will explore these intriguing questions in the next section, inviting you to delve deeper into the world of endocrinology.

Why Male Sex Hormone Levels Increase

When considering the production, transport, and metabolism of steroid hormones, including male sex hormones (androgens), the causes of elevated androgen levels can be categorized into four main groups:

1. Excess androgen production

2. Deficiency of androgen-binding proteins

3. Impaired androgen metabolism and utilization

4. Impaired androgen elimination from the body

The sources of androgens differ between non-pregnant and pregnant women, as do the levels of various male sex hormones. Therefore, it is important to discuss these aspects separately. First, let's examine cases of **hyperandrogenism** — elevated male sex hormone levels in women outside of pregnancy.

It's important to note that while every woman may experience periods of elevated androgen levels at some point in her life, hyperandrogenism is not as common as it is often portrayed. Only about 5–8% of women have consistently high levels of male sex hormones. The condition is most frequently observed during adolescence (up to 21–22 years of age), as a side effect of certain medications, or in response to stress, which can also lead to irregular menstrual cycles.

It is crucial to take a comprehensive approach when evaluating hormone test results. This involves determining which specific androgens are elevated, in what form (bound or free), and how this affects the female body biologically and symptomatically.

Excess Androgen Production

Androgen overproduction can be mild or severe. Marked elevations require urgent medical attention, as they not only cause noticeable symptoms but may also indicate the presence of a dangerous ovarian or adrenal tumor. Any rapid increase in male sex hormone levels warrants immediate investigation.

Ten types of tumors (eight ovarian and two adrenal) can produce male sex hormones. Although androgen-producing tumors are rare, about 30% of them are malignant. Ultrasound can detect ovarian or adrenal masses but cannot determine whether they are hormonally active.

Another cause of elevated androgen levels in non-pregnant women is **congenital adrenal hyperplasia (CAH)** — specifically, hyperplasia of the adrenal cortex. Less commonly, **acquired adrenal cortical hyperplasia** can also be responsible.

There are two forms of CAH: classical and non-classical, each presenting with different symptoms. All forms of congenital adrenal hyperplasia stem from enzyme deficiencies due to genetic mutations.

Five primary types of adrenal cortical hyperplasia exist, along with over twenty other less common variants. Diagnosis follows specialized protocols, including measuring specific substances in blood serum and, less frequently, urine. The combination of hormone and metabolite imbalances varies by CAH type. The most common deficiencies involve *21-hydroxylase* (an autosomal recessive disorder) and *11α-hydroxylase*. A precise diagnosis is critical, as not all forms of the condition can be managed with medication.

Deficiency of Androgen-Binding Proteins

Another frequent cause of hyperandrogenism is a deficiency in sex hormone-binding globulin (SHBG), the protein responsible for binding and regulating free androgens. When SHBG levels are high, bound testosterone increases, which is not harmful but can lead to misinterpretation of lab results; if only total testosterone is measured, the results may appear falsely elevated.

SHBG levels naturally increase during pregnancy, with estrogen use, combined oral contraceptive (COC) use, and hyperthyroidism. Conversely, SHBG is reduced by androgens, synthetic progestins, glucocorticoids, growth hormone, insulin, and ACTH. Hypothyroidism and obesity can also lower SHBG levels, leading to increased free testosterone. Some synthetic progestins are used to treat mild to moderate hyperandrogenism by lowering free androgen levels.

Impaired Androgen Metabolism

Hyperandrogenism can also result from defective androgen metabolism, meaning that the body does not properly break down and eliminate these hormones.

Androgen metabolism requires specific enzymes, and a deficiency in these enzymes can cause normal androgen production to result in excessive hormone accumulation.

These enzyme deficiencies (enzymopathies) are typically congenital and genetically determined, though they may also be acquired. Under normal conditions, most circulating testosterone is converted in the liver into androstenedione and etiocholanolone, binding with glucuronic and sulfuric acids for elimination. Liver diseases can disrupt this process, leading to androgen accumulation and, consequently, hyperandrogenism.

Androgen metabolites are excreted in the urine as 17-ketosteroids (17-KS). However, only 20–30% of 17-KS in urine originates from ovarian androgens, while most come from adrenal androgens. Stress, which elevates cortisol levels, can also increase 17-KS excretion, sometimes leading to a misdiagnosis of adrenal dysfunction.

Hyperandrogenism is not just a laboratory finding but a condition that may present with various clinical symptoms. Elevated androgen levels can be associated with numerous conditions, so it is essential to focus not only on hormone levels but also on a patient's symptoms, complaints, and the results of other diagnostic tests.

Manifestations of Hyperandrogenism

The manifestation of hyperandrogenism is a complex interplay of a woman's age, the level of male sex hormones, and the duration of their influence. This complexity underscores the need for a thorough understanding and careful evaluation, as androgens affect multiple organs, and the changes are not limited to ovarian function.

In female fetuses, excessive androgens can lead to changes in the external genitalia, particularly clitoral enlargement and fusion of the labia minora. Fetuses are susceptible to both excess and deficiency of male sex hormones. Interestingly, in male fetuses, the absence of androgens leads to underdevelopment of the male genitalia, testes, and prostate, and the newborn may later develop along a female phenotype.

In adolescent girls, hyperandrogenism is marked by:

- Increased body hair growth combined with hair thinning on the head (alopecia)

- Acne

- Clitoral enlargement

- Increased skin oiliness

- A deepening, lower-pitched voice

- Delayed menstruation (the first period may be absent until a later age)

- Increased muscle mass

- Obesity, since androgens affect fat metabolism

In women who have completed puberty, hyperandrogenism often manifests as *hirsutism*, occurring in 70–80% of cases. Hirsutism refers to excess terminal hair — thick, coarse, pigmented hair. There are three types of hair:

- Vellus hair – delicate, soft, and unaffected by male sex hormones,

- Bristle hair – forms eyebrows and eyelashes and grows inside the nostrils and ears,

- Terminal hair – covers the scalp, as well as the underarm, pubic, and external genital areas.

Since bristle and terminal hairs are sensitive to androgens, their growth increases with hyperandrogenism.

Before concluding that a woman has hyperandrogenism, it is crucial to evaluate family history. The presence of other "hairy" women in the family (mother, sister, aunts) is a significant factor in diagnosing hyperandrogenism. This emphasis on comprehensive patient assessment will make the audience feel the need for a holistic approach to diagnosis.

Misdiagnosis of hyperandrogenism can lead to unnecessary hormonal treatment and potential risks. Young women taking hormonal medications or certain drugs may experience mild elevations in testosterone, usually bound or total testosterone. In such cases, it is crucial to avoid a hasty diagnosis of hyperandrogenism and to conduct further evaluation to ensure precision in practice.

Hirsutism as a pathological condition appears and progresses rapidly in cases of true hyperandrogenism. Androgens, in addition to their role in hair growth, also regulate sebum production. Increased skin oiliness often accompanies hirsutism due to this regulation. Acne vulgaris also develops due to excess androgens, as Propionibacterium acnes bacteria multiply more actively, leading to inflammation of the skin and hair follicles. Although there is ongoing debate about whether acne is a sign of hyperandrogenism, more than 70% of women with acne have been found to have elevated androgen levels in their blood.

Another manifestation of hyperandrogenism in women is menstrual cycle irregularity, which may lead to a lack of ovulation and infertility. The higher the androgen levels, the more likely menstrual cycle disturbances will be. Therefore, further evaluation, including androgen level testing, is required when menstruation stops.

Hyperandrogenism is a hallmark of polycystic ovary syndrome (PCOS), which will be discussed separately in the chapter on endocrine disorders common in women.

In addition to these disorders, elevated androgens are associated with insulin resistance and an increased risk of type 2 diabetes, particularly in women approaching menopause. They are also linked to lipid metabolism disorders (*dyslipidemia*), high blood pressure (*hypertension*), and vascular diseases. Hyperandrogenism increases the risk of cardiovascular disease, which is a significant concern for women's health.

The presence of symptoms characteristic of elevated male sex hormone levels requires medical evaluation, which may range from simple to complex and involve multiple tests. These tests help determine the source of hyperandrogenism — ovaries, adrenal glands, or other tissues. Common tests include blood tests to measure androgen levels, imaging tests to visualize the ovaries and adrenal glands, and sometimes, more invasive tests to sample tissue for further analysis. However, this does not mean all possible tests must be conducted on every woman without proper clinical indications.

17-Hydroxyprogesterone

All steroid hormones break into other compounds and are typically excreted as *17-ketosteroids*. 17-Hydroxyprogesterone (17-OHP, 17-HPG) is a derivative of progesterone and other steroid hormones. It's important to note that its levels naturally increase during pregnancy, which is a normal physiological process and not a cause for concern.

In non-pregnant women, an elevation in 17-OHP levels, particularly a 17-OHP level of 6.05 nmol/L or higher, may signal the presence of testosterone-producing tumors or non-classical congenital adrenal hyperplasia (CAH), most commonly due to 21-hydroxylase deficiency. This underscores the need for further evaluation using an ACTH stimulation test, highlighting the potential health issues associated with elevated levels.

In many countries, the standard practice of newborn screening for 17-hydroxyprogesterone is a crucial step in the early detection of congenital adrenal hyperplasia (CAH) at birth. This underscores the importance of early intervention and management of this condition.

Deficiency of Male Sex Hormones

While much is known about excess androgens, the deficiency of male sex hormones, particularly hypoandrogenism, remains largely underexplored. **There are no established minimum androgen levels for women, and androgen deficiency is far more pronounced in men.** This underexplored area holds the potential for discoveries and insights.

It is believed that low androgen levels in women may lead to a range of symptoms, including drowsiness, fatigue, reduced muscle mass, loss of libido, lack of motivation, and low mood. However, these symptoms can also occur with deficiencies of other hormones or because of various medical conditions such as anemia, depression, and autoimmune diseases.

Most commonly, *hypoandrogenism* occurs with age, particularly in postmenopausal women, as well as after ovary removal ovarian insufficiency (including cases induced by chemotherapy, pelvic radiation, or estrogen therapy). *Hyperprolactinemia* may be associated with both elevated androgens (as seen in PCOS) and low androgen levels. Essentially, any condition that impairs ovarian function can disrupt androgen production.

Another potential cause of hypoandrogenism is adrenal dysfunction, particularly *adrenal insufficiency*. The adrenal glands play a crucial role in androgen production, and any dysfunction in these glands can decrease androgen levels, contributing to hypoandrogenism.

Diagnosing androgen deficiency is a complex task, as there are no reliable tests or defined reference values for the minimum levels of androgens in women. The peak of testosterone levels in the early morning suggests that hormone testing is best conducted at this time. The day of the menstrual cycle is generally not critical, although testosterone levels tend to rise before ovulation. Testosterone and other hormone levels are best tested for the most accurate results between days 8 and 20 of the menstrual cycle. This complexity underscores the need for further research and development in this area.

It's important to note that **no standard androgen deficiency treatment exists**. While testosterone creams are often prescribed to postmenopausal and reproductive-age women, it's crucial to understand that existing testosterone formulations contain doses designed for men. As a result, testosterone replacement therapy in women remains extremely rare, highlighting the urgent need for more treatment options in this area.

2.5.5. Female Sex Hormones

Male sex hormones are important for women, but a woman without **female sex hormones** is simply unimaginable. Most estrogens (a general term for female sex hormones) are produced in the ovaries during follicular maturation, while a smaller portion is synthesized in the adrenal glands.

Interestingly, a woman's body can never have zero estrogen levels, even after ovary removal or complete ovarian failure. The ovaries contain enormous follicles that, even dormant, can still produce a certain amount of female sex hormones, which is usually sufficient for the body. Even during menopause, when very few follicles remain in the ovaries, estrogen production continues. **Despite declining estrogen levels, no woman has ever physically transformed into a man due to estrogen deficiency.**

There are more than 20 types of estrogens, but three main ones receive the most attention:

- **Estrone** (E1) – A weak form of estrogen that becomes the dominant estrogen after menopause.

Specific amounts of estrone are stored in muscle, fat, and other tissues. Estrone can convert into estradiol.

- **Estradiol** (E2) – The most potent and abundant estrogen, produced primarily by the ovaries. It is 1.25 to 5 times stronger than estrone and is often referred to as 17β-estradiol. Estradiol is the dominant estrogen in reproductive-age women and plays a significant role in hormone-dependent conditions such as endometriosis, endometrial cancer, and fibroid growth. A woman's body produces between 70 and 500 mcg of estradiol daily.

- **Estriol** (E3) — Like estrone, estriol is a weak estrogen, primarily a breakdown product of estradiol. During pregnancy, estriol levels rise significantly, along with estradiol. However, unlike estrone, estriol cannot convert back into estradiol or estrone.

Female sex hormones are classified as potent steroid hormones with both beneficial and harmful effects. Their association with the development of certain cancers places estrogens in the category of carcinogens — substances linked to malignant disease formation.

Only about 3% of estradiol circulates freely in the bloodstream, meaning it is not bound to proteins. Sixty percent is bound to albumin, while the remaining 37% is bound to SHBG (sex hormone-binding globulin).

In recent years, the impact of estrogens on various organ systems has been studied intensively, as estrogen receptors have been found in numerous tissues and cells throughout the body. The number of estrogen receptors fluctuates during the menstrual cycle, and these variations are closely related to changes in progesterone receptor levels.

Estrogen levels decline with high dietary fiber intake, especially in middle-aged and premenopausal women. Diets rich in fiber are believed to reduce β-glucuronidase activity in the large intestine, leading to impaired estrogen reabsorption. Fiber can also decrease fat and cholesterol absorption, partly due to more frequent bowel movements.

Measuring Estrogen Levels

Estrogens, the primary female hormones, are complex to measure. Disruptions in estrogen production typically manifest first as menstrual irregularities. For instance, if ovulation does not occur, estrogen levels may be low, but anovulatory women do not transform into men. In other words, **critically low estrogen levels are exceedingly rare**.

What should be kept in mind when testing estrogen levels? Since estradiol is the dominant estrogen, it is usually measured only. Like all steroid hormones, estradiol exists in the blood in bound and free forms.

When evaluating estrogen levels, it's crucial to consider a range of factors. These include age, the day of the menstrual cycle, pregnancy, lactation, and other conditions. Each of these factors can significantly influence estrogen levels.

Estradiol levels are most measured in cases of infertility, menstrual irregularities, menopause, and issues related to sexual maturation. In the latter case, specialized estrogen panels, which include estrone measurements, are often used.

Estradiol levels are typically measured on the third day (or in the early days) of the cycle to evaluate the hormonal profile during the menstrual cycle. To confirm ovulation, estradiol should be tested during its pre-ovulatory peak (2–3 days before ovulation), when levels increase significantly — by 500–1000% compared to baseline levels at the start of the follicular phase. During the luteal phase of the cycle, estrogen levels drop considerably. This drop, combined with very low progesterone and estradiol levels, triggers "withdrawal bleeding" — the menstrual period.

Monitoring estradiol fluctuations is critical to making decisions about ovulation stimulation for IVF and other assisted reproductive technologies. In cases of chronic anovulation, where follicles fail to mature for serious underlying reasons, artificial ovulation stimulation may be ineffective. Often, these women require donor eggs for IVF. Anovulatory cycles become more frequent with age, making it increasingly difficult for older women to produce the required number of eggs for IVF.

When evaluating estrogen levels, three parameters are considered:

- Free estradiol levels.

- Total estradiol levels (the sum of free and bound estradiol).

- The ratio of free to bound estradiol.

Estradiol levels can be measured in serum and plasma, with varying results depending on the sample type. Seldom is estradiol tested in saliva or urine; such tests currently lack practical application.

Low Estrogen Levels

Low estrogen levels are more common than elevated levels, but this condition is often a form of *physiological hypoestrogenism*. For example, during each menstrual cycle, low estradiol levels occur just before menstruation, which may lead to symptoms such as vaginal dryness and itching. This premenstrual state creates favorable conditions for fungal growth, so *candidiasis* often flares up during this time. However, when a woman presents to her doctor with complaints of discomfort, itching, or burning before her period, and no abnormalities are found in vaginal swab tests, the cause is often *physiological premenstrual hypoestrogenism*. There is no specific treatment for this condition, but hormonal contraceptives may be offered to women who are not planning a pregnancy.

Another period of physiological hypoestrogenism occurs postpartum, particularly during breastfeeding, when menstrual cycles have not yet fully resumed. While ovulation may occur as early as six weeks after childbirth, most women experience their first menstruation a few months after delivery. In non-breastfeeding women, cycles typically return within 3–4 months, whereas breastfeeding mothers often resume menstruating after 5–6 months. Even then, cycles may be irregular due to elevated prolactin levels during breastfeeding and other factors such as sleep deprivation, fatigue, thyroid disorders, weight fluctuations, or stress. Menstrual cycles may be absent for months during breastfeeding, sometimes until weaning. During this period of irregular ovulation, postpartum women may show signs of hypoestrogenism.

Physiological hypoestrogenism also occurs in postmenopausal women, but its impact on health is more significant than at other life stages. Estrogen deficiency is associated with an increased risk of cardiovascular disease, and higher mortality rates from heart attacks and strokes have also been observed in younger women who develop hypoestrogenism due to hypothalamic dysfunction.

Hypoestrogenism does not only cause vaginal symptoms but may also lead to painful urination, often mistaken for cystitis or other urinary tract disorders. Skin dryness and increased wrinkle formation are also common.

It's important to distinguish between physiological and pathological hypoestrogenism. The former, which is a natural part of the body's processes, can occur after ovarian failure, whether due to surgical removal of the ovaries, premature ovarian insufficiency (POI), high androgen or progesterone levels, or the use of medications that suppress ovarian function. The latter, however, is a result of a disruption at the level of the hypothalamic-pituitary-ovarian axis, which regulates ovarian function.

High Estrogen Levels

Understanding the causes of hyperestrogenism, an elevated level of estrogen in the blood, is crucial. The most common reason is hormonal ovarian tumors, with less frequent occurrences from tumors of the adrenal glands and other estrogen-producing tissues.

Early detection of estrogen-producing tumors, particularly granulosa-theca cell tumors, is key. These tumors are the most common source of excess estrogen, with up to 70% of them being hormonally active. Estrogen-producing tumors account for about 2% of all ovarian tumors, and around 10% of such tumors may develop in pregnant women, complicating the diagnosis due to physiological *hyperestrogenism* during pregnancy.

Although these tumors produce hormones, the most frequent complaint among such women is discomfort in the lower abdomen. The causes of ovarian tumors remain unknown, but it is believed that specific genes may play a role in the development of hormone-producing tumors.

Another common cause of hyperestrogenism is *ovarian hyperstimulation syndrome*, which occurs after the use of ovulation-stimulating drugs. As many women now plan pregnancies at a later age (after 35 years old), they increasingly require assisted reproductive technologies, leading to a significant increase in the frequency of ovarian hyperstimulation syndrome.

A scarce condition is *aromatase excess syndrome* or *familial hyperestrogenism*, which occurs due to a genetic defect. The aromatization process is necessary for the synthesis of estrogens from androgens. If, for some reason, the activity of the aromatase enzyme increases, the amount of estrogen produced by the ovaries also rises.

To the surprise of many women, a hyperestrogenic state can occur while taking hormonal contraceptives or hormone replacement therapy (HRT) due to an excess of exogenous (external) estrogens. Less commonly, hyperestrogenism may result from liver disease (cirrhosis), as the liver is actively involved in estrogen metabolism. The liver plays a crucial role in metabolizing and eliminating excess hormones from the body. When the liver is compromised due to cirrhosis, it may not be able to effectively metabolize estrogen, leading to its accumulation in the body.

Although female sex hormones are crucial for the body (without them, a woman wouldn't be a woman), an excess of estrogens can manifest with various symptoms:

- Menstrual cycle disturbances

- Ovulation suppression

- Lower androgen levels

- Uterine and breast enlargement

- Vaginal bleeding

In men, an excess of estrogen leads to *gynecomastia*, in which breast tissue enlarges. Other symptoms in men may include decreased libido, erectile dysfunction, and feminization of body features such as reduced body hair and increased fat deposition in the hips and breasts.

An excess of estrogens requires treatment, which can be medicinal or surgical, depending on the cause.

2.5.6. The Impact of Nutrition on Ovarian Hormone Levels

Earlier chapters have mentioned that steroid hormones, including sex hormones and progesterone, are synthesized from cholesterol. Cholesterol is a type of fat partly obtained from food and produced within the body. It serves as a precursor for synthesizing these hormones, highlighting the crucial role of dietary fats in hormone production.

A woman's diet directly influences hormone production, particularly sex hormones and progesterone, because all steroid hormones require adequate cholesterol intake from food. Additionally, normal fat levels in blood plasma and tissues are essential for the absorption and metabolism of sex hormones.

A balanced intake of essential nutrients is crucial and empowering for every woman's health (just as it is for men). By understanding and managing their diet, women can take control of their hormonal balance and overall well-being.

Many women restrict their diet to maintain or achieve a desired body shape. They often resort to strict diets, excessive use of chemical or natural weight-loss supplements, extreme physical activity, or trendy exotic diets, depriving themselves of vital nutrients. The result is almost always the same: menstrual cycle disturbances. Many doctors refer to this as a 'hormonal imbalance' and treat it with hormonal contraceptives without investigating the actual cause or explaining to the woman that she needs to change not just her diet but also her mindset — to realize that she is becoming an enemy to her own body.

Dieting and weight loss have a profound effect on sex hormones and progesterone levels. Studies have shown that weight loss due to intense physical activity (exercise) significantly lowers progesterone and estrogen levels.

Since progesterone and sex hormones are fat-soluble substances, consuming fats or fat-soluble vitamins (E, A, D) enhances their absorption. Conversely, lacking fats reduces the body's ability to absorb hormones from internal and external sources. Foods rich in fats improve hormone absorption. Research has shown that drinking whole milk (which contains a certain percentage of fat) increases progesterone and estrogen levels in the blood. At the same time, a low-fat or fat-free diet reduces progesterone levels by more than 50% compared to women with a regular diet. Interestingly, some experiments have shown that a potassium-deficient diet increases progesterone concentration in rodents and men (though no studies have been conducted on women).

Excessive exercise combined with a low-fat diet can significantly lower progesterone and estrogen levels, leading to severe ovarian dysfunction and disrupted ovulation.

It has also been observed that women suffering from malnutrition, especially during winter when food is scarce, are more likely to experience anovulatory cycles. Anovulatory cycles refer to menstrual cycles where ovulation does not occur, which can lead to fertility issues and other health concerns.

Fiber Intake and Hormone Absorption

Obsession with diets, detox regimens, and so-called cleansing of the intestines, gallbladder, and lymphatic system seriously interferes with the body's natural processes. Such interventions usually lead to negative consequences rather than health improvements. One such trend is excessive fiber consumption.

Fiber belongs to the carbohydrate group, but unlike simple carbohydrates (sugars), it is not broken down or absorbed in the human body. In plants, fiber acts as a structural component, and depending on its chemical composition, fibers vary in thickness and length. Examples include cellulose (used to make paper), artificial rayon, and cotton. Wood fiber is widely used in various industries.

Animal-derived fibers include hair, fur, wool, and silk. Though asbestos is widely known, it is a mineral fiber, and there are many other natural mineral fibers. Both natural and synthetic fibers have been used for centuries in industry and everyday life.

Plant-based fibers, primarily found in vegetables, grains, and fruits, are obtained through food. Although *polysaccharides* are not fully absorbed, they are essential for healthy intestinal function, helping the body eliminate digestion byproducts. Fiber acts as a mesh that traps undigested food particles, toxins, and metabolic waste and stimulates intestinal motility, aiding food movement through the digestive tract.

The amount of fiber in the diet influences rectal function and the timely elimination of wasted food. A healthy digestive process depends mainly on the fiber content of food. This is why many nutritionists, dietitians, and general practitioners recommend fiber intake for all individuals. In constipation or digestive disorders, fiber is often prescribed in various forms — from powders, tablets, and compressed bars to fiber-enriched foods such as grain and nut bars, oat-based mixtures, and fiber-fortified drinks.

Today's primary issue is the overreliance on pharmaceutical supplements, where natural products are mechanically and chemically processed into pills, capsules, and powders. The health industry often prioritizes selling supplements over educating people about balanced nutrition. Instead of encouraging fresh fruit and vegetable consumption, the market is flooded with fiber supplements and other nutrients in pill or powder form. Understanding the importance of a balanced diet can empower individuals to make informed choices about their health.

It has been well-established that fiber benefits people with cardiovascular disease, digestive disorders, and diabetes. Increased fiber intake has been shown to reduce the risk of colorectal and even breast cancer. As a result, older adults, who often have various chronic conditions, limited mobility, poor lifestyle habits, excess weight, and a tendency to overeat, have embraced high-fiber diets.

However, excessive fiber consumption also has negative consequences, including adverse effects on female hormonal balance.

Research has shown that high fiber intake is linked to lower levels of sex hormones and progesterone, increasing anovulatory cycles, especially in young women. Excessive fiber intake can disrupt ovulation, a fact that is often overlooked by medical professionals when addressing menstrual irregularities.

Women who consume excessive fiber, particularly those in their mature and premenopausal years, often experience a decrease in estrogen levels. High-fiber diets are believed to reduce β-glucuronidase activity in the large intestine and impair estrogen reabsorption. Additionally, fiber can reduce fat and cholesterol absorption, partly due to more frequent bowel movements.

Women who overconsume fiber often have low follicle-stimulating hormone (FSH) and luteinizing hormone

(LH), which are crucial for folliculogenesis. In women with healthy ovarian function, these hormonal fluctuations may be temporary and self-regulated, meaning anovulatory cycles occur only occasionally. However, in women already experiencing menstrual irregularities, excessive fiber intake worsens the problem.

Additional risk factors in such women include low body weight (low BMI), intense physical activity, and extreme dietary restrictions.

Alcohol and Hormones

The effects of alcohol consumption on women's bodies across different ages have been extensively studied over the past half-century and even earlier. Many of these studies were conducted as part of government-level programs in various countries, aiming to determine minimum safe alcohol doses, given that alcohol consumption is deeply ingrained in the traditional cuisines of many cultures worldwide.

Significant research has been dedicated to understanding the impact of alcohol on female reproductive function. This includes its effects on sex hormone levels, progesterone, fertility, and the onset of menopause. These findings are crucial for women's health and should be widely known.

Studies have shown that moderate alcohol consumption (100 ml per week) slightly reduces conception rates and increases the risk of endometriosis.

Observations of healthy couples trying to conceive their first child over six months yielded the following results: consuming 100 g of alcohol per week reduced conception rates by half compared to those consuming only 10–50 g of alcohol. This means that for a couple trying to conceive, the chances of getting pregnant are significantly lower if either partner consumes more than 100 g of alcohol per week.

A comparative analysis of smoking, alcohol consumption, and their combination also revealed interesting findings.

- The monthly conception rate for women who neither smoked nor drank alcohol was just over 24%.

- For those who smoked but did not drink alcohol, it dropped to nearly 22%.

- Alcohol consumption, regardless of smoking, proved to be a significant factor in reducing female fertility.

One study focused on women with ovulatory cycles, which are menstrual cycles where ovulation occurs, who consumed more than 90 g of alcohol per week. Their monthly conception rate dropped to just 11%. In this study, alcohol intake was limited to days 14–21 of the menstrual cycle, the period when conception and implantation likelihood is highest. Yet, the impact of alcohol on fertility was undeniable.

Other researchers examined the effects of long-term alcohol consumption (up to 10 years). They found that even moderate alcohol intake exacerbated infertility problems by increasing the frequency of anovulatory cycles, which are menstrual cycles where ovulation does not occur, thereby reducing the chances of conception.

It's important to note that a key limitation of all these studies was the inconsistency in measurement units — some expressed alcohol intake in grams, others in milliliters, and variations in types of alcoholic beverages and duration of consumption.

Interestingly, in some countries where alcohol is traditionally part of daily meals (such as Italy, Spain, and France), no clear link was observed between occasional or moderate alcohol intake and fertility levels.

The impact of alcohol consumption on hormone levels, a topic of significant research and debate, has been studied in both menstruating and postmenopausal women. This research, which considers the amount of alcohol consumed, ranging from acute intoxication to chronic alcoholism, is of utmost importance in understanding the potential health implications of alcohol use.

Heavy alcohol consumption significantly increases estradiol levels in the blood, which is explained by alcohol's effect on opioid receptors in the hypothalamus. This stimulation enhances the pituitary gland's LH, FSH, and prolactin secretion. The most pronounced effect of alcohol occurs during the pre-ovulatory phase (late follicular phase) and the early implantation period (second half of the luteal phase). This is due to alcohol altering the balance of liver enzymes responsible for metabolizing estradiol into estrone, as the same liver enzymes are also required for alcohol detoxification. As a result, more estradiol remains in circulation since its breakdown in the liver is impaired.

Regular alcohol consumption leads to elevated levels of various estrogens (estradiol, estrone, and estriol) in both blood plasma and urine. It has been observed that biologically active estradiol levels increase before ovulation in all women who consume alcohol regularly and in moderate amounts. However, in cases of lower alcohol intake, some women experience a decrease in estradiol levels.

In postmenopausal women, alcohol raises estrogen levels even more significantly than in women of reproductive age.

Understanding the hormonal effects of alcohol consumption is not only of scientific interest but also has practical implications for healthcare. For instance, the finding that alcohol increases estrogen and male sex hormone levels in women has a direct impact on the management of hormonal medications, such as hormone replacement therapy (HRT) and hormonal contraceptives.

Alcohol significantly elevates estrogen levels in women using hormonal contraceptives and HRT. However, despite the high levels of exogenous estrogens, their absorption and elimination may be disrupted, leading to enhanced side effects of relative hyperestrogenism.

Several studies have shown that alcohol does not affect progesterone levels during the follicular phase or mid-luteal phase, even though theoretically, an imbalance in enzymes involved in progesterone synthesis and metabolism should also interfere with pregnenolone-to-progesterone conversion.

Studies on the effects of alcohol on progesterone levels in early pregnancy have not been conducted due to ethical concerns, given alcohol's known teratogenic effects. However, researchers have created a simulated pregnancy state in non-pregnant women by administering human chorionic gonadotropin (hCG) during specific days when hCG naturally appears in the blood during early pregnancy. The findings, which showed that alcohol lowered progesterone levels in these women, suggest potential implications for embryo implantation and early pregnancy health.

Other studies on women taking oral contraceptives and HRT confirmed that alcohol significantly reduces progesterone levels in the blood.

Laboratory experiments have also examined the direct effect of alcohol on placental cells and their ability to synthesize progesterone. The results showed that alcohol interferes with cholesterol transport into placental cells, preventing progesterone production. The amount of alcohol required to cause these changes corresponded to a blood alcohol concentration of 0.10–0.20%, equivalent to 1.5–3 glasses of wine or 110–230 ml of vodka.

2.5.7. Smoking and Ovarian Hormones

The detrimental effects of smoking on human health and its role in the development of various diseases, including lung cancer, have long been established. In women who smoke, fertility levels are significantly lower, and egg quality is poorer, leading to a reduced success rate of in vitro fertilization (IVF). This alarming trend necessitates a higher number of embryos, almost twice as many, to achieve pregnancy. This can be attributed to the direct toxic effects of nicotine and other harmful components of tobacco on reproductive cells, a concerning issue that needs immediate attention.

Smoking women are also at an increased risk of ectopic pregnancy, are more likely to have multiple pregnancies, and face a higher likelihood of preterm birth.

Interestingly, in young women who smoke, before ovarian aging begins (before the ages of 25–27), fertility appears to be slightly increased. Studies have shown that smokers exhibit heightened progesterone receptor activity in the endometrium, making them more sensitive to progesterone. This increased sensitivity might explain the higher implantation rates observed in young smoking women, which could have implications for fertility treatments and reproductive health management in this population.

Surprisingly, smokers also have a lower incidence of endometrial cancer and endometriosis compared to non-smokers. What could explain this phenomenon? Research indicates that smoking, particularly in older women, leads to an overall reduction in estrogen levels, thereby limiting endometrial growth. Since both endometriosis and endometrial cancer are largely estrogen-dependent conditions, lower estrogen levels may contribute to their reduced prevalence in smokers.

Other studies suggest that prolonged smoking does not significantly alter levels of estrogen, progesterone, or sex hormone-binding globulin (SHBG). However, some women experience a slight decrease in progesterone levels and an increase in estradiol levels during the second phase of the menstrual cycle. The reliability of these findings remains uncertain, and further research is needed in this area.

Another theory attributes the lower incidence of endometrial cancer and endometriosis in smokers to the effects of nicotine and other tobacco compounds on the ovaries. These substances may accelerate ovarian aging, reduce the reserve of eggs, and consequently lower estrogen production. The relative increase in progesterone levels further suppresses endometrial growth. Women with endometriosis typically exhibit reduced progesterone receptor numbers and activity, both in the uterus and in ectopic endometrial lesions.

Because smokers have heightened progesterone receptor activity, the prevalence of endometriosis is lower among them. However, it would be erroneous to conclude that smoking provides any meaningful protection against endometrial cancer or endometriosis, as this so-called "protective effect" is negligible compared to the overall harm smoking inflicts on the body, including the ovaries.

Cigarette smoke contains more than 4,000 chemical compounds, with even one capable of influencing progesterone receptors and activating genes involved in endometrial growth and differentiation. Therefore, the focus should not be on encouraging smoking but rather on identifying substances that can provide therapeutic benefits for the endometrium, such as potential drugs or treatments that mimic the effects of these substances without the harmful side effects of smoking.

Even among women with low estrogen levels—such as those experiencing anovulatory cycles or amenorrhea—the risk of endometrial cancer remains elevated. This is because such women also have low progesterone levels due to the absence of ovulation and, consequently, no corpus luteum formation. Endometrial hyperplasia, which arises in anovulatory cycles, results from an imbalance between estrogen and progesterone, even when both hormones are at low levels. It is unlikely that a minor reduction in estrogen levels would protect smokers from developing hyperplasia. In perimenopausal women, fluctuating estrogen levels, unopposed by adequate progesterone production due to infrequent or absent ovulation, can also contribute to the development of endometrial hyperplasia.

2.5.8. Understanding Ovarian Reserve

Since we are discussing the ovaries and the hormones they produce, it is important to mention **ovarian reserve**, as this term is often misused. Many women seeking medical help after unsuccessful attempts at conception or pregnancy loss undergo testing to assess their ovarian reserve.

What is an ovarian reserve, and why is it so important? Each woman is born with a set supply of germ cells (oocytes) in small follicles within the ovaries, which is determined during fetal development while she is still in her mother's womb. This supply continuously diminishes as germ cells naturally perish, with the loss rate fluctuating throughout a woman's life.

Several waves of *accelerated oocyte loss* have been identified, the most notable occurring during puberty (sexual maturation) and the premenopausal period (from approximately ages 37–38 until menstruation ceases). These periods are crucial as they mark significant decreases in the ovarian reserve, which can impact a woman's fertility.

What determines oocyte loss? This is a genetically programmed process that cannot be controlled at will or influenced by a woman's feelings. However, several factors can significantly impact it:

- Surgical procedures on the ovaries and other pelvic organs, including laparoscopic surgeries that disrupt ovarian blood supply.

- Use, particularly misuse, medications that stimulate oocyte maturation or impair microcirculation in the pelvic organs.

- Radiation and chemotherapy.

- Any condition affecting blood supply or nerve function in the ovaries and pelvic organs.

- Harmful habits, mainly smoking, which disrupt microcirculation in ovarian tissue.

- Genetic mutations like those in the **FMR1** gene may arise spontaneously or be inherited.

  Every woman should remember the following:

o **Lost ovarian reserve cannot be restored—what is lost forever.**

o **There is no medical treatment or method capable of halting ovarian depletion or slowing the rate of oocyte loss.** On the contrary, certain medications and incorrect treatment regimens can accelerate oocyte loss (for example, frequent interruptions in hormonal contraceptive use).

o **Hormonal contraceptives and hormone replacement therapy do not provide "rest" for the ovaries, do not rejuvenate them, and do not preserve or increase ovarian reserve.**

o **As oocytes are lost, especially under negative external influences, the quality of remaining eggs deteriorates, and genetic mutations become more frequent.**

During the maturation of a single egg, approximately 70 follicles perish. In the presence of additional factors affecting oocyte maturation, a woman may lose up to 100 follicles per month.

Even today, the concept of 'ovarian reserve' remains elusive, with no universally accepted methods for its accurate assessment. While several tests and techniques exist, none have emerged as the definitive solution, underscoring the need for further research and development.

One approach is measuring *follicle-stimulating hormone* (FSH), which directly influences follicular growth during the final stage of their development. FSH levels are regulated by estradiol, produced by the follicles, and *inhibin B*, a specific protein also synthesized within them. If follicles fail to grow, levels of these substances decrease, triggering a compensatory rise in FSH. This mechanism is known as *negative feedback*. Therefore, elevated FSH levels (>18–20 IU/L) are often associated with diminished ovarian reserve.

While FSH testing is a primary tool in reproductive medicine for assessing ovarian response to artificial stimulation, it has its limitations. A poor response to stimulation, indicated by a significant increase in FSH levels, may suggest a less favorable prognosis for natural conception. In such cases, in vitro fertilization (IVF) with donor eggs may be recommended. However, it's important to note that **a single FSH measurement, used solely for evaluating ovarian reserve, has limited practical**

value due to its fluctuating levels. Therefore, repeated testing over several months is necessary for a more accurate assessment.

A single FSH measurement, especially when used solely to evaluate ovarian reserve, offers limited practical value. Its levels fluctuate from cycle to cycle in each woman and may not accurately reflect the actual ovarian reserve. This underscores the need for more comprehensive and repeated testing over several months for a more accurate assessment.

Anti-Müllerian hormone (AMH) is a protein produced by small follicles. Follicular development progresses through several stages — from primordial to antral and then dominant follicles. AMH is secreted by granulosa cells of growing follicles. Each year, a woman develops between 20 and 150 growing follicles (0.05–2 mm in size), but these cannot be detected using standard diagnostic methods. Therefore, AMH levels are often correlated with the number of antral follicles.

It's important to note that the claim that *antral follicle count* or AMH levels accurately reflect ovarian reserve has yet to be scientifically validated. While AMH levels remain relatively stable throughout the menstrual cycle, whether they are directly linked to follicles smaller than 2 mm remains unclear.

AMH levels do not predict a woman's future ability to conceive. However, AMH testing is used in infertility treatment, where low AMH levels indicate a poor ovarian response to stimulation. This could be due to incorrect treatment approaches, including misdiagnosis or actual ovarian reserve depletion.

AMH is not a predictor of early menopause.

Ultrasound can visualize and count follicles measuring 2–10 mm in both ovaries. *Antral follicle count* (AFC) is linked to AMH levels. However, approximately half of these follicles will not continue to grow and will undergo *atresia* (degeneration). **Ultrasound cannot determine whether a follicle is growing or atretic, as they all appear identical on imaging.**

Another issue is the lack of standardized guidelines for counting follicle sizes: some recommendations suggest counting follicles 2–5 mm, others 2–8 mm, and others 2–10 mm. This inconsistency can lead to misleading conclusions and incorrect infertility treatment strategies.

AFC is primarily used to determine ovarian response to stimulation, including for IVF. If AFC is below 7, the ovaries are expected to have a weak reaction to stimulation, leading to a poor prognosis.

When using AFC to determine ovarian response to stimulation, it's crucial to consider the whole picture. Trial ovarian stimulation can help determine whether visible follicles are sensitive to FSH and respond by differentiating between growing and atretic follicles. If most follicles are atretic, stimulation will be ineffective. In combination with AMH testing, AFC has only limited prognostic value in predicting pregnancy outcomes.

Modern reproductive medicine relies on only three biomarkers in infertility assessment: *AMH, inhibin B, and FSH*. Low AMH and inhibin B levels, along with elevated FSH (in the follicular phase), are considered potential indicators of infertility due to ovarian dysfunction or decline.

Recent research has revealed that the biomarkers commonly used in infertility assessment, such as AMH, inhibin B, and FSH, do not necessarily correlate with fertility in women aged 30–44 who have no history of infertility and have not actively tried to conceive for at least three months. This highlights the need for age-specific assessment methods in reproductive medicine.

Similarly, FSH measurements showed no difference in conception rates over 6- and 12-month periods between women with normal FSH levels and those with>10 mIU/mL.

Inhibin B levels also had no impact when measured in the early follicular phase — pregnancy rates were identical in both groups.

If a woman has not attempted pregnancy for at least 6–12 months, measuring AMH, FSH, or inhibin B is not a reliable method for assessing her fertility potential. On the contrary, such testing may cause unnecessary psychological distress and lead to excessive and unwarranted medical interventions.

Can progesterone levels determine ovarian reserve in women with infertility? It's important to note that measuring progesterone levels in isolation does not provide a complete picture of ovarian reserve. Progesterone and estrogen levels, while relatively stable throughout most of a woman's life, do not necessarily reflect ovarian reserve. This is particularly true during the premenopausal and menopausal periods. As a result, using progesterone levels as a sole indicator for evaluating ovarian reserve, especially in the context of IVF preparation, is not a practical approach and is rarely performed.

While several methods are available to assess ovarian reserve, none, whether used individually or in combination, have been proven to be consistently accurate or reliable for predicting a woman's fertility potential. It's crucial to interpret test results within a broader clinical context, including the couple's infertility history, partners' medical examinations, and other relevant analyses. This comprehensive approach is essential for a more accurate assessment of fertility potential.

While age is a crucial factor in fertility assessment, it is not the only one. For instance, if a woman has high FSH levels, low AMH and AFC levels, and a history of ovarian surgery for cyst removal, the prognosis is likely unfavorable. These factors and age should be considered in a more nuanced understanding of fertility assessment. Such findings carry less prognostic weight in younger women than in older women, highlighting the need for a comprehensive approach to fertility assessment.

When it comes to fertility assessment, there is no one-size-fits-all approach. The evaluation should always be individualized, considering each patient's unique circumstances and medical history.

2.6. Adrenal Glands

The adrenal glands have long fascinated doctors and researchers due to their complex structure, the variety of hormones they produce, their unique innervation, and the vital functions they perform for the body. These endocrine glands consist of two primary components — the cortex (10%) and the medulla (90%), each responsible for producing entirely different hormones. Dysfunction of the adrenal glands can be life-threatening.

The adrenal glands, first described by Bartolomeo Eustachio in 1552 as *glandulae renibus incumbents*, have a rich historical significance. Their close anatomical relationship with the kidneys was emphasized, and even renowned anatomists like Leonardo da Vinci and Galen had previously overlooked them. However, their immediate classification as glands suggests their glandular nature was correctly identified. In 1845, German embryologist and anatomist Emil Guschke was the first to distinguish the two distinct regions of the adrenal glands — the cortex and the medulla.

The study of adrenal function has been ongoing for nearly a century, following the discovery of the hormones they produce. Over the last decade, research has primarily focused on two crucial areas: the impact of adrenal hormones on fetal growth and development and their role in the human stress response. This continuous research keeps us informed about the latest developments in the field.

It is important to mention prenatal stress, which refers to a woman's physiological reaction to pregnancy and its complications. As women in developed countries are now conceiving and giving birth later in life and less frequently, pregnancy complications have become more common. Some physicians in the 18th and 19th centuries recognized the negative impact of stress on pregnancy and mentioned it in their writings. However, scientists did not take this topic seriously until the early 21st century. Research has since confirmed that stress increases the risk of pregnancy loss, particularly in the early stages, and is associated with a higher incidence of complications. However, there is a crucial distinction between stress affecting the body of an adult woman and stress directly impacting the developing embryo or fetus.

Epigenetics explores the influence of external and internal factors on the fetus as a future adult. Studies have demonstrated a link between prenatal stress and cardiovascular diseases in adult men whose mothers experienced stress during pregnancy, particularly in cases of pregnancy-induced hypertension.

Acknowledging the complexity of the term' prenatal stress' is essential, as there is no precise definition of this condition. Emotional fluctuations, anxiety, and fear of pregnancy loss are common among almost all pregnant women and inevitably trigger increased adrenal hormone levels. This complexity highlights the challenges in defining and understanding prenatal stress.

From the earliest weeks of pregnancy, the fetal adrenal glands function as a factory for androgen production. By 8 weeks, cortisol synthesis is already occurring in the embryo. Since the trophoblast-placenta system produces an enormous amount of progesterone, some converted into androgens, cortisol plays a protective role, particularly in female fetuses, by preventing excessive testosterone exposure that could disrupt genital development. This protective role of cortisol in fetal development is a crucial aspect of prenatal health that needs to be understood.

Sexual differentiation under hormonal influence occurs between weeks 7 and 12, a period often referred to as the window of *sexual differentiation*, during which the external genitalia develop. After 12 weeks, the fetal adrenal glands produce two androgens in large quantities — DHEA and DHEAS — which can be converted into female sex hormones in the placenta, a crucial process for fetal development. The fetus and placenta produce up to 90% of estriol and 50% of estrone and estradiol, which circulate in the mother's bloodstream. However, the precise role of steroid hormones in fetal development remains incompletely understood.

In adults, the adrenal glands produce glucocorticoids, mineralocorticoids, and androgens from a common precursor — cholesterol. The most well-known adrenal hormone is cortisol, often called the stress hormone. It is frequently described in a negative light, with claims that it damages blood vessels, contributes to cardiovascular disease, raises blood pressure, and disrupts the function of many organs. It is sometimes called the "king of stress." However, the reality is more nuanced.

Adrenal androgens are unique because their increase signals the onset of puberty in both girls and boys. These androgens, particularly DHEA, play a significant role in the development of secondary sexual characteristics and the maturation of the reproductive system during puberty. Understanding this role is crucial for comprehending the physiological changes during this life stage.

Interestingly, adrenal androgen production varies with age. After 30 years, their levels gradually decline, reaching their lowest point during adrenopause. Unlike *menopause* in women or *andropause* in men, *adrenopause* does not signify the cessation of androgen production but rather its reduction to minimal levels. This phenomenon remains poorly understood, and little is known about the age of onset or factors influencing adrenopause.

Previously, the adrenal glands were believed to be the only source of glucocorticoids and mineralocorticoids. However, research has shown that these hormones are also synthesized in the intestines, skin, lymphatic system, brain, and possibly heart and blood vessels. The physiological significance of hormone production in these organs remains unclear.

2.6.1. Glucocorticoids

The adrenal cortex functions as a factory for producing a group of hormones collectively known as corticoids or corticosteroids, which include *glucocorticoids* and *mineralocorticoids*. The adrenocorticotropic hormone (ACTH), secreted by the pituitary gland, is key in stimulating adrenal cortex function.

The name "glucocorticoids" reflects their connection to glucose metabolism, as these hormones increase blood sugar levels. Stress plays a significant role in the development of diabetes, with numerous cases reported where severe stress leads to metabolic disturbances. Glucocorticoids stimulate gluconeogenesis in the liver, promoting glucose production from fats and proteins.

Why does glucose level rise when glucocorticoid levels are elevated? This is a protective response to stress, as glucose is the most accessible and efficient energy source, readily used by all cells. Acute, short-term stress increases overall energy levels, improving alertness, motor function, and coordination, enhancing survival in humans and animals. However, chronic, prolonged stress depletes energy reserves and reduces survival capacity. The liver's ability to generate additional energy via cortisol-driven glucose production helps the body endure stress with minimal harm. However, energy and nutrient reserves are not infinite — chronic stress can ultimately lead to disease and even death.

When discussing stress, it is crucial to recognize that it is not limited to external stressors (challenges in daily life, work, or relationships). It also includes a person's lifestyle (physical activity, thought patterns, malnutrition, overeating, interpersonal conflicts) and illnesses, especially those that are sudden, acute, or life-threatening — the more severe the illness, the higher the stress hormones produced by the body.

A distinct condition related to stress is shock, which can manifest in various ways and affect multiple organ systems. Hemodynamic shock, for instance, arises from circulatory failure and fluid imbalance and poses a serious risk of death. Glucocorticoids help the body cope with shock by improving blood supply to the heart, brain, and lungs, essential for survival.

The most important glucocorticoid is cortisol, historically referred to as *hydrocortisone.* If you have encountered medications called hydrocortisone, you might recall that this hormone is crucial in reducing inflammation, particularly in conditions such as rheumatoid arthritis and autoimmune diseases. Cortisol achieves this by suppressing the immune system, which is responsible for the inflammation. Glucocorticoids are also used to treat asthma, as they suppress allergic reactions and facilitate organ transplant acceptance by preventing immune rejection.

As mentioned earlier, cortisol plays a beneficial role in short-term stress. However, under chronic stress, it becomes harmful, accumulating in excess and negatively impacting multiple organs. You may have noticed that during times of anxiety, depression, or distress, there is a strong urge to eat constantly. This is because an initial spike in blood glucose triggers a rise in insulin levels. While fats can initially be converted into glucose, prolonged stress has the opposite effect, promoting the conversion of sugars and proteins into fats, leading to fat accumulation — primarily in the abdomen, buttocks, and thighs. This condition is sometimes called *Cushing's syndrome*, though in most cases, it is not a valid form of the syndrome caused by excess cortisol production. A more accurate term is *"metabolic syndrome,"* which reflects a broader pattern of metabolic dysfunction, including high blood pressure, high blood sugar, excess body fat around the waist, and abnormal cholesterol levels.

Metabolic syndrome is more common in middle age when additional risk factors, such as a sedentary lifestyle, poor diet (high-calorie intake), and harmful habits (smoking, alcohol consumption), further contribute to metabolic imbalances.

Like all steroid hormones, cortisol binds to proteins, primarily corticosteroid-binding globulin (CBG or transcortin), while approximately 10–15% of cortisol binds to albumin. Only free cortisol is biologically active and capable of binding to cellular receptors. Under normal, non-stress conditions, only 5% of cortisol remains free, but stress significantly increases free cortisol levels. Free cortisol is a form of cortisol that is not bound to proteins and can exert its effects on the body. Increased free cortisol levels during stress are a key part of the body's response to stressors.

Interestingly, a balance exists between bound and free cortisol, preventing excessive hormonal damage to tissues. However, this equilibrium is influenced by body temperature and the body's acid-base balance (pH).

Cortisol levels in women depend on estrogen levels, which increase the production of transcortin, leading to higher total cortisol levels. The use of estrogen-containing medications (such as combined oral contraceptives and COCs) also raises cortisol levels, and this effect can persist for several weeks after discontinuation. To assess cortisol and other steroid hormones accurately, hormonal contraceptives containing estrogens should be discontinued for at least six weeks before testing.

Regrettably, current cortisol measurement methods overlook the crucial distinction between bound and free cortisol. Total cortisol, the most measured form in serum, does not accurately reflect the hormone's bioactivity, potentially leading to misleading conclusions. Therefore, it's imperative to remember that the measurement of free cortisol is paramount!

High cortisol levels are observed in adrenal cortex tumors, as well as in cases of excessive use of medications that increase cortisol levels, particularly during prolonged glucocorticoid use. In such cases, Cushing's syndrome develops. If a tumor produces cortisol, this is called endogenous Cushing's syndrome, whereas if glucocorticoids are taken as medication, this is referred to as exogenous Cushing's syndrome.

There is also *Cushing's disease*, which occurs when an excess of adrenocorticotropic hormone (ACTH) is produced by the pituitary gland, usually due to a tumor in this gland.

Adrenal adenoma is the most common cause of Cushing's syndrome. This is a hormonally active tumor, but it is benign.

Cushing's syndrome, a rare disorder, is characterized by rapid weight gain and fat deposits in specific body areas while other parts remain thin. Blood pressure often rises, bone mass decreases (osteoporosis), the skin develops purple stretch marks and bruises, and muscle mass declines. People suffering from this syndrome may experience changes in their emotional state and libido. It's important to note that Cushing's syndrome is uncommon and has distinct symptoms.

In women, high cortisol levels due to stress, just like in Cushing's syndrome, disrupt ovulation. Menstrual cycles become irregular, and in some cases, they disappear for some time. I have already mentioned hypothalamic or stress-related amenorrhea earlier in this book. This stress-induced disruption of the menstrual cycle occurs due to increased cortisol levels and the shutdown of the reproductive program. In a state of stress, the body cannot focus on conception and pregnancy maintenance, as its priority is self-preservation and survival. This is precisely why pregnancy losses increase in stressful conditions.

In recent years, scientists have shown great interest in the effect of glucocorticoids on psycho-emotional states, psychosomatic disorders, and the development of mental illnesses such as depression and anxiety disorders. However, there is still very little data of practical significance.

Cortisol deficiency leads to *Addison's disease*. This infrequent condition develops due to adrenal damage, including cases caused by autoimmune processes, where antibodies attack adrenal tissue. Symptoms include weakness, fatigue, dizziness, weight loss, muscle weakness, and skin darkening.

Addison's disease was named after Thomas Addison, an English scientist and physician, who described adrenal insufficiency in 1855 in 11 patients, all of whom died. Post-mortem examinations revealed adrenal atrophy.

Surgeries to remove the adrenal glands were performed on animals and humans for many years, beginning in the late 19th century. The first adrenal tumor removal was conducted in 1905. However, for a long time, the role of the adrenal glands was not well understood, even though most animals died after adrenal removal, and more than 30% of humans did not survive these interventions. It was only with the discovery of cortisone in 1934, which began to be used as hormone replacement therapy that the concept of adrenal insufficiency became scientifically established.

There are many myths surrounding hormones, and this book is dedicated to debunking these myths, offering scientific explanations for the various processes in which hormones produced by the human body are involved.

It's crucial to address the emergence of a non-existent diagnosis, often called *'adrenal fatigue syndrome.'* This term, seemingly coined by some practitioners, lacks any scientific basis or legitimacy in the medical field. There are no established diagnostic criteria, necessary examinations, or proven treatments for this syndrome. It's essential to be cautious and informed about such unsubstantiated medical claims.

This fictional diagnosis is exploited to prescribe various drugs — ranging from hormones (which are particularly dangerous, as they are taken without medical indication) to substances that are not even medications, with no proven efficacy or safety. This made-up diagnosis is most abused in countries with weak healthcare systems, where there is little regulation of medical practice and poor oversight of physicians and medical institutions.

2.6.2. Mineralocorticoids

Mineralocorticoids, particularly aldosterone, are pivotal in regulating the body's water and electrolyte balance. They are the second type of steroid hormone produced by the adrenal cortex.

Despite being discovered relatively late, between 1953 and 1956, aldosterone's role in sodium metabolism is paramount. It plays a critical role among several substances involved in sodium metabolism, and its significance is on par with other steroid hormones.

When delving into corticosteroids, it's crucial to understand the complexity of the *renin-angiotensin-aldosterone system* (RAAS). This intricate hormonal system controls mineralocorticoid production. *Renin*, a specialized enzyme the kidneys produce, responds to changes in blood pressure, circulating blood volume, and serum sodium and potassium concentrations. It acts on angiotensinogen, converting it into angiotensin I, which is further transformed into angiotensin II. This final product, angiotensin II, stimulates the adrenal glands to produce aldosterone.

Kidney diseases associated with impaired renal blood flow (such as renal artery stenosis) often lead to high blood pressure. This type of hypertension is commonly referred to as renin-dependent (renal) or *renovascular hypertension*. It is highly resistant to antihypertensive drugs and is accompanied by disruptions in sodium and water excretion. Renovascular hypertension is associated not only with elevated blood pressure but also with abnormal aldosterone production.

Aldosterone affects the kidneys' nephrons and influences sodium absorption in the intestines. A deficiency of this hormone can lead to renovascular hypertension and a life-threatening loss of essential minerals, including sodium and potassium. Low mineralocorticoid levels in the blood can lead to heart attacks and cardiac arrest.

Practically nothing is known about aldosterone's role in women's health.

2.6.3. Catecholamines

The adrenal glands produce several vital substances with hormonal activity. I am sure that many have heard of *adrenaline* and *noradrenaline*. It is common to hear people say that someone who is overly "nervous" has too much adrenaline in their blood. When people engage in extreme sports, they often crave adrenaline to feel happy.

Indeed, the body produces several hormones that play a crucial role as *neurotransmitters*, transmitting signals in the central nervous system and helping regulate motor function, emotions, cognition, memory formation, and endocrine gland function. These include adrenaline (epinephrine), noradrenaline (norepinephrine), and *dopamine*, which are synthesized in the *adrenal medulla*.

Previously, we discussed cortisol, the hormone of chronic stress. Let's focus on how the body reacts to acute stress, such as fear. This is a reaction every adult can describe, having experienced it more than once. A sudden, sharp stress often causes a rapid heartbeat, faster breathing, and an initial sensation of cold followed by sweating. Blood pressure first rises, then drops. There may be abdominal discomfort and an urge to urinate. And, of course, the legs feel weak, making standing difficult. Adrenaline and noradrenaline are crucial in these reactions, releasing first and initiating the body's *fight-or-flight response*. Their rapid breakdown means their effects are short-lived, with the body quickly returning to equilibrium.

In such reactions, cortisol does not play the leading role — adrenaline and noradrenaline are released first, and cortisol appears later. However, since catecholamines break down quickly, their effects are short-lived. Within minutes, a person recovers, heart rate and breathing return to normal, and only the memory of the fright remains. If the stress factor persists longer, cortisol and catecholamines are also released.

Adrenaline and noradrenaline act in a specific ratio, maintaining a balance that, if disrupted, can lead to neurological and psychiatric disorders. The role of catecholamines in brain function and overall physiology continues to be studied, including through animal models. Experiments in mice have shown that dopamine deficiency leads to motor impairments, reduced movement, and poorer signal memory retention.

Since catecholamine release is often synergistic, meaning they are released together, and their effects are interdependent, it is difficult to isolate their individual effects. It is also challenging to determine precisely which processes each hormone controls. However, it is known that:

174

- Noradrenaline is involved in long-term memory formation, skill acquisition, and learning from multiple sources of information.

- Dopamine is responsible for emotion regulation, feelings, and emotional memory.

Epinephrine (adrenaline) is considered the most critical catecholamine, as it plays a key role in the body's fight-or-flight response. This physiological reaction occurs in response to a perceived harmful event, attack, or threat to survival. It is released in any adverse situation, such as fear, anxiety, shock, or stress. No organ or tissue in the human body that catecholamines do not affect. They are critical for activating the body's survival mechanisms, often called the fight-or-flight response. In any adverse situation, such as fear, anxiety, shock, or stress, adrenaline (epinephrine) is released, preparing the body to confront or flee the threat. This crucial role in the body's protective systems is why catecholamines can be called protection hormones, as they influence the function of all endocrine glands and the production of other hormones.

Catecholamines do not directly affect reproductive function (although they may contribute to erectile dysfunction). However, because they play a crucial role in the stress response, they can indirectly influence factors that suppress germ cell maturation and disrupt the menstrual cycle. Several studies have confirmed that **chronic stress contributes to pregnancy loss at any stage, fetal growth restriction, and preterm birth**.

While testing for various catecholamines is rarely performed due to their rapid breakdown and elimination from the body, the research on these hormones is vast and continually expanding. Thousands of scientific and clinical studies worldwide continue to explore their role in human physiology—from birth to old age. The past decade alone has seen nearly 100,000 scientific papers published on catecholamines and their involvement in metabolism, obesity, learning, neurodegenerative diseases, memory disorders, attention regulation, and cardiovascular disease. This ongoing research keeps the field dynamic and full of potential for discoveries.

We will not delve into a detailed discussion of catecholamines' full significance. Still, we can draw an important conclusion: all diseases stem from nerves because many hormones are released!

2.7. Thyroid Gland

In previous chapters, I mentioned TSH, the pituitary hormone that regulates the function of the thyroid gland. The thyroid gland is also an endocrine organ that produces hormones.

Did you know that the first endocrine gland to develop in a human embryo is the thyroid gland? By day 22 after conception, the future thyroid begins forming in the pharyngeal region, and by day 49, a primitive gland with developing follicles appears in front of the trachea. By week 11, the thyroid starts accumulating iodine and synthesizing thyroxine (T4). However, the fetus remains highly dependent on maternal thyroid hormones because its thyroid does not produce sufficient hormone levels until the second trimester of pregnancy.

The thyroid gland is the largest in newborns (1–2 grams) and adults (20–30 grams). However, with age, the gland decreases in size, and functional abnormalities develop. By age 60, 40% of individuals show structural changes in the thyroid (cysts, nodules, tumors). By 75–80 years, more than 30% of people experience thyroid dysfunction. Over time, the gland accumulates lymphocytes, and in nearly 50% of older women, antibodies to thyroid hormones appear in the blood.

The two main thyroid hormones are thyroxine (T4) and triiodothyronine (T3), which require the synthesis of iodine, selenium, boron, and several other trace elements. T4 is always produced in larger quantities than T3, with a blood concentration ratio 14:1. T3 is four times more biologically active than T4 but has a half-life of only one day, whereas T4 remains in the bloodstream for 5–7 days.

Approximately 99.9% of circulating thyroxine is bound to plasma proteins: 85–90% binds to thyroxine-binding globulin (TBG), while about 10% binds to transthyretin and albumin.

The thyroid gland, one of the oldest known glands, has a rich historical significance — references to goiter treatment with iodine-rich seaweed in Chinese medicine date back to 1600 BCE. Every ancient civilization has left records mentioning the thyroid gland and its disorders. Its prominent location in the body makes its enlargement easy to notice. The Roman writer Celsus described goiter in 15 CE, calling it bronchocele (neck tumor). Interestingly, for several centuries in Europe, goiter was treated with a burnt sponge, referring to a marine or freshwater animal consumed orally.

The history of thyroid study and treatment is long and fascinating, full of scientific breakthroughs and anecdotal remedies. In the 16th century, Paracelsus, a Swiss physician and alchemist, was the first to suggest that thyroid diseases might be linked to mineral deficiencies in drinking water. His pioneering work laid the foundation for modern understanding of the thyroid gland and its disorders.

For a long time, the thyroid was believed to primarily moisten the trachea and play a cosmetic role in women. An enlarged thyroid was considered an alarming sign; something husbands were advised to notice — since their wives would become more irritable, emotional, and moody. Indeed, thyroid disorders have always been more common in women, both in ancient times and today, making it fair to call it a 'female gland.' The truth is thyroid dysfunction significantly impacts emotional well-being. Depending on the type of disorder, women may experience increased tearfulness, irritability, mood swings, aggression, apathy, or emotional indifference.

The first recorded thyroidectomy (surgical thyroid gland removal) occurred in 1884. This landmark event marked the beginning of surgical interventions for thyroid disorders. The successful removal of the thyroid gland paved the way for further research and advancements in endocrine surgery. But could a surgeon receive a Nobel Prize for removing an organ? It turns out — yes! Swedish surgeon Theodor Kocher won the Nobel Prize in 1909 after performing over 2,000 such surgeries (at the time, postoperative mortality was 5%).

Thyroxine was first isolated in 1914, but synthetic hormone production only began in 1926. This innovation made hormone replacement therapy possible for individuals who had no thyroid gland or whose thyroid function was insufficient.

To fully describe the role of the thyroid gland, one would need another book as large as this one — and indeed, many such books already exist. However, I am sure you will be surprised to learn that the primary consumer of thyroid hormones is muscle tissue.

When T4 levels are excessively high, as seen in *hyperthyroidism*, muscle motor activity decreases, and electrolyte and energy metabolism disrupt oxidation and glucose utilization. Prolonged exposure to high T4 levels leads to muscle mass loss. Additionally, muscle relaxation time is shortened, meaning the heart beats more frequently but does not fully relax between contractions, preventing proper recovery. Conversely, thyroid hormone deficiency prolongs relaxation time, impairing blood circulation.

Thyroxine affects cellular structures such as mitochondria, regulates protein synthesis and breakdown, influences tissue sensitivity to catecholamines, and affects antioxidant enzyme levels, capillary growth, muscle fiber differentiation, and cerebral blood circulation.

Over the past decade, an extensive body of research has emerged on thyroid hormones and their role in the brain and central nervous system. These hormones play a critical and irreplaceable role in CNS development and function, starting from the embryonic stage. Without sufficient thyroxine, proper brain formation does not occur. This is why thyroid function in pregnant women and those planning pregnancy receives significant medical attention today.

Thyroxine regulates neural cell architecture (*cytoarchitecture*), nerve fiber growth, and *myelination*. A deficiency or excess of thyroid hormones can cause irreversible damage to nerve cells, disrupting neuronal organization, biochemical function, and viability. These irreversible processes can begin in early childhood and even before birth at the embryonic level.

Regarding women's health, normal thyroid function is crucial for germ cell maturation. Women with thyroid disorders frequently experience menstrual cycle irregularities, uterine bleeding, and infertility.

Let's discuss some thyroid diseases.

2.7.1. Thyroid Function Screening

For an extended period, thyroid problems can remain compensated and asymptomatic, making early detection challenging. There are no universal guidelines for thyroid disease screening, but it is recommended for the following high-risk groups:

- Pregnant women

- Women over the age of 50–60

- Individuals with type 1 diabetes

- Patients with any autoimmune disease

- Individuals with a history of neck irradiation

These categories are considered at high risk for developing hypothyroidism.

Endocrine professional societies recommend screening all women starting at age 35 and repeating the test every five years.

The screening process typically commences with the measurement of thyroid-stimulating hormone (TSH) levels, a crucial step. In most cases, this is sufficient. However, if TSH levels are found to be above or below the normal range, further testing of **free thyroxine (T4)** and, less frequently, **triiodothyronine (T3)** is recommended.

Several types of antibodies are produced in autoimmune thyroiditis, particularly in hypothyroid conditions. The most clinically relevant tests measure **anti-thyroid peroxidase (anti-TPO) antibodies** and **anti-thyroglobulin (anti-Tg) antibodies** to determine whether the disease is autoimmune. However, it's important to note that repeat antibody testing holds little practical value once a positive antibody result has been detected and should be used cautiously.

Moreover, antibody levels do not always correlate with disease severity. Mildly elevated antibody levels can be associated with severe symptoms, while high antibody levels may not present with any complaints. However, studies have shown a correlation between high anti-TPO levels and an increased risk of infertility, miscarriages, and early pregnancy loss. In such cases, levothyroxine therapy is recommended, and while its efficacy is limited, it has been observed to significantly improve conception rates and pregnancy outcomes, offering hope to patients.

The **TSH stimulation test** is primarily used in older women and men to assess the function of the pituitary and hypothalamus, providing a clear understanding of their role in the process.

2.7.2. Thyroid Disorders

As mentioned, the thyroid gland can be called the "female gland," as its disorders most frequently occur in women. This gender disparity in thyroid diseases becomes apparent as early as adolescence.

Thyroid disorders can be conditionally divided into the following groups:

- **Hypothyroidism** – decreased thyroid hormone production (hypothyroid condition).

- **Hyperthyroidism** – increased thyroid hormone production (hyperthyroid condition).

- **Autoimmune inflammation of the thyroid** – thyroiditis, which may occur with increased, decreased, or normal hormone production.

- **Thyroid cysts and tumors** – including benign growths, thyroid cancer, hormone-producing tumors, and non-hormone-producing tumors.

This classification is somewhat arbitrary, as the causes of thyroid disorders vary widely.

Dysfunctional thyroid disorders are complex and act like a 'copycat monkey' mimicking many other diseases. The symptoms of hypothyroidism and hyperthyroidism are highly diverse, affecting multiple organ systems, making them easily confused with different conditions. This complexity underscores the need for specialized knowledge and skills in diagnosing and managing thyroid disorders.

For example:

- Patients with hyperthyroidism often complain of heart palpitations (tachycardia) and chest pain, which may be mistaken for cardiovascular disease.

- Irritability, tearfulness, and sleep disturbances can be confused with depression.

- Swelling of the skin and generalized weakness may suggest metabolic disorders or systemic diseases.

Doctors only examined the thyroid gland for a long time when it visibly enlarged, forming a goiter, and caused discomfort. Today, however, early assessment of thyroid function is crucial in newborns, children, adolescents, adults, pregnant women, and the elderly to ensure early diagnosis and effective management.

When diagnosing thyroid disorders, it is crucial to conduct a comprehensive evaluation, considering the woman's age and overall health, especially when interpreting TSH levels. Though less practical, measuring T4 and T3 levels is an important part of this thorough evaluation and is usually performed when TSH abnormalities are detected.

Hypothyroidism

A deficiency of thyroid hormones, or hypothyroidism (hypothyreosis), occurs more frequently than hyperthyroidism. It is most observed in women, usually between 30 and 50, although it can develop at any age. On average, between 1.4% and 2% of women suffer from various forms of hypothyroidism.

Hypothyroidism was first described in 1912 by the Japanese physician Hakaru Hashimoto, to whom we also owe the identification of *Hashimoto's disease* or *Hashimoto's thyroiditis*. This autoimmune condition is characterized by lymphocytic infiltration (accumulation of lymphocytes) in the thyroid tissue. As a result, the gland enlarges and often becomes painful, and there is a deficiency of thyroxine. However, lymphocytic infiltration of the thyroid gland is not always a disease; it also occurs naturally with age. In women over 60–70, infiltration of varying degrees is observed in nearly half of all cases.

Hypothyroidism's TSH level is above the reference range (usually greater than 4 mIU/L). Some mistakenly believe that an elevated TSH level is a sign of hyperthyroidism, where there is an excess of T4. On the contrary, TSH increases in hypothyroidism.

Complaints do not always accompany hypothyroidism. Often, it can be asymptomatic for an extended period. A high TSH level in the absence of symptoms or clinical manifestations, with normal levels of T4 and T3, is referred to as *subclinical hypothyroidism*. There is much debate among doctors regarding this condition, particularly concerning the need for hormone replacement therapy. However, detecting this condition early is crucial, especially for those planning pregnancy and for pregnant women, as pregnancy hormones suppress thyroid function. To this day, we do not know what role subclinical hypothyroidism plays in non-pregnant women and men. An elevated TSH level may require further examination of the thyroid gland and other organs.

It's crucial to note that certain medications can suppress thyroid function. Therefore, it's vital to thoroughly assess a patient's medical history before considering hormone therapy.

Hypothyroidism can present with various symptoms. The most common include:

- Weakness, lack of energy, drowsiness
- Decreased appetite
- Weight gain (often due to fluid retention)
- Dry skin
- Hair loss
- Insomnia
- Cold intolerance, chills
- Muscle pain
- Emotional instability, depression
- Memory impairment
- Vision disturbances
- Numbness in the legs and arms
- Menstrual irregularities
- Apparent infertility
- Sore throat and difficulty swallowing (if the thyroid gland is enlarged)

More than fifty other complaints and symptoms can be added to this list. Their manifestation depends on the severity of thyroid dysfunction, although TSH, T4, and T3 levels may not always correspond to the severity of the disease. It's important to understand that the body's reaction to hypothyroidism is always individual, making each person's experience unique.

It is believed that determining TSH levels is sufficient for diagnosis. If TSH levels are elevated, the next step is to determine the level of free T4 and the free thyroxine index. Low levels of free T4 characterize hypothyroidism.

Determining T3 is not recommended in most cases. Why? Primary hypothyroidism (developing for the first time in a person's life) presents with an elevated TSH level. In response, the body tries to produce more T4, meaning a larger amount of T4 is converted into T3. Therefore, at the beginning of the disease, TSH is elevated, T4 may be within the normal range or low, and T3 remains normal. However, the TSH level is always the primary indicator when prescribing treatment and monitoring its effectiveness.

A thyroid ultrasound is recommended in cases of throat pain and discomfort, thyroid enlargement, a family history of thyroid disease, and other situations. Additional examinations, including those using radioactive iodine, are conducted strictly as indicated. If nodules are present, a biopsy is required to rule out thyroid cancer.

Treatment of hypothyroidism is carried out using synthetic thyroid hormone medications (levothyroxine, Euthyrox, and others), known as hormone replacement therapy. A complete hormone dose can be prescribed immediately to people without other underlying diseases. In older individuals, a gradual increase in thyroxine dosage is recommended, starting with a quarter or half dose and increasing over 4–6 weeks after rechecking TSH levels. Clinical improvement is usually observed within 3–5 days after the start of treatment, providing hope and optimism for those undergoing therapy.

Hyperthyroidism

Hyperthyroidism encompasses several thyroid disorders of various origins, all characterized by excessive hormone production. The thyroid gland, a small, butterfly-shaped organ located at the base of the neck, plays a crucial role in metabolic processes, including regulating body temperature, heart rate, and energy levels. An overproduction of thyroid hormones often leads to a condition known as *hypermetabolic syndrome* or *thyrotoxicosis* (thyrotoxic syndrome). The most common forms of thyrotoxicosis include diffuse toxic goiter (Graves' disease), toxic nodular goiter (Plummer's disease), and toxic adenoma.

The connection between thyroid gland enlargement and hyperthyroidism was first described in 1786 by the English provincial physician Caleb Parry. His name also appears in medical classifications as part of Parry-Romberg syndrome, although his publication on this topic came much later, in 1825. Almost simultaneously, in 1835, Irish physician Robert Graves and 1840 German physician Karl Adolph von Basedow described the condition now known as *Graves' disease* or *Basedow's disease*, also called *Parry's disease*.

Dr. Graves observed enlarged thyroid glands in three women, one of whom, a 20-year-old girl, exhibited hysterical behavior, pronounced tachycardia, pale skin, and large, protruding eyes that she could not fully close even during sleep.

Thyrotoxicosis manifests differently depending on a person's age and the presence of other systemic diseases. In younger individuals, hyperthyroidism often presents with psycho-emotional symptoms such as anxiety, excessive sensitivity, hyperactivity, irritability, anger, and hysteria. Hand tremors are also typical. In older individuals, hyperthyroidism primarily affects the cardiovascular system, causing high blood pressure, tachycardia, shortness of breath, and heart pain. Electrocardiograms in such patients may show various abnormalities, including different types of fibrillation. It's important to note that these symptoms may not always be present, and the absence of these symptoms does not rule out hyperthyroidism.

Regardless of the underlying cause, hyperthyroidism is most associated with the following symptoms:

- Nervousness, anxiety, irritability
- Excessive sweating
- Heat intolerance
- Increased motor activity
- Hand tremors
- Muscle weakness
- Heart palpitations
- Warm, moist skin
- Eye changes, such as prominent, protruding eyes giving a fixed stare; eyelids may not fully close
- High blood pressure
- Rapid heartbeat (tachycardia)
- Increased appetite
- Weight loss ("food burns off quickly")

- Menstrual irregularities

Unlike hypothyroidism, hyperthyroidism does not significantly affect ovulation and the menstrual cycle. If menstrual cycles become less frequent and periods become lighter, this is usually due to weight loss, hyperactivity, or a negative psycho-emotional state. Menstrual disturbances manifest as lighter and sometimes prolonged spotting over several days. Compared to hypothyroidism, hyperthyroidism has less impact on conception and pregnancy maintenance.

Doctors measure TSH, free thyroxine, the free thyroxine index, and triiodothyronine levels to diagnose hyperthyroidism. In hyperthyroidism, TSH is below normal, T4 is typically elevated, and T3 may be normal or increased. A condition known as subclinical hyperthyroidism is also recognized, in which TSH is below normal while T4 and T3 remain within normal ranges. However, this diagnosis has little clinical significance and is debated among physicians. Some argue that it may be a precursor to overt hyperthyroidism, while others believe it may not necessarily lead to the development of hyperthyroidism.

Testing for thyroid antibodies is generally not recommended in hyperthyroid cases. Thyroid peroxidase antibodies (TPO) are found in only 8% of people with Graves' disease. However, other types of antibodies may be detected, such as thyrotropin or thyroid-stimulating immunoglobulin (TSI), TSH receptor antibodies (TRab), and long-acting thyroid stimulator (LATS), often collectively referred to as thyroid-stimulating antibodies (TSab). These antibodies are present in nearly 80% of people with Graves' disease and help differentiate different types of thyrotoxicosis.

189

Treatment depends on the patient's condition and the severity of symptoms. It can be conducted in either inpatient or outpatient settings, using various medications. Some forms of therapy are contraindicated during pregnancy and in women planning to conceive. Surgical removal of the thyroid gland is considered a radical treatment option and can be performed at any age, including during pregnancy, when indicated.

Thyroiditis

Thyroiditis is rarely considered a distinct thyroid disease by doctors, primarily because the inflammation of this organ has not been mentioned in medical textbooks for a long time. An enlarged and painful thyroid gland can indicate goiter or other conditions.

Thyroiditis can develop as an independent disease or occur against the background of pre-existing thyroid dysfunction. Most often, thyroiditis is observed in cases of hypothyroidism.

There are three main types of thyroiditis.

• **Bacterial thyroiditis** is more common in cases of thyroid gland malformation, where bacteria from the upper respiratory tract can infiltrate the gland. Typically, bacterial thyroiditis is caused by *Staphylococcus aureus*, various strains of streptococci, and pneumococci. However, the inflammatory process may involve human mucous membranes and skin bacteria.

• **Viral thyroiditis** is a complication of a systemic viral infection, most commonly in children suffering from influenza, measles, infectious mononucleosis, *Coxsackie* virus infection, acute respiratory viral infections (ARVI), and other illnesses. Even a common cold can lead to thyroiditis. Viral thyroid involvement is more frequently observed in individuals carrying the human leukocyte antigen HLA-Bw35, although the exact role of this antigen remains unclear. This form of thyroiditis typically arises during childhood.

• **Chronic autoimmune thyroiditis** is one of the most common types of thyroiditis and is characterized by the production of antibodies against the body's thyroid tissue. It is termed *chronic* because it represents an ongoing inflammatory process without infection, with alternating periods of exacerbation and remission. The level of antibodies does not necessarily reflect the severity of the inflammatory process or thyroid dysfunction.

Thyroiditis can either impair thyroid function or leave it unaffected. However, thyroiditis with reduced gland function is the most observed form. The gland may enlarge two to three times its standard size or even more. This condition is often referred to as *goiter*.

The causes of autoimmune thyroiditis are numerous, but the disease is so complex and resistant to pharmaceutical intervention that there are still no definitive explanations for why it develops.

Depending on symptom severity, thyroiditis can be classified as acute, subacute, or chronic. Acute thyroiditis requires anti-inflammatory treatment. Subacute or subclinical thyroiditis may be asymptomatic; in most cases, the thyroid gland returns to normal within 2–7 months without treatment. Chronic autoimmune thyroiditis in adults typically presents with recurrent exacerbations and remissions, with frequency influenced by various factors, including stress, hormonal contraceptive use, and steroid medications. The normalization of thyroid function in such cases can take several years.

Graves' disease and Hashimoto's disease, the most common chronic autoimmune thyroid disorders, are challenging to treat and require continuous monitoring of thyroid function. This emphasizes the importance of vigilance and care in managing these conditions.

Graves' disease, mentioned earlier, predominantly affects women, occurring eight times more frequently than in men, and is associated with hyperthyroidism. Hashimoto's disease, on the other hand, is characterized by decreased thyroid function, although periods of hyperthyroidism may also occur. Initially, this type of thyroiditis was called lymphocytic thyroiditis, autoimmune thyroiditis, or lymphatic adenoid goiter. Women are affected 15–20 times more often than men. It is believed that genetic factors contribute to its development. The human leukocyte antigen (HLA) also plays a significant role in thyroiditis onset. Antibodies can be detected several years before any clinical signs of thyroid dysfunction appear.

Since autoimmune thyroiditis most frequently affects women, there is a clear connection between sex hormones and the disease's development. Before puberty, autoimmune thyroiditis is extremely rare in children, and its incidence is similar in boys and girls. However, with the onset of puberty and menarche, the incidence among girls and women increases significantly. This increase is believed to be due to the influence of sex hormones, particularly estrogen and progesterone, on the immune system and the thyroid gland.

Additional doses of progesterone can trigger hyperthyroidism in non-pregnant women, whereas progesterone deficiency combined with high estrogen levels (even if only in relative excess) contributes to goiter and hypothyroidism. Therefore, thyroid function should be evaluated before prescribing progesterone, and any existing abnormalities should be addressed.

Hormonal contraceptives protect the thyroid gland, with estrogen playing a beneficial role in maintaining thyroid health. Estrogen can enhance the sensitivity of thyroid cells to thyroid-stimulating hormone (TSH), thereby promoting the production of thyroid hormones. In contrast, progesterone increases the levels of anti-thyroid antibodies and the risk of developing thyroiditis. It can also influence the levels of thyroid hormones, potentially leading to hyperthyroidism or hypothyroidism.

The reason progesterone increases the risk of some autoimmune conditions while reducing the risk of others remains unknown. However, it is likely related to various substances interacting differently with progesterone, notably different classes and subclasses of antibodies.

2.7.3. Thyroid Disorders and Pregnancy

For a long time, the role of the thyroid gland in pregnancy remained unexplored. However, as I have repeatedly emphasized, this endocrine organ is crucial for normal egg maturation, conception, and pregnancy maintenance. I have also discussed the importance of the thyroid gland in pregnancy in my book "*9 Months of Happiness*".

Hyperthyroidism is uncommon during pregnancy, occurring in only up to 0.4% of cases, whereas hypothyroidism is detected much more frequently (2–3%). Progesterone, which significantly increases during pregnancy, suppresses thyroid function.

Pregnancy affects autoimmune thyroiditis: the more frequently a woman becomes pregnant and gives birth, the higher her risk of developing this condition. In turn, thyroiditis negatively impacts pregnancy. Thyroid antibodies can cross the placenta and affect the embryo, particularly its thyroid tissue and brain. It is well established that women with autoimmune thyroiditis, especially those with reduced thyroid function, have a higher rate of spontaneous pregnancy loss and miscarriage compared to healthy women. In a small number of cases, Graves' disease may subside during pregnancy, but it often flares up again after childbirth.

Postpartum thyroiditis is much more common than thyroid disorders occurring before or during pregnancy, affecting 4–10% of women. This condition is recognized as a distinct diagnosis typically identified within the first year after childbirth. Postpartum thyroiditis is often asymptomatic but can progress to chronic thyroiditis.

Hyperthyroidism is particularly dangerous in the second half of pregnancy. It increases the risk of preeclampsia, preterm birth, pregnancy loss, and placental abruption. Newborns of mothers with hyperthyroidism may develop congenital heart failure. However, the most critical risk for the mother is thyroid storm (thyrotoxic crisis), a life-threatening condition requiring urgent treatment due to the high risk of mortality.

Hypothyroidism is more common and is also associated with numerous complications. In the first half of pregnancy, hypothyroidism can lead to miscarriage. In the second half, hypothyroidism, especially autoimmune forms, may contribute to preeclampsia, placental abruption, pregnancy loss, and preterm birth. Additionally, it can cause maternal heart dysfunction, anemia, and hemorrhages during and after childbirth. Pregnancies complicated by hypothyroidism are associated with a higher incidence of fetal and neonatal abnormalities, including low birth weight, congenital anomalies, poor neurological development, and congenital thyroid disorders.

Maternal thyroid hormones are believed to play a crucial role in fetal brain development, as the fetus does not begin producing its thyroid hormones until 10–12 weeks of gestation. Antibodies that cross the placenta and enter fetal circulation can negatively affect fetal development.

At the same time, treatment for thyroid disorders during pregnancy may also pose risks to the developing fetus, potentially leading to iatrogenic fetal hypothyroidism. This underscores the need to carefully monitor medication dosages and TSH levels, ensuring that expectant mothers and healthcare professionals are aware and prepared for the potential challenges.

Pregnancy is a state of physiologically increased antibody production, affecting almost all classes of antibodies. Up to 15% of pregnant women have thyroid autoantibodies, and in some cases, these levels can rise significantly. A 300% increase or more in antibody levels has been linked to the development of goiter and thyroid dysfunction in the fetus, necessitating ultrasound monitoring of fetal thyroid size and cardiac function due to the high risk of fetal heart dysfunction. Even if the mother has never undergone a thyroid evaluation, persistent fetal tachycardia (heart rate exceeding 160 beats per minute) is a reason to assess maternal thyroid function.

An experienced endocrinologist who understands how the function and condition of the thyroid gland change during pregnancy should manage the treatment of thyroid disorders during pregnancy.

2.7.4. Thyroid Nodules and Thyroid Cancer

The thyroid gland can develop cysts and tumors, some of which may be malignant. Since it is impossible to determine the exact nature of a cystic or tumor-like formation without analyzing the tissue structure, such findings are often called "nodules." While this term is not entirely accurate from a medical standpoint, it has become widely accepted by doctors and patients.

Recently, there have been reports of an increasing number of thyroid tumors, but this does not necessarily reflect an actual rise in cases. Thyroid ultrasound was rarely performed in the past, whereas today, it is a standard part of preventive health screenings in many countries. As a result, more thyroid nodules are being detected.

Although thyroid enlargement occurs in 15% of people, nodules are found in only 3–7% of cases. Most nodules are benign and can arise for various reasons, including iodine deficiency or inflammation. Cysts may be *true cysts* containing fluid without additional tissue growth (*thyroid cysts*) or develop from old adenomas. Most commonly, tumor-like tissue overgrowth is accompanied by fluid accumulation, in which case the formation is referred to as a *thyroid adenoma*. The suffix "-oma" denotes a tumor, although these formations may contain malignant cells in rare cases.

Another condition known as nodular goiter occurs when cystic structures are found within the thyroid tissue. Naturally, the most significant concern with any thyroid formation is whether it could be cancerous.

Doctors first raised alarms about the increasing incidence of thyroid dysfunction and cancer after the Chornobyl nuclear disaster in 1986. This catastrophic event revealed the strong link between radioactive iodine exposure and thyroid cancer. The most alarming consequence was the rise in cancer cases among children and adolescents. It is estimated that up to 10,000 cases of thyroid cancer may have developed in children exposed to radioactive iodine during the disaster, though the actual number could be higher. Many of the affected zone's population relocated to various cities and villages across the former USSR. However, only workers involved in disaster cleanup efforts were systematically monitored for health conditions, while most of the affected population received little to no medical follow-up. Additionally, the long latency period between radiation exposure and cancer development was often overlooked.

For years, the long-term effects of the Chornobyl disaster were disputed. However, when the Fukushima nuclear accident occurred in Japan in 2011 following a massive earthquake and tsunami, a similar surge in thyroid cancer among children was observed, further reinforcing the connection between radiation exposure and thyroid malignancies.

Thyroid cancer is classified as a rare malignancy and is more frequently observed in families with a genetic predisposition or cases where other endocrine gland cancers are present. This type of cancer occurs more commonly in men, even though benign thyroid tumors and cysts are more frequently diagnosed in women. One of the most significant risk factors is radiation exposure, particularly radiation affecting the head and neck region.

There are several types of thyroid cancer, with the most common being papillary (80%), followed by follicular, anaplastic, and medullary carcinomas. Rarely, thyroid lymphomas and sarcomas may also occur.

Early detection of thyroid cancer significantly improves treatment outcomes, making early diagnosis critical. Understanding the steps to detect it in time empowers you to take control of your health.

Your physician can help assess your risk level (high or low) for thyroid cancer, providing you with the guidance and reassurance you need. High-risk individuals should be prioritized for regular thyroid ultrasound (US) screenings. The frequency of these screenings, tailored to your level of risk and the presence of nodules in the thyroid gland, ensures you are being cared for and monitored. Although thyroid cancer is more common in men, increased attention should be given to children and adults under 30 or over 60 years old.

Rapid nodule growth and/or the onset of symptoms such as difficulty swallowing, hoarseness, or a persistent cough require urgent evaluation. Pain is more commonly associated with inflammation or bleeding into the nodule than malignancy. However, any new or concerning symptoms should be promptly discussed with a healthcare professional. If necessary, a doctor may recommend a fine-needle biopsy of the nodule to assess for malignancy.

Any changes in the neck area, discomfort, or new symptoms warrant a medical consultation—this is the key to early diagnosis and effective treatment of thyroid conditions.

2.7.5. Does a Thyroid Diet Exist?

A balanced diet is essential for many organs, including the thyroid gland. Iodine and selenium are crucial for thyroxine synthesis, the hormone produced by the thyroid gland. Iodine deficiency is known to be associated with hypothyroidism, as the thyroid gland needs iodine to make thyroxine. Similarly, selenium is essential for converting thyroxine into its active form, triiodothyronine, and reducing the risk of autoimmune thyroid diseases.

Since thyroid dysfunction is common, particularly in women, numerous diets claiming to improve thyroid function have emerged and continue to gain popularity. However, it is essential to acknowledge that different thyroid disorders require different approaches, meaning there is no universal "thyroid diet" that fits all conditions.

Hypothyroidism and hyperthyroidism are opposite conditions, and both may involve autoimmune reactions with antibody production. Thyroid tumors, on the other hand, have no proven link to diet.

Until recently, iodine supplementation was widely recommended for pregnant and breastfeeding women, with doses significantly higher than current guidelines. However, true iodine deficiency is rare in developed countries. It is estimated that around 1 billion people worldwide may be at risk of iodine deficiency, but this primarily applies to populations in low-income countries.

Today, iodine is present in many fortified foods, including iodized salt, seafood (such as seaweed and fish), certain flour-based products, and grains. However, food manufacturers rarely list the iodine content on labels, as there are no regulatory requirements for iodine dosage in fortified products.

Another challenge is the lack of clear recommendations for iodine intake, as previous standards have been significantly revised in recent years. Currently, it is estimated that:

- Adults need 150 mcg of iodine per day.

- Pregnant women require 220 mcg daily.

- Lactating women should receive up to 290 mcg per day.

The recommended doses of iodine supplementation were much higher in the past. Additionally, the iodine content in foods has increased, so most people do not suffer from iodine deficiency today.

In health food stores and pharmacies (including online retailers), dietary supplements marketed as "thyroid support" contain iodine and other ingredients. Many of these supplements provide iodine doses that exceed the recommended daily intake by several times, or even several hundred times, posing a serious health risk. **Excess iodine can worsen thyroid dysfunction, particularly in those with autoimmune thyroiditis, often leading to flare-ups.**

There is also speculation about iodine deficiency in drinking water in certain regions, but this is misleading. Humans obtain iodine from multiple sources, not just water. In the past, endemic goiter was frequently linked to iodine deficiency ("endemic" refers to a condition characteristic of a specific geographical area or population). Historically, some villages had higher rates of hypothyroidism than other regions. However, several factors were overlooked, including low migration rates in the past, leading to isolated communities with a higher prevalence of genetic predisposition due to intermarriage. While local geological factors can influence water quality and mineral concentrations, iodine deficiency today is far less common, as modern diets are diverse and abundant.

Interestingly, people who take extra iodine supplements due to concerns about iodine deficiency often develop thyroid dysfunction due to iodine overdose, particularly if they already have underlying thyroid conditions. While some individuals may need iodine supplementation, their daily intake should not exceed 500 mcg.

Many supplements also contain spirulina, which is often promoted as a "superfood" for the thyroid. However, its effectiveness has not been scientifically proven.

Over the past 10–20 years, the global market has been flooded with tens, if not hundreds, of thousands of dietary supplements. Among them are so-called goitrogens — substances believed to suppress thyroid function. Some recommend goitrogens for hyperthyroidism, while endocrinologists and dietitians warn that they should be avoided in hypothyroidism, especially in large amounts.

Many cruciferous vegetables and soy products are labeled "goitrogenic" because they may inhibit iodine metabolism and suppress thyroid hormone production. However, these foods also contain beneficial nutrients, including potential anti-cancer compounds.

The most mentioned goitrogenic foods include:

- Cabbage (white, red, and savoy)
- Broccoli
- Brussels sprouts
- Radish
- Cauliflower
- Kale (curly leaf cabbage)
- Bok choy
- Other leafy green vegetables

This does not mean people with thyroid dysfunction should eliminate these vegetables. Cabbage and radish are highly beneficial. It is generally recommended that they be consumed in moderation, particularly for individuals with hypothyroidism.

There is no established maximum daily intake of cruciferous vegetables that would cause thyroid harm. Most studies on goitrogens have been conducted on healthy individuals using excessively high quantities of these vegetables. Furthermore, the combined effect of different vegetables in a varied diet has not been well studied. The negative impact of goitrogens is most observed in people with metabolic disorders or in older adults. Consuming 1–2 kg of raw cruciferous vegetables daily is not justified for improving health.

Overall, no clinical evidence confirms cruciferous vegetables' actual harm or benefit for thyroid function.

Another trendy food that has gained popularity in Western markets is soy milk, tofu, soy sauce, and miso. Despite limited scientific research and a lack of evidence-based medicine supporting their claims, soy contains isoflavones, which are often overhyped as miraculous compounds.

Some researchers suggested that soy isoflavones may inhibit thyroid peroxidase, an enzyme essential for thyroid hormone production. Theoretically, excessive soy intake was thought to contribute to hypothyroidism, making it potentially harmful for people with thyroid dysfunction. However, studies show that soy consumption in healthy individuals living in iodine-sufficient areas does not negatively impact the thyroid. The effect of soy on people with existing thyroid disorders has not been studied, meaning that soy and soy-based foods can be consumed but should not be overused.

As I have previously mentioned, selenium is essential for thyroid hormone production. The recommended daily intake is 55 mcg for all adults, including pregnant and breastfeeding women, and this amount is usually obtained through food. Selenium is abundant in seafood, organ meats, grains, bread, fish, and eggs. Endocrinologists sometimes recommend selenium supplementation (100–400 mcg per day), particularly for autoimmune thyroiditis. Selenium supplementation is often long-term — at least 6 months.

Certain "thyroid support" supplements also contain magnesium, copper, and zinc, but their roles in thyroid function remain unproven. All recommendations regarding these minerals are theoretical and lack solid clinical evidence.

There is widespread misinformation about coffee and its supposed adverse effects on the thyroid. In reality, coffee does not impact thyroid function, nor does tea or alcohol. However, coffee may reduce thyroxine absorption in people undergoing hormone replacement therapy for hypothyroidism.

The gluten-free diet is another fad that has become fashionable in the last decade. Many supermarkets now sell gluten-free products at significantly higher prices. I mention this because many people, including patients, follow trendy diets, believing they will improve their health. Studies show that over 63% of dieters think their diet will make them healthier, while the opposite is often true. The worst part is that these diets are frequently promoted by non-medical individuals and even some doctors with little knowledge of nutrition and metabolism.

A gluten-free diet is a medical necessity for individuals with celiac disease, a severe condition affecting about 1% of the population. However, for

people without gluten sensitivity, eliminating gluten provides no health benefits.

Evidence-based medicine has shown that a gluten-free diet:

- Does not reduce cardiovascular disease risk (it may slightly increase it).

- Leads to deficiencies in folic acid, vitamins B12 and D, calcium, iron, zinc, magnesium, and fiber.

- Increases the risk of diabetes and does not lower metabolic syndrome risks.

- Raises levels of toxic heavy metals (arsenic, mercury, copper, cadmium) in the blood and tissues.

No scientific evidence supports the effectiveness of any "thyroid diet."

2.8. The Parathyroid Glands

Many people are unaware that their body contains four tiny but crucial glands known as the parathyroid glands. As the name suggests, they are located next to the thyroid gland. Their size is so small (3–4 mm in diameter) that they are difficult to detect even using ultrasound.

Even the most renowned anatomists of the past struggled to identify these glands. The first description of the parathyroid glands was provided by Sir Richard Owen, a British physician, anatomist, and curator of the Natural History Museum, but not in a human — he discovered them in a rhinoceros that had died at the London Zoo in 1850. Between 1877 and 1880, Ivar Sandström, a 25-year-old medical student and future physician, was the first to identify the parathyroid glands in humans during his anatomical studies. He was astonished by the variability in their location relative to the thyroid, a factor that remains a challenge for surgeons today. This was the last anatomical discovery in medicine.

Even modern medical publications should focus more on the essential function of the parathyroid glands rather than just their anatomical localization. This understanding is crucial, especially during thyroid gland removal surgery.

The role of the parathyroid glands remained unknown until the early 20th century when French physiologist Eugène Gley linked muscle convulsions to thyroid removal surgery. For a long time, thyroidectomy (thyroid removal) was performed along with the parathyroid glands, sometimes resulting in unexplained patient deaths. In 1907, after a patient died from severe bone softening, doctors discovered significantly enlarged parathyroid glands, leading to the hypothesis that these glands influence bone health.

The parathyroid glands play a crucial role in calcium metabolism, essential for maintaining healthy bones. They produce **parathyroid hormone** (PTH), or parathormone, which has several key functions.

- It increases calcium levels in the blood by promoting calcium release from bones.

- It enhances calcium absorption from food in the intestines.

- It helps retain calcium in the bloodstream by acting on the kidneys to reduce calcium excretion.

Thus, the two primary targets of PTH are bones and kidneys.

Another unique function of PTH is converting vitamin D into its active form, which is essential for bone health and many other organ functions.

Calcium, vitamin D, and bones — these words are most associated with osteoporosis, a condition that primarily affects postmenopausal women. However, the exact involvement of the parathyroid glands in osteoporosis remains unclear.

The most common disorder related to parathyroid function is *hyperparathyroidism,* in which the glands overproduce PTH. This leads to excess calcium in the blood (hypercalcemia) and bone tissue destruction (osteodystrophy).

Approximately 1 in 100 people (or 1 in 50 women over the age of 50) develop a parathyroid tumor, which can result in hyperparathyroidism — a condition characterized by excessive PTH production. In older women, this can worsen osteoporosis, significantly increasing the risk of heart attacks, strokes, and other complications. In most cases, surgical removal of the tumor is necessary.

Parathyroid cancer is sporadic, but it is difficult to diagnose in its early stages.

Hypoparathyroidism (a condition where too little PTH is produced) is also rare and typically occurs after thyroid surgery, mainly if performed by an inexperienced surgeon. Overall, very little is known about the impact of parathyroid hormone on women's health, including its effects on pregnancy and fetal development.

Chapter 3. The Menstrual Cycle and Hormones

The menstrual cycle is a pivotal aspect of a woman's life and the foundation of her reproductive health. This biological process, which begins at puberty, marks the transformation of a girl into a young woman and later into an adult woman.

Although the name suggests that menstruation (periods) follows a cyclic pattern, **menstruation itself does not determine the regularity of the cycle**. I have developed a **philosophical law of women's health**, which I frequently share in seminars, lectures, and public discussions. This law, which I call 'Ovulation is primary; menstruation is secondary,' is a fundamental principle that guides our understanding of the menstrual cycle. I already mentioned it at the beginning of this book, but I will repeat it here once again:

Ovulation is primary; menstruation is secondary.

What does this principle mean? The entire process of sexual maturation in both women and men is aimed at the development of reproductive cells. In women, these are oocytes (egg cells), and their maturation process is called *folliculogenesis*. The release of a mature egg from the follicle is *ovulation*. In men, reproductive cells are spermatozoa, which mature through *spermatogenesis* and are released through *ejaculation*.

Although a woman's egg reserve is formed during the embryonic period, which is the early stage of development before birth, these eggs undergo certain stages of division before reaching full maturity. The final phase of their development begins with the establishment of menstrual cycles. Since oocyte maturation is closely linked to hormone production, a woman's hormonal profile depends on her age and physiological state, such as pregnancy or lactation, which we will discuss further.

3.1. How a Woman's Hormonal Profile Changes Across Different Life Stages

A woman's hormonal background is a marvel of nature, but it remains one of its great mysteries. Women are unique in the animal world, but they experience hormonal and reproductive processes that function like any other species.

As discussed in previous chapters, multiple endocrine organs regulate the female body, producing around 50 hormones that influence the menstrual cycle — from oocyte maturation to menstrual bleeding.

Hormone levels fluctuate throughout the day (as mentioned earlier, many hormones are secreted in a pulsatile manner) and throughout the menstrual cycle. These fluctuations influence tissues, organs, and overall health.

During my medical training, surgeons recommended performing surgeries in the first half of the menstrual cycle. This practice was not fully understood regarding endocrinological mechanisms at the time. However, based on better tissue healing and less severe inflammatory reactions after menstruation, their rationale underscores the practical importance of understanding the menstrual cycle for surgical timing.

And they were right! Due to growing follicles, the rising estrogen levels in the first phase of the cycle promote better wound healing after surgical incisions, reduce tissue swelling, and help form higher-quality scars. Additionally, performing surgery in the first phase of the cycle eliminates any risk of interfering with an undiagnosed pregnancy since a woman cannot be pregnant at this stage.

Hormone levels also change with age, a topic we will explore in more detail next.

3.1.1. Strange Phenomena in Newborns

When a child is born, parents, doctors, and nurses focus primarily on growth, development, feeding, and activity. Hormone levels are rarely tested, as there is usually no need for such evaluations. However, newborns may exhibit unusual signs seldom described in parenting books in the first few weeks of life. These are typically attributed to maternal hormones entering the baby's bloodstream before birth and exerting effects after delivery.

In my book *Growing Up Strong: A Guide to Girls' Health and Well-Being*, which explores the formation of the female body from birth to puberty, I discuss many of these hormonal changes, including those occurring in infants. However, since many of you may not have read that book, I will briefly mention these changes here to help illustrate the uniqueness of the human body, particularly the female body.

Starting as early as 7–8 weeks of pregnancy, the placenta becomes the primary hormone-producing organ for the developing fetus. A little later, the fetus produces some hormones, demonstrating hormonal independence from the mother's endocrine system. By this stage, the mother's ovaries become functionally inactive, and placental hormones greatly influence the woman's body more than her ovarian hormones.

The placenta is the leading producer of progesterone, which is converted into estrogens, testosterone, and other steroid hormones. As pregnancy progresses and progesterone production increases, estrogen, and androgen levels also rise dramatically—so much so that they far exceed the levels found in non-pregnant women. It is not entirely known how much of these placental hormones are used by the fetus, but it is estimated that at least one-quarter to one-third is absorbed, though the actual amount may be higher. Interestingly, the concentration of these hormones in the fetal environment (amniotic fluid and fetal tissues) is significantly higher than in the mother's bloodstream. Essentially, the fetus exists in a hormone-rich "solution."

Thus, we can conclude that by the end of pregnancy, the fetus receives mainly nutrients from the mother, while the placenta and the fetus produce its hormones. We are not discussing cases where maternal hormonal imbalances occur before conception or early pregnancy when maternal hormones can influence embryonic development. However, for most steroid hormones, including estrogens, testosterone, and progesterone, the fetus relies on its placental source rather than the mother's endocrine system.

Immediately after birth, steroid hormone levels in the newborn are incredibly high — higher than those found in any healthy adult. Most laboratories do not have standardized newborn hormone reference values, especially during the first two months of life. In one sense, a newborn is hormonally inactive, meaning many endocrine glands remain immature and require months or even years to function fully. However, at birth, the baby's blood is still saturated with placental hormones, rapidly breaking down and being eliminated from the body after delivery.

The most intense breakdown of steroid hormones occurs within the first 24 hours of life. After that, the rate of hormone elimination slows down gradually. For example, before delivery, the mother's plasma progesterone levels range from 45 to 400 ng/mL (average: 130 ng/mL). In the umbilical cord blood of a newborn, progesterone levels are much higher, ranging from 440 to 2000 ng/mL (average: 1030 ng/mL). Twelve hours after birth, progesterone drops to 20 ng/mL. By the end of the first day of life, it declines further to 16 ng/mL. By day three, it reaches 8 ng/mL.

Similarly, estriol levels drop sharply in the newborn's blood after birth. Another hormone, cortisol, which is derived from placental progesterone (in adults, cortisol is produced by the adrenal glands), also decreases significantly. Since steroid hormone levels in newborns are initially very high, the levels of their metabolic byproducts are also elevated. One of these is 17-hydroxyprogesterone (17-OHP). Immediately after birth, 17-OHP levels in umbilical cord blood range from 10,000 to 30,000 ng/L. Within 24 hours, 17-OHP decreases to 1,000 ng/L. For the rest of life, it rarely exceeds 2,000 ng/L. Thus, newborns experience a rapid decline in placental steroid hormones in the first hours and days after birth.

This sharp hormonal drop explains several common newborn symptoms, including swelling of the labia and hymen, vaginal discharge, breast engorgement, and even nipple discharge (neonatal milk).

In newborn girls, this hormonal withdrawal causes temporary genital swelling and redness. In some cases, girls develop clear vaginal discharge (physiological leukorrhea) or even light blood-stained discharge resembling a menstrual period. These pseudo-menstrual secretions usually last no more than 2–3 days and are entirely normal. It is not just the labia that become swollen — the hymen also thickens and turns pale pink, sometimes forming folds that protrude from the vaginal opening. In most cases, swelling of the vulva and hymen resolves within 2–4 weeks, though in some infants, it persists for longer.

Apart from genital changes, both boys and girls may experience breast enlargement, which is also linked to hormonal fluctuations, particularly the drop in prolactin levels. After birth, maternal progesterone and prolactin levels drop, triggering lactation in the mother when the baby begins suckling. Interestingly, similar hormonal shifts occur in newborns. In the first five days of life, serum prolactin levels in newborns range from 100 to 500 µg/L. By two months, prolactin drops to 5–70 µg/L. Between 12 months and puberty (11–13 years), prolactin levels stabilize at 2.5–25 µg/L.

During the first days after birth, a rapid drop in prolactin — along with falling progesterone levels — triggers a breast reaction like that seen in postpartum women. The newborn's breasts swell, and in some cases, they may produce a milky secretion. Unlike in the maternal body, where suckling maintains lactation, the newborn has no ongoing breast stimulation, and their

213

mammary glands remain undeveloped. Therefore, these hormonal effects disappear within a few days.

All these hormonal symptoms in newborns usually resolve quickly. Even if they persist for several weeks, if the baby is healthy, growing normally, and showing no other symptoms, there is no need for concern. This rapid resolution of symptoms should instill a sense of relief and confidence in parents and healthcare professionals, knowing that these changes are part of a normal process and do not indicate any underlying health issues.

3.1.2. The Hidden Stage of Puberty

It is often assumed that puberty begins in adolescence when girls start menstruating and boys experience their first nocturnal emissions (pollution). However, the actual onset of puberty, marked by hormonal changes, occurs long before the visible signs of maturation appear (such as secondary sexual characteristics) and well before the first menstrual period — menarche. This hidden stage of puberty, often overlooked, is a crucial aspect of child development that we aim to shed light on in this article.

Many medical sources indicate that adolescence is not simply the period from 13 to 16 years old, as it is often described. In reality, puberty begins around the ages of 11–12 and continues until 20–21, marking the completion of sexual maturation.

Beyond the noticeable physical changes in boys and girls, there is an initial, hidden period when puberty truly begins on a hormonal level. Two important processes often go unnoticed in descriptions of child development, yet they serve as the primary triggers of puberty:

- **Gonadarche** – the activation of the pituitary gland and increased gonadotropin production.

- **Adrenarche** – the rise in androgen (male sex hormone) levels in the blood.

The growth hormone also plays a significant role in these changes.

The first surge of gonadotropins (FSH and LH) occurs as early as three months of age in both boys and girls due to the drop in placental hormone levels (progesterone and estrogens) that were transferred from the mother during pregnancy. In girls, these gonadotropin levels remain elevated for the first 1–2 years of life, whereas in boys, they normalize by six months. After this period, gonadotropin levels gradually decrease but fluctuate until around four years old, when a mild increase is observed. Unlike in adults, pulsatile secretion of gonadotropins is not well established in young girls until the menstrual cycle fully matures, which happens closer to 19–22 years old.

Around the ages of 10–11, when puberty begins to manifest outwardly, the hypothalamus initiates the secretion of gonadotropin-releasing hormone (GnRH) during sleep, stimulating an increase in gonadotropins and estrogens. The LH-to-FSH ratio fluctuates constantly, remaining unstable for a long time. This gonadotropin surge does not immediately lead to full egg maturation, which is why, for an extended period, girls may menstruate without ovulating. As a girl ages, the connection between the hypothalamus, pituitary gland, and ovaries strengthens, gradually regulating the hormonal cycle.

There is no direct link between the rise in gonadotropins (gonadarche) and the increase in androgens (adrenarche) — these are autonomous processes in growing children. However, as a child matures, gonadotropin secretion becomes more rhythmic, adopting a pulsatile pattern and synchronizing with sex hormone production, including progesterone.

The transition from chaotic gonadotropin release to a structured pulsatile rhythm marks the onset of the first menstrual period (menarche) in girls and the first spontaneous ejaculation (spermarche) in boys, commonly referred to as nocturnal emissions (pollutions).

An increase in male sex hormones (androgens) in both girls and boys during the prepubertal and pubertal periods is known as *adrenarche*. Many parents, and even some doctors, are unaware of this phenomenon. As a result, when elevated androgen levels are detected in girls, they may mistakenly undergo unnecessary medical treatment.

In children, the first androgens to increase are androstenedione, dehydroepiandrosterone (DHEA), and dehydroepiandrosterone sulfate (DHEA-S), all produced by the adrenal cortex. Laboratory tests can detect rising androgen levels as early as six, though these increases occur between 7 and 8 years old in most children.

Elevated androgen levels can persist throughout puberty, which is why concerns about oily skin, acne, and irregular menstrual cycles in girls should be carefully evaluated. It's important to note that in most cases, these are part of normal physiological development, reassuring parents and caregivers about the natural progression of puberty.

Adrenarche is observed only in humans, chimpanzees, and gorillas but is absent in other species.

Increased androgen levels affect the entire child's body, particularly the brain. This hormonal surge is believed to stimulate the development of the prefrontal cortex, a region of the brain associated with higher cognitive functions and emotional regulation. Androgens also play a crucial role in the maturation of brain tissue. In recent years, scientists and medical researchers have closely studied the relationship between hormonal fluctuations and mental health disorders in adolescents.

Androgens also influence body hair growth, particularly in the axillary (underarm) and pubic areas.

The hormonal phase of puberty — the earliest stage of sexual "awakening" — often remains unnoticed, yet it is the first and most critical step in the maturation process. Genetic and external factors such as nutrition, physical activity, stress levels, socioeconomic conditions, and family relationships influence this stage.

3.1.3. Adolescence

Adolescence is considered one of the most complex and contradictory periods, involving physiological, psycho-emotional, and cognitive changes. The appearance of secondary sexual characteristics accompanies the increase in hormone levels. Around 7–8, breast development (thelarche) and pubic hair growth (pubarche) begin.

Numerous studies in pediatrics and related sciences have shown that the age at which the first visible signs of puberty appear depends on many factors but is primarily determined by genetic, ethnic, and racial characteristics. For example, in Black girls, puberty begins 1–1.5 years earlier than in Caucasian girls.

Some girls may develop pubic hair as early as 4–6 years old, and nipple or breast enlargement can also occasionally be observed at such a young age. If no other signs of puberty or hormone-secreting tumors are present, these findings are not considered symptoms of precocious puberty and do not require treatment.

A child's pubertal development is influenced by nutrition and physical activity. In overweight or underweight girls, the thelarche phase may go unnoticed. Athletic girls may experience delayed breast development, as excessive physical activity can suppress the natural progression of puberty.

It is also essential to know that breast growth is often asymmetrical, which is usually normal. Many women retain unequal breast sizes throughout their lives. Suppose an adolescent notices this difference; explaining that such variations are not harmful and do not require correction is essential. Some women may choose to undergo plastic surgery to correct asymmetry, but such procedures should not be performed during adolescence (before the age of 20–21), as breast development may continue.

Modern girls tend to develop larger breasts at a faster rate, as evidenced by the increasing number of breast reduction surgeries (mammoplasty). The reasons for this trend remain unknown, but some hypothesize that the widespread use of antibiotics and hormones in modern food production contributes to accelerated breast growth.

Adolescence also includes a growth spurt in most girls between 10 and 14. During this period, a girl's height may increase by 6–8 cm per year, less than in boys. This growth surge typically lasts two years. Body weight also increases, with an average gain of about 2 kg annually.

The most significant milestone in female puberty is the onset of menstruation (menarche). In the past, and some cultures even today, menarche was considered a sign of a girl's readiness for marriage and childbirth.

The first period typically occurs two years after the onset of thelarche. Around 10% of girls begin menstruating at age 11, while 90% experience their first period by 13.8 years old. By 15 years old, 98% of girls have started menstruating. In 60% of cases, menstrual cycle patterns are genetically determined.

It is believed that body weight, height-to-weight ratio, and body fat percentage play a crucial role in the onset of menarche. A girl's (and a woman's) body weight is essential for establishing menstruation and regular cycles. This is because of energy metabolism and adipose (fat) tissue, which are actively involved in the metabolism and absorption of sex hormones.

The critical weight for menarche is approximately 48 kg, while the minimum fat percentage needed is 17% of body weight (some sources suggest 21–22%).

During the first three years after menarche, cycles generally last 28–35 days, but over time, they become shorter, more regular, and more frequently accompanied by complete ovulation. Normal cycle length fluctuations in adolescents are as follows:

- First year after menarche: 23–90 days (average: 32 days)

- Fourth year: 24–50 days

- Seventh year: 27–38 days

Most girls do not establish regular menstrual cycles until at least 18 months after their first period. After two years, cycles usually become not only regular but also ovulatory. However, 50% of adolescents experience anovulation (absence of ovulation) for the first three years. The later menarche occurs, the longer it takes for ovulatory cycles to become established.

3.1.4. Reproductive Period

The term "reproduction" was rarely used in popular science literature and was primarily associated with animal breeding. However, with the development of reproductive medicine, which aids people in having children, this term has become widely accepted not only among medical professionals but also among the public.

"Reproduction" refers to the process of producing offspring, which is why reproductive organs or the reproductive system encompass the structures responsible for the production of sex cells, conception, and pregnancy.

In the past, women married early (14–16 years old) and immediately took on their expected duties, with childbearing as the primary focus. Reliable contraception was unavailable, and the idea of birth control was generally disregarded. Among many cultures, menstruation was not considered a regular occurrence because women rarely experienced it. Instead, they were frequently pregnant, gave birth, breastfed, and then repeated the cycle. By the age of 35, many women had given birth to 7–14 children, yet most did not live long enough to experience menopause, which typically occurred around 37–39 years old. A healthy woman was, therefore, defined not by the presence of menstruation but by continuous cycles of pregnancy and breastfeeding.

Modern women, especially those in developed countries, approach reproduction very differently. Many marry around 30, planning their first — and often only — pregnancy between 30 and 35. Many women consider having children, particularly a second child, after age 40. This shift in reproductive priorities has been driven by socio-economic factors: the rising cost and duration of education, increasing living expenses, higher consumer expectations, and evolving perceptions of family and women's societal roles. These changing societal norms have significant implications for reproductive health, influencing the age at which women choose to have children, and the potential risks and complications associated with pregnancy at different ages.

But does nature align with these changing priorities? Unfortunately, practical knowledge about human reproduction is rarely taught in schools. Understanding the mechanics of sexual intercourse is crucial, but it's equally important to educate students on the origins of menstruation, the formation of the menstrual cycle, the factors influencing conception and pregnancy, and the optimal age for childbearing. This knowledge empowers individuals to make informed decisions about their reproductive health.

The reproductive period refers to the age at which a woman can conceive, carry, and give birth to a child. Today, with menstruation beginning earlier (around 11–12 years old) and menopause occurring later (at 52–54 years old), a woman theoretically has 40–43 years available for childbearing. However, this figure is misleading, as menstrual cycles alone do not guarantee fertility.

Human reproductive capability depends on the maturation of fully functional sex cells, including genetically viable ones, the openness of the fallopian tubes, a healthy uterine lining, and the absence of conditions that could lead to serious pregnancy complications.

During adolescence, ovulation occurs irregularly, and the body is still growing and developing. While the genetic material in egg cells remains intact mainly and less affected by environmental and internal factors, pregnancy complications are still more common at this age.

The optimal period for conception is between the ages of 20 and 30. This is when natural fertility rates are highest, miscarriage rates are lowest, genetic material is still in good condition, and most women have good overall health. Awareness of this age range and its benefits can help individuals make informed decisions about their reproductive health. It's a period that carries the lowest risks of complications for both mother and child, making it an ideal time for conception.

After the age of 30, fertility gradually declines, while the risk of miscarriage begins to rise. Until age 35, these changes occur slowly, and many women can still conceive without difficulty. However, between 35 and 38–39, about half of couples will seek medical assistance for conception, though most will still conceive without the need for reproductive technologies. Beyond 38–39, as the final wave of accelerated egg loss begins, conception becomes increasingly challenging. Genetic defects in reproductive cells become more pronounced, leading to a higher risk of pregnancy loss and congenital abnormalities in offspring.

After the age of 40, most women require the assistance of reproductive medicine as pregnancy complications increase significantly.

It's a fact that we all age from the moment we're born. A one-year-old looking at photos from when they were just one or two months old might exclaim, "Oh my, I've aged so much! I was tiny, only 3 kg, and now I weigh nearly 10 kg. I've grown; I've aged." To ten-year-olds, forty-year-olds seem ancient, while adults perceive their aging with fluctuating emotions — one moment lamenting how "old" they are, the next insisting they still feel 25. But who indeed remembers their feelings and sensations from when they were 25?

Women may use makeup or even undergo plastic surgery to enhance their appearance, but **no one can smooth the "wrinkles" of internal organs, including the ovaries. And since the ovaries are among the first organs to age, there is no way to "rejuvenate" them.** Yet, plenty of charlatans promote so-called ovarian rejuvenation through various dubious methods. In reality, ovaries cannot be made younger — though one can certainly waste a lot of money and even risk harming one's health in the attempt.

Because ovaries contain all their follicles from birth, there are rare, almost anecdotal cases of pregnancy occurring at both extremes of reproductive age — girls as young as 7–8 and women in menopause. While the number of follicles decreases dramatically with age, some women still experience sporadic ovulations from the remaining few. This explains the documented cases of spontaneous conception during menopause.

Nature, however, is indifferent to a woman's career, professional achievements, wealth, or possessions. **The human body follows natural laws, and extending life expectancy does not equate to extending reproductive capacity.** It's important to be aware of these natural limitations and plan accordingly.

Some scientists argue that physiological adaptation to new living conditions takes centuries or even millennia — these are evolutionary changes. Although advancements in living conditions, nutrition, and medicine have nearly doubled human lifespans over the past 150–200 years, the natural limitations of reproduction remain unchanged.

While we can't change the natural limitations of reproduction, there is hope for the future. Over the next 50–100 years, the window for natural conception may extend by another year or two, much like the age of menopause has gradually increased. Moreover, medical advancements will allow for earlier detection of genetic abnormalities and pregnancy complications, improving outcomes for future generations.

3.1.5. Menopause

The gradual decline of reproductive function accompanies the aging process in women. The visible aspect of this decline is the cessation of menstruation, while the invisible aspect is the cessation of egg maturation (anovulation).

Menopause is defined as the period beginning one year after the cessation of menstruation (amenorrhea) due to anovulation. If a woman undergoes a hysterectomy for any reason, she will no longer menstruate, but if her ovaries remain intact, her hormonal balance may persist for a considerable time. That is why when we talk about menopause, we often mean hormonal menopause.

Among European women, the term *climacteric* is more commonly used to describe the cessation of menstruation. It's important to understand the difference between climacteric and menopause. Climacteric often refers to the hormonal changes that occur in the first 5–6 years after menstruation stops. Menopause, on the other hand, is a single moment — the cessation (*pause*) of menstruation. The following period is called postmenopause, but since this term is long, people often refer to it simply as menopause. This knowledge of terminology can help you better understand discussions about menopause and reproductive health.

The term *menopause* (*la Ménopause*) first appeared in 1816, when it was introduced by the French gynecologist de Gardanne. In 1839, another French physician, Dr. Meunier, published the first book on menopause. The concept of *climacteric syndrome* (*climax*) emerged in 1899 in an article titled *Epochal Madness*, where symptoms observed in postmenopausal women were described as climacteric insanity. The word "climax" has since acquired multiple meanings in everyday speech.

The period between ages 45 and 54, when hormonal fluctuations become frequent, estrogen levels decline, and fertility drops sharply is called *perimenopause* or *pre-climacteric phase.*

Over the past century, both the age of menopause onset and life expectancy have significantly increased. In the 18th–19th centuries, the average lifespan for women was 35–37 years (for men, 40–45 years), meaning many women never reached menopause. Since ovarian function typically declined after 37–39 years, menopause occurred at a much younger age than today.

Seventy to eighty years ago, early menopause was defined as the cessation of menstruation (and ovulation) after age 40 because, at that time, 90% of women over 40 were already menopausal. This diagnostic criterion for early menopause remains unchanged in medicine today.

The typical age range for menopause is 40–60, but most women stop ovulating and menstruating by 51–52. However, the trend is shifting, and more women now continue menstruating until 52–54.

It is essential to understand that menstrual cycles change significantly after 40. More cycles occur without ovulation (anovulatory cycles); by this age, up to six ovulatory cycles per year are considered normal. The older the woman, the less frequently ovulation occurs. Menstrual cycles also tend to shorten, often lasting less than 26 days, which is linked to insufficient corpus luteum function and reduced progesterone production.

Doctors and patients often ask whether menopause can be predicted. Clinical studies have shown an interesting pattern: **the interval between the end of natural fertility (ability to conceive without reproductive technologies) and menopause is about 10 years.** The

226

challenge lies in determining individual fertility. For example, if a woman at 35 years old is using contraception because she has already had children, it is impossible to assess her natural fertility. Similarly, a woman who is not sexually active falls outside menopause predictions.

There are two types of menopause: natural and artificial. *Natural menopause* occurs when ovarian function gradually declines. *Artificial menopause* is caused by medical intervention — either through drugs that suppress ovulation or surgical removal of the ovaries. Even natural menopause can be masked using hormonal contraceptives or hormone replacement therapy (HRT). **A woman taking HRT or birth control pills may experience regular withdrawal bleeding, mistakenly believing she is still menstruating, even though her ovaries may have already stopped functioning due to age**.

Studies conducted among women who do not use contraception, meaning those who rely on their natural fertility, have shown that the average age of infertility (sterility) is 41 years. It is important to emphasize that this is an average, not an absolute number. In other words, by 41, most women can no longer conceive. This finding supports the existence of the 10-year transition period leading up to menopause, which, on average, occurs at 51 years. This transition period, which begins around the age of 40, is characterized by a gradual decline in fertility and the onset of menopausal symptoms.

The timing of menopause is genetically determined, meaning it is programmed into a woman's genes, though several factors can accelerate its onset. There is a strong genetic link in families where early menopause is common — six times stronger than in families where menopause occurs at a standard age. The mother-daughter inheritance pattern is observed in 50% of menopause cases, but the correlation is even stronger between sisters, especially twins. However, little is known about the specific genes involved in menopause onset. So far, scientists have identified 17 candidate genes potentially linked to ovarian decline and climacteric changes, but these genes remain insufficiently studied.

The onset of natural menopause can be predicted by measuring FSH levels and antral follicle count. An elevated FSH level in the first phase of the cycle, combined with irregular menstrual cycles, has long been considered a precursor to menopause. More recently, the AMH (Anti-Müllerian Hormone) test has been introduced as a predictor of menopause. AMH levels increase during adolescence, remain relatively stable from 20–25 years, and then gradually decline with age. Approximately five years before menopause, AMH levels drop so low that they are nearly undetectable in the blood. This moment, when AMH becomes unmeasurable, is considered a key predictor of menopause onset. However, as laboratory technology improves and tests become more sensitive, AMH measurement may lose its practical significance shortly. It's important to note that while the AMH test is a promising tool for predicting menopause, it is not a definitive indicator and should be used in conjunction with other tests and clinical evaluations.

Modern medicine remains highly disorganized in its understanding of hormonal changes during menopause and the effects of hormone replacement therapy (HRT) on women's health. This confusion stems from the lack of an accurate animal model that replicates human menopause.

Additionally, there is an overwhelming variety of hormonal treatments, including synthetic progestins, used by menopausal women for various reasons.

Although menopause is associated with a decline in sex hormones and progesterone levels, it is not a disease but a natural aging process. However, this stage of life can be accompanied by unpleasant symptoms, including:

- Irregular menstruation
- Vaginal dryness
- Hot flashes
- Night sweats
- Insomnia
- Chills
- Mood swings
- Weight gain
- Breast changes
- Thinning hair and increased skin wrinkling

Many other signs of aging are associated with hormonal decline, but it's important to remember that not every woman experiences all of them. **The severity of symptoms is highly individual, depending on biological factors and psychological perception.** In many cases, psychosomatic responses play a dominant role in how a woman experiences menopause. Each woman's experience is unique and should be respected.

Analysis of menopausal issues across different regions of the world shows that cultural, religious, and ethnic attitudes toward menopause strongly influence the level of suffering women report. In many Eastern cultures, where menopause is respected as a natural transition, unpleasant symptoms are less common. In contrast, in societies where women are conditioned to fear menopause, being warned about hot flashes, loss of femininity, and aging skin, negative perceptions contribute to more significant distress. The widespread use of anti-menopause treatments, many of which lack scientific proof of effectiveness, further reinforces this fear. In most cases, the placebo effect dominates because psychosomatic factors outweigh physiological ones.

Unfortunately, in many developed countries, especially among white populations, menopause has been turned into a monster that must be fought continuously. The commercial industry plays a massive role in this, profiting from selling anti-aging treatments, medications, and hormones.

Menopause deserves closer attention, as women today live longer than ever, with average life expectancy reaching 70–80 years. This means that a third or even half of a woman's life is now spent in menopause. My upcoming book, explicitly dedicated to this topic, will provide more in-depth information on the climacteric period.

3.2. What is the Menstrual Cycle

In previous chapters, I discussed sexual development, the onset of the first menstruation, and the fact that the menstrual cycle takes time to establish itself. To truly appreciate the profound impact of this process, let's delve into the menstrual cycle, the intriguing fluctuations in hormone levels, and the factors that determine this delicate hormonal balance, all of which are integral to the overall harmony of a woman's life.

The classic description of the menstrual cycle, a marvel of nature, is that it consists of two phases, estrogen and progesterone, separated by ovulation and menstruation. However, modern gynecology and reproductive medicine divide the cycle into more detailed phases, corresponding to significant hormonal and tissue-level changes. To fully grasp the processes occurring in a woman's body, the 28–30-day menstrual cycle, which is considered the normal duration for most women, can be broken down into the following phases:

- **Early follicular phase** (EF) – Days 1–8 from the start of menstruation. Estrogen levels gradually increase, progesterone remains very low, and follicles begin to grow.

- **Late follicular phase** (LF) – Days 9–13. Estrogen reaches its peak, triggering a rise in FSH and LH, while the dominant follicle continues to develop.

- **Pre-ovulatory period** (PO) – Days 14–16. Estrogen levels drop sharply while progesterone and 17-OHPG start to rise.

- **Ovulation** – A rapid rupture of the dominant follicle and the release of a mature egg from the ovary.

- **Early luteal phase** (EL) – Days 15–23. Progesterone rises sharply, reaching its peak, with a slight increase in estrogen. The corpus luteum begins to form.

- **Late luteal phase** (LL) – Days 23–30. Progesterone and estrogen levels decline rapidly while 17-OHPG increases. The corpus luteum regresses if conception and implantation do not occur.

Progesterone plays a key role during the pre-ovulatory period, the early luteal phase, and if pregnancy occurs, it remains crucial throughout the late luteal phase.

3.3. What is Ovulation and Why is it Important

The ovaries contain follicles, each housing a primary oocyte (egg cell). Whether a follicle can contain more than one oocyte is one of the many mysteries in reproductive biology that continue to intrigue scientists.

During puberty and throughout the reproductive years, only a tiny fraction of follicles begins to grow, and an even smaller number (just 300–400 out of several million) will fully mature and reach ovulation, releasing a viable egg from the ovary. This rarity underscores the complexity and precision of the process.

3.3.1. How Egg Cells Mature

The process of follicular growth and maturation is called *folliculogenesis*. Follicles are categorized based on maturity, with nearly all starting as *primordial follicles* from birth. These tiny structures, measuring just 0.03–0.05 mm and about the size of a grain of sand, are invisible to the naked eye and cannot be detected on ultrasound.

Activating primordial follicles is a complex, tightly regulated process that begins at puberty. Once activated, it triggers the rapid growth of follicular structures and is irreversible, underscoring its significance in the reproductive process.

If a follicle is not dominant, it undergoes *atresia*, shrinks, and the oocyte degenerates. **More than 99% of all follicles present at birth will never reach ovulation and instead die through this process.**

In the final two weeks of an oocyte's life, it undergoes final maturation, a process regulated by gonadotropins, a type of hormone that stimulates the growth and function of the gonads, culminating in ovulation. However, the exact mechanisms that control the initial activation of primordial follicles remain unknown.

Once activated, follicles begin to grow, passing through several stages — *primary, secondary, early antral, and antral follicles.* Even at this stage, their size does not exceed 2 mm. Their growth is influenced by follicle-stimulating hormone (FSH), though FSH does not directly regulate them, so the growth process remains slow.

Approximately 70 primary follicles begin to grow at the start of a new cycle. Of these, around 60 follicles reach the secondary follicle stage (Class 1), followed by 50 early antral follicles (Class 2) over the next 25 days. Within 20 days, 20 follicles continue developing into antral follicles (Class 3), but only about 10 will respond to FSH and continue growing. Eventually, within 14 days, one follicle will fully mature and ovulate, while the rest will undergo atresia and die.

Under the influence of FSH, antral follicles begin to grow. However, in most natural menstrual cycles, only one dominant follicle emerges, reaching a size of 2 cm, at which point ovulation usually occurs.

The dominant follicle typically appears in the first third of the follicular phase, usually right after menstruation ends. However, in older women, the dominant follicle may emerge earlier, sometimes even at the end of the previous cycle's luteal phase, just days before menstruation begins.

The journey from primary follicle to pre-antral follicle is a complex process that unfolds over four months; reaching 2 mm in size (antral follicle stage) requires another two months. Granulosa cells within the follicle undergo intricate division and multiplication during this period. This means that any factors that affect the hypothalamic-pituitary-ovarian axis over six months can disrupt this delicate process of follicular maturation, potentially leading to anovulatory cycles or amenorrhea (absence of menstruation).

The highest conception rates are observed when the mature follicle reaches approximately 21 mm. Larger follicles are more prone to aging or post-luteinization, which disrupts the balance of steroid hormones. Progesterone becomes the dominant hormone in such follicles, leading to premature luteinization—where the follicle transforms into a corpus luteum without ovulating.

The table below compares follicle sizes and growth periods across different mammals:

SPECIES	PRE-ANTRAL FOLLICLE (µM)	GROWTH PERIOD (DAYS)	MATURE FOLLICLE (MM)
Mouse	100–200	10–12	0.5–0.6
Pig	150–300	40–50	3–10
Sheep	180–250	40–50	3–10
Cow	180–250	40–50	4–9
Human	180–250	≥90–180	17–20

Thus, the follicular growth period in women, from the pre-antral stage to ovulation, is significantly more extended than in other mammals. This prolonged growth period is one of the unique aspects of human reproduction, contributing to women's longer pre-ovulatory period than other mammals.

During the first five days of the menstrual cycle, progesterone and estrogen levels are at their lowest, allowing the endometrium to shed and exit the uterus. FSH and estrogen levels gradually increase throughout the first phase, although they fluctuate with intermittent rises and dips. However, progesterone remains consistently low until the end of the follicular phase. FSH levels also decline by this time but begin to rise again around days 21–22, triggering the growth of new follicles in the ovaries.

Interestingly, despite very low progesterone levels in the bloodstream during the follicular phase, the situation within the follicles is entirely different.

As early as the 1960s, researchers discovered that **progesterone levels in the maturing follicle before**

ovulation are significantly higher than in the bloodstream. In 1954, Dr. Zandler measured progesterone concentrations in blood, follicular fluid, the corpus luteum, and the placenta, finding that progesterone levels in the follicle were hundreds of times higher than in the blood of a pregnant woman in the second and third trimesters. However, this crucial data was ignored for nearly 40 years.

Modern studies have revealed that progesterone concentration in follicular fluid is 6,100 times higher than estradiol levels and 16,900 times greater than testosterone levels. Interestingly, these hormone ratios remain stable regardless of follicle maturity before ovulation.

Before ovulation, despite high progesterone levels within the follicle, there is a delicate hormonal balance between estrogen and progesterone. This balance is crucial for regulating the menstrual cycle. However, after ovulation, the dynamics change. Estradiol levels in the follicular fluid now depend on testosterone rather than progesterone, marking a shift in the hormonal environment within the follicle.

Another surprising discovery is that progesterone and testosterone levels in follicular fluid remain constant throughout the cycle. In contrast, estrogen levels fluctuate significantly — with larger follicles (10–15 mm in diameter) showing lower estrogen concentrations. Additionally, no correlation has been found between steroid hormone levels and the amount of follicular fluid, nor has it been found whether the follicle's oocyte was successfully fertilized. **Surprisingly, small follicles produce as much progesterone as larger ones.**

These findings have reshaped our understanding of folliculogenesis and challenged the hormonal theory of follicular maturation. They confirm that progesterone is the primary steroid hormone produced during follicular growth, which can later be converted into androgens and estradiol under gonadotropin influence. This also explains why, during pregnancy, when steroid hormones are essential for fetal development, the placenta produces large amounts of progesterone, which converts into estrogens and testosterone, which also increase during pregnancy.

3.3.2. Ovulation

Ovulation, a complex and intriguing event, begins when the follicle grows beyond 2 cm and ruptures. This seemingly instantaneous event follows specific stages, with the rupture taking about 7 minutes on average.

Approximately 8–10 minutes before ovulation, a portion of the granulosa layer, which likely contains the egg cell, begins to detach. The follicle shrinks slightly, and blood flow in the surrounding vessels increases, a change detectable via Doppler ultrasound.

Despite detailed studies on the stages of ovulation, the mechanism of follicular rupture and the breaking of the ovarian wall remains unclear. Immediately after the follicle ruptures, its walls collapse, and due to a sudden drop in intrafollicular pressure, the released follicular fluid exits the ovary, leading to the rupture of small blood vessels. The cavity left behind quickly fills with blood, and additional bleeding occurs from damaged ovarian blood vessels at the rupture site.

There are different opinions regarding the size a follicle must reach to rupture. In most cases, ovulation occurs when the follicle measures 2–3 cm, though 2.1–2.5 cm is the most typical size for follicular rupture.

Ovulation plays a crucial role in a woman's reproductive life, especially for those trying to conceive. Progesterone alone does not trigger ovulation — if progesterone levels are too high in the first phase of the menstrual cycle or if it is administered externally, ovulation may be inhibited.

Progesterone levels in the bloodstream remain very low throughout the follicular phase, yet ovulation cannot occur without it. Substances that suppress progesterone production or block progesterone receptors can also inhibit ovulation. If progesterone receptors are absent in the ovaries, ovulation does not occur.

The role of progesterone in both inhibiting and stimulating ovulation is a complex and vital aspect of the process. A rise in 17-α-hydroxyprogesterone (17-OHPG) is believed to be the first sign of impending ovulation, occurring 12 hours before the surge in luteinizing hormone (LH) — the hormone most used to predict ovulation.

The LH surge, a key event before ovulation, has long been a mystery. Its discovery and understanding have enlightened us about the foundation for ovulation predictor tests and its exact role in ovulation. 20% of women's LH rise begins at 4:00 AM, while the remaining 80% starts at 8:00 AM. This clear time-based pattern is linked to the circadian rhythm of cortisol. In women, plasma cortisol levels peak around 4:00 AM, aligning with LH rising at this time in some cases. In others, LH increases at 8:00 AM, when cortisol levels peak again. In other ovulating mammals, the LH surge may occur at different times of day but remains closely linked to circadian (daily) fluctuations in corticosteroids.

Estrogens can also trigger an LH surge, but this process is gradual and prolonged, as estrogen levels rise steadily without sudden spikes. Low progesterone levels before ovulation were previously believed to contribute to the LH surge. Still, when ovariectomized animals and humans were stimulated with estrogen alone, no LH peak occurred, regardless of the estrogen dose. Instead, LH levels increased gradually, without surges. This is why, in women with polycystic ovary syndrome (PCOS), estrogen stimulation of the pituitary gland leads to chronically elevated LH levels rather than a distinct pre-ovulatory surge.

Studies in humans and animals have revealed a strong link between a brief progesterone rise and the LH peak. In rats, there is a 14-hour delay between the progesterone rise and the LH surge. In women and rhesus macaques, the progesterone rise and LH surge interval is approximately 12 hours.

There has been some confusion regarding the timing of ovulation following the LH surge. Many medical textbooks, ovulation test kits, and gynecological guides state that ovulation occurs within 24–48 hours after the LH surge.

Ovulation tests work by detecting a threshold LH concentration in urine or other bodily fluids, but every woman's LH pattern is unique. Some women may reach the required LH level two days before ovulation, while in others, LH levels may be too low for detection yet still high enough to trigger ovulation. Due to these variations, commercial ovulation tests frequently produce false positives and false negatives.

Understanding why the interval between LH rise and ovulation varies is important. The two primary reasons are:

1. Some sources measure the interval from the start of the LH increase.

2. Others measure it from the LH peak — the hormone's highest concentration.

A 1980 WHO report stated that follicular rupture occurs 32 hours after the start of the LH rise and 17 hours after the LH peak. Other studies found that the LH rise can begin up to 40 hours before ovulation, while in some cases, it may be slightly delayed. However, follicular rupture often happens approximately 17 hours after the LH peak.

Unfortunately, many early studies failed to consider the post-LH rise in progesterone levels or did not explain this phenomenon.

Interestingly, progesterone receptor activation begins at least 4 hours after the LH surge and reaches its maximum effect around 8 hours after the gonadotropin peak.

During infertility treatments, particularly ovulation induction protocols, the timing of follicular rupture after the LH peak can be delayed. Viable oocytes have been retrieved up to 36 hours after the LH peak.

A highly delicate, short-lived phase exists between the LH surge and the subsequent progesterone rise. Any disruption during this window can lead to anovulation, resulting in a luteinized unruptured follicle (LUF) — a condition in which the follicle fails to rupture and goes through the *luteinization* (becomes corpus luteum).

If progesterone levels fail to rise after the LH surge, ovulation will not occur. This is because the activity of enzymes responsible for breaking down the ovarian wall at the follicular rupture site depends on progesterone elevation. Some women may have deficiencies in these enzymes, leading to infertility.

Experiments have shown that anti-inflammatory medications, particularly nonsteroidal anti-inflammatory drugs (NSAIDs) such as ibuprofen and aspirin when taken in the pre-ovulatory phase, can cause anovulation by inducing luteinization without follicular rupture. When taken in the luteal phase, these medications may disrupt endometrial quality and impair embryo implantation.

Besides the LH rise before ovulation, there is also a rise in FSH levels. The exact role of this FSH peak in the ovulation process is an area of ongoing research. It is suspected to be necessary for follicular rupture. Interestingly, in women with a short luteal phase, the FSH surge before ovulation is either minimal or absent.

3.3.3. The Corpus Luteum and Its Role

The female body has several sources of progesterone. In non-pregnant women, the ovaries, primarily the corpus luteum, are the leading producers of this hormone. As previously mentioned, progesterone is synthesized in the adrenal glands and, less commonly, in other tissues.

What is the corpus luteum? During ovulation, the follicle ruptures, releasing the egg cell into the abdominal cavity near the opening of the fallopian tube. Meanwhile, the ruptured follicle rapidly fills with blood, forming what is known as a *hemorrhagic body* (*corpus haemorrhagicum*).

On ultrasound, a hemorrhagic body can resemble ovarian bleeding, often leading to misdiagnosis as an ovarian hemorrhage or apoplexy, prompting unnecessary surgical intervention.

The formation of the hemorrhagic body, or blood-filled follicle, is a complex process that occurs within 1–2 minutes after ovulation despite the relatively small follicle. The follicle expands 12–14 minutes after rupture, reaching approximately 20% of its pre-ovulatory size.

While the egg cell travels through the fallopian tube, the ruptured follicle undergoes a transformation known as **luteinization**, during which it becomes the corpus luteum (yellow body).

The corpus luteum comprises three cell types: granulosa-lutein, theca-lutein, and K-cells. The first two types, sometimes called large and small granulosa cells, are responsible for hormone production. Large lutein cells produce estrogens, possibly under the influence of FSH, while small lutein cells synthesize progesterone and androgens.

The corpus luteum shares its blood supply with the dominant follicle. As progesterone levels rise, the endometrium becomes plusher and more vascularized, creating an optimal environment for implantation.

Luteinization involves the formation of new blood vessels (*vascularization*), cell growth (*proliferation*), and accumulation of lipids and lutein, which give the corpus luteum its yellow color.

Granulosa cells self-regulate, producing follicular inhibin, which influences FSH secretion. These cells also contain numerous LH receptors, but high estrogen and *luteinization inhibitor* (LI) levels in follicular fluid prevent premature luteinization.

When the pre-ovulatory LH surge occurs, several key changes take place in the follicle:

- *Meiosis* resumes in the oocyte (a critical step in egg cell maturation).

- Enzyme activity shifts from estrogen production to progesterone synthesis.

- Follicular rupture occurs, marking ovulation.

Granulosa cell proliferation begins before ovulation, as LH levels rise during the pre-ovulatory period. However, this process is gradual and does not interfere with ovulation. **Once the egg is released, luteinization intensifies, leading to the formation of the corpus luteum.**

Without pre-ovulatory LH and FSH surges, the corpus luteum will be incomplete and fail to produce sufficient progesterone.

Lutein, the pigment responsible for the corpus luteum's yellow coloration, is a carotenoid also found in green plant leaves, which plays a role in photosynthesis. In animals, lutein is stored in fat cells, giving fat its yellow tint.

A yellowish skin tone results from lutein in skin cells, particularly subcutaneous fat layers.

Can a corpus luteum form without ovulation? This phenomenon is known as *luteinized unruptured follicle syndrome* (LUFS). This condition occurs in some infertile women, though it is relatively rare.

Under the influence of LH, small lutein cells (theca-lutein cells) produce progesterone. Meanwhile, large lutein cells, derived from granulosa cells, contain prostaglandin receptors (PGF2α), which play a role in corpus luteum regression (*luteolysis*) if pregnancy does not occur.

Seven days after ovulation, the corpus luteum reaches an average size of 1.5 cm, though it can grow to 3–3.5 cm. At this point, it produces maximum levels of progesterone, which can be confirmed by measuring progesterone levels in the blood.

If pregnancy occurs, the corpus luteum must continue producing progesterone to support implantation and maintain early pregnancy. The uterus sends biochemical signals to the corpus luteum in multiple ways:

- hCG (human chorionic gonadotropin) secretion by the trophoblast
- Anti-luteolytic factors
- Neuroendocrine reflex mechanisms

In humans, hCG secretion by the trophoblast is considered the primary signal that sustains corpus luteum activity.

If pregnancy does not occur or implantation fails, the corpus luteum ceases its function around day 24 of the cycle (10 days after ovulation), initiating luteolysis. Prostaglandin 2α (PGF2α) is believed to play a key role in this process. Luteolysis is the process of the corpus luteum's regression, which leads to a decline in progesterone production and the initiation of the menstrual cycle.

Prostaglandins are produced by uterine tissues in most primates, including humans. It is also suspected that the ovaries themselves generate PGF2α, which contributes to corpus luteum suppression and regression via *apoptosis* (programmed cell death).

By day 26 of the cycle (28-day cycle), progesterone, estradiol, and inhibin levels drop significantly, triggering withdrawal bleeding — *natural menstruation*. This marks the end of the corpus luteum's function in the current cycle, highlighting its crucial role in regulating the menstrual cycle and fertility.

Due to their structural and functional relationship, ovarian follicles and the corpus luteum should not be viewed as separate entities but rather as sequential stages of follicular development. The follicle's granulosa cells transform into granulosa-lutein cells, while theca cells become theca-lutein cells.

If pregnancy does not occur, the corpus luteum begins to regress around day 21, progesterone production declines, and the ruptured follicle is replaced by a scar-like structure —the *corpus albicans* (white body).

If pregnancy does occur, hCG levels rise with implantation, stimulating corpus luteum function, and it transitions into the corpus luteum of pregnancy. **Around 7–**

8 weeks of gestation, the corpus luteum gradually loses its role as the primary progesterone producer, with the developing placenta taking over. By 8–10 weeks, the decline in hCG levels reflects this transition.

The classic model of corpus luteum regulation describes hypothalamic-pituitary control via LH secretion. However, this is only one level of regulation. An autonomous regulatory mechanism at the corpus luteum level can temporarily sustain hormonal activity in hypothalamic-pituitary signal deficiencies or brief LH shortages.

It is essential to understand that the corpus luteum is not a separate, isolated structure fundamentally distinct from follicles. Regarding hormonal function, the corpus luteum is very similar to the mature ovarian follicle, making it an essential continuation of the follicular phase rather than an entirely new entity.

3.4. Factors Affecting the Menstrual Cycle

The menstrual cycle regulation has been described extensively in textbooks and medical publications, with the hypothalamic-pituitary-ovarian system playing a central role. However, when doctors diagnose *"hormonal imbalance"* or, at best, the slightly more specific but equally vague *"ovarian dysfunction,"* the focus tends to remain solely on the *ovaries*.

The hypothalamic-pituitary-ovarian system is a marvel of interconnectedness. It is a complex network of endocrine glands, including the brain and the ovaries, which function as endocrine glands and reproductive organs. This system involves numerous biochemical substances, cellular interactions, and tissue structures. Understanding this system reveals how everything in the body is interconnected, making it impossible to isolate ovarian function as an independent process or consider the ovaries as standalone organs.

If attention is placed solely on the ovaries, the critical connections between these organs and the nervous system, the brain, and other endocrine glands may go unnoticed.

The theory of menstrual cycle regulation was first formulated in the 1960s, though the concept of a biphasic cycle had been known long before that. The traditional explanation, still found in many medical textbooks, is simplified: estradiol increases in the first phase, progesterone in the second, and gonadotropins rise mid-cycle. This gonadotropin surge (FSH and LH) responded to falling estradiol levels, which signaled the pituitary gland via a *negative feedback* loop.

However, menstrual cycle regulation is based not only on negative feedback but also on positive feedback mechanisms. **Both negative and positive feedback loops govern the regulation of all hormones in the female body, creating a delicate balance between these interactions and the hormones they influence.**

Negative feedback refers to the self-regulation of hormone levels by suppressing further hormone production. For example, when the ovary synthesizes estradiol, its levels in the blood increase. At the same time, estradiol binds to receptors in the endometrium and other target organs. The tissues send signals to reduce hormone levels when these receptors become saturated. These signals reach the brain (hypothalamus and pituitary gland), leading to decreased production of gonadotropins (FSH and LH), stimulating estradiol synthesis.

Positive feedback functions in the opposite way. High estradiol levels stimulate the pituitary gland to release LH, which triggers progesterone production. As a result, estradiol suppresses FSH production (negative feedback), but upon reaching a certain threshold, it stimulates LH production (positive feedback), which promotes progesterone synthesis.

The hypothalamic-pituitary system produces gonadotropins, which are regulated by stimulating and inhibiting factors. Several key factors influence gonadotropin production, including:

- Age and stage of development, including puberty
- Ovarian function and folliculogenesis stage
- Energy balance and metabolism
- Body composition (weight-to-height ratio)
- Circadian (daily) and circannual (seasonal) rhythms
- Stress and emotional activity
- Cognitive function (how the brain processes, transforms, analyzes, and stores information)

Beyond these biological factors, it is crucial to consider the pathways through which the hypothalamus and pituitary gland communicate with the ovaries and other reproductive organs. These signals travel through neurohumoral pathways, specifically neurovascular cells, responsible for transmitting electrical impulses and regulating cerebrospinal fluid exchange. Any disruption in these communication pathways can impair ovarian function and disrupt the entire reproductive system.

Irregular menstrual cycles are not a diagnosis — they are merely symptoms that may occur under normal and pathological conditions. More than 300 diseases and conditions can be associated with menstrual irregularities. Therefore, it's important to consider lifestyle factors such as diet, work schedule, rest patterns, stress levels, and coexisting medical conditions like thyroid disorders or gastrointestinal diseases when assessing the cause of cycle irregularity.

It is always essential to take a comprehensive approach when evaluating a woman's health in an irregular cycle. Does it cause significant discomfort? Is she trying to conceive? Is she interested in contraception? Only after evaluating these factors can an appropriate management strategy be chosen, emphasizing the importance of a holistic approach to reproductive health.

Chapter 4. Women's Diseases and Hormones

It's crucial to understand that hormones play an important role in almost every disease. Even a common cold triggers a stress response in the body, activating the adrenal glands and other endocrine organs to enhance immune defense. In our previous chapters, we have delved into numerous diseases that are intricately linked to dysfunctions of the endocrine system, underscoring the importance of your study in endocrinology.

Often, distinguishing between endocrine and systemic diseases is nearly impossible because dysfunction occurs at multiple levels of the body's structure and function. For example, diabetes mellitus is classified as endocrinopathy, which is a term used to describe an endocrine disorder, yet its impact on multiple organs also places it in the category of systemic diseases.

Additionally, when discussing various hormones, we have repeatedly highlighted their complex effects on multiple tissues and organs, often complicating accurate diagnosis.

In the female body, all physiological processes are intricately governed by hormonal fluctuations, primarily those of the ovaries. Moreover, several conditions are directly and significantly influenced by a woman's hormonal balance. This chapter will delve into some of the most notable examples, highlighting the importance of your understanding of female physiology.

4.1. Polycystic Ovary Syndrome (PCOS)

Polycystic ovary syndrome (PCOS) is considered not only an endocrinopathy but also a complex genetic disorder. The term itself is outdated, as it was initially based on ovarian appearance, whereas ovarian size and structure are not the primary factors in diagnosing the condition.

For a long time, diagnostic criteria for PCOS varied due to disagreements between American and European physicians. However, efforts have been made to reach a consensus and establish international diagnostic standards.

European specialists traditionally focused on ultrasound imaging of the ovaries, whereas American doctors emphasized laboratory assessments of hormone levels and other biochemical markers. As a result, the prevalence of PCOS depends on the diagnostic criteria used, ranging from 4% to 21%.

Two-thirds of women with PCOS experience metabolic disorders, including metabolic syndrome, which significantly increases the risk of developing type 2 diabetes and cardiovascular diseases.

4.1.1. Signs of PCOS

The following signs characterize polycystic ovary syndrome (PCOS):

Physical manifestations:

- Irregular menstrual cycles (cycles shorter than 21 days or longer than 35 days, fewer than nine cycles per year), most commonly *oligomenorrhea*.

- Lack of egg maturation (anovulation).

- Excessive hair growth (hirsutism).

- Acne.

- Obesity.

   Biochemical markers:

- Elevated levels of male sex hormones (hyperandrogenism).

- Increased luteinizing hormone (LH) levels.

- Elevated lipid levels (hyperlipidemia).

- Increased insulin levels (hyperinsulinemia).

The differences in diagnostic approaches have led to significant challenges in identifying PCOS:

- *National Institute of Child Health and Human Development Conference* (1990): Defined hyperandrogenism and menstrual irregularities due to anovulation as mandatory diagnostic criteria.

- *Rotterdam Consensus* (2003): Added polycystic ovarian morphology on ultrasound as a diagnostic criterion.

- *Androgen Excess–PCOS Society* (2006): Emphasized hyperandrogenism as the primary feature.

- *The National Institutes of Health* (2012): Recommended classifying PCOS *phenotypes*, recognizing nine subtypes based on symptom combinations.

Elevated levels of male sex hormones remain the most critical diagnostic marker for PCOS.

In September 2018, a group of physicians proposed simplifying PCOS diagnosis by focusing on four key criteria: oligomenorrhea, hirsutism, elevated androgen levels, and increased anti-Müllerian hormone (AMH) levels. Ultrasound findings were suggested as supplementary rather than primary diagnostic criteria.

Additionally, new reference values were proposed for assessing PCOS-related indicators:

1. Free testosterone: ≥1.89 nmol/L, androstenedione: ≥13.7 nmol/L, DHEAS: ≥8.3 µmol/L.

2. Antral follicle count: ≥21.5 follicles in each ovary.

3. Right ovary volume: ≥8.44 cm³ (the right ovary is always larger than the left).

4. AMH levels: ≥37.0 pmol/L.

This combination of markers demonstrates over 80% specificity for PCOS. However, AMH alone has proven impractical as a sole diagnostic criterion and should not be used independently. The proposed diagnostic criteria are currently under discussion in medical circles.

4.1.2. Ultrasound Findings in PCOS

Polycystic ovarian morphology is observed in 62–84% of women aged 18–30 years and 7% of women aged 40–45 years. However, many physicians performing and interpreting ultrasounds are unfamiliar with the specific ultrasound markers of PCOS and may diagnose it solely based on the absence of a dominant follicle.

During anovulatory cycles or when ovulation is delayed (cycles longer than 28 days), a dominant follicle may not be visible in the first two weeks. Given that ovaries naturally have a follicular (cystic) structure, polycystic ovarian morphology is frequently detected as a variant of normal anatomy. For this reason, many specialists suggest renaming PCOS to metabolic syndrome rather than focusing on ovarian morphology.

The ESHRE/ASRM consensus defines the following ultrasound criteria for PCOS:

- 12 or more follicles measuring 2–9 mm in each ovary (new recommendations: more than 21–25).

- Ovarian volume greater than 10 cm^3.

- "String of pearls" appearance of follicles.

- Thickened ovarian capsule.

It is important to emphasize that ultrasound findings alone are not sufficient for diagnosing PCOS and should not be used as the primary diagnostic criterion.

4.1.3. Characteristics of Hormonal Imbalances

Are all women with hyperandrogenism candidates for a PCOS diagnosis? After all, elevated levels of male sex hormones are also associated with menstrual irregularities.

It turns out that 15–20% of women with high androgen levels do not have PCOS. As mentioned in previous chapters, the causes of elevated testosterone vary. In PCOS, testosterone levels are usually not more than three times the normal range (increased by about 40%), and DHEAS levels typically remain below 8 mmol/mL. Women with PCOS may experience acne, hirsutism, and alopecia, but these symptoms alone are not definitive for diagnosis.

A key feature of PCOS is *insulin resistance*, which is present in most patients. Insulin directly disrupts ovulation by stimulating androgen production in ovarian follicles and indirectly by suppressing the synthesis of gonadotropin-releasing hormones in the hypothalamus. Elevated LH levels further stimulate androgen production, while a deficiency in FSH prevents the proper conversion of androgens into estrogens. This impairs follicular growth and suppresses ovulation.

Although diagnosing insulin resistance is complex, as discussed in earlier chapters, body mass index (BMI) can help predict its presence. Obesity is found in 75% of women with PCOS, and 50% of cases may involve a genetic defect in insulin receptors. This explains why hyperinsulinemia is also common in PCOS. Additionally, type 2 diabetes is frequently observed in families of women with PCOS, further suggesting a hereditary influence on metabolic processes.

4.1.4. Hereditary Factors in PCOS

PCOS predominantly affects women with excess weight, although both overweight and underweight conditions can disrupt menstrual cycles. In 50% of PCOS cases, obesity is moderate. With nearly 100 factors influencing metabolism, pinpointing the exact level at which metabolic dysfunction occurs is challenging. Modern medicine considers multiple parallel mechanisms involved in PCOS development.

Studies show that:

- Up to 70% of PCOS cases have a hereditary link.

- Up to 50% of sisters of affected women exhibit hyperandrogenism (half of them also have PCOS).

- Brothers of women with PCOS tend to have elevated DHEA-S levels.

- Genes such as FBN3 and HSD17B6 may contribute to PCOS development.

- PCSK9 and its polymorphisms are not associated with PCOS.

- Variants rs505151AA and rs562556GG are linked to increased lipid levels.

- Variant rs562556AA is associated with elevated testosterone levels.

Overall, research is examining nearly 100 genes potentially involved in PCOS development.

Interestingly, PCOS is the only condition associated with amenorrhea that does not lead to bone loss or osteoporosis.

It is crucial to remember PCOS is a diagnosis of exclusion. It cannot be determined from a single test, a single ultrasound, or a single consultation.

Moreover, it is a lifelong condition requiring ongoing management.

4.1.5. Progesterone Levels in PCOS

Since most cycles in PCOS are anovulatory, progesterone deficiency is often caused by the absence of normal cycle phases.

Women with PCOS tend to produce more progesterone in response to the accelerated LH pulse frequency, which is why LH levels are often elevated in this condition. However, due to a lack of synchronization between gonadotropins and sex hormone production, fluctuations in LH secretion also contribute to low progesterone levels.

Progesterone insufficiency in PCOS is secondary, as the first phase of the menstrual cycle is already disrupted. This leads to a slightly higher rate of spontaneous pregnancy loss compared to healthy women. While this remains a debated topic, many physicians prescribe progesterone supplementation after assisted reproductive treatments to support the luteal phase in women with PCOS.

4.1.6. Proper Interpretation of Diagnostic Results

In the past, many women viewed doctors as infallible figures—some still do. However, blind trust in medical professionals has gradually diminished, and patients increasingly seek second opinions. Modern medical education leaves much to be desired. The vast availability of knowledge and rapid advancements in science, while making information more accessible, have not significantly changed the public's perception of the medical profession. Being a doctor is still considered prestigious and financially rewarding but improving one's expertise depends mainly on individual motivation. As a result, the global decline in medical training quality is becoming evident.

Doubt in physicians' competence drives many women to seek additional information online. However, 90–95% of internet sources contain outdated, misleading, or false information. Schools and universities do not teach students how critical it is to assess the credibility of medical information.

Diagnosing PCOS requires a deep understanding of hormonal processes in both health and disease. It also requires a comprehensive evaluation, meaning test results can sometimes appear contradictory. To avoid reliance on questionable sources, let's clarify key points in interpreting PCOS test results:

- Testosterone levels may be within the normal range in some PCOS cases.

- Some oral contraceptives (OCPs) lower serum testosterone levels, so testing should be done at least three months after discontinuing hormonal contraceptives.

- Testosterone is only mildly elevated in PCOS. If levels exceed 7 nmol/L, ovarian or adrenal tumors should be ruled out.

- DHEA-S levels in PCOS are usually normal or slightly elevated. If levels are significantly high, an adrenal tumor should be excluded.

- Urinary free cortisol levels in PCOS are generally normal but may sometimes be elevated. If cortisol exceeds twice the upper normal limit, Cushing's syndrome should be ruled out.

- Mild cortisol elevation requires additional tests (dexamethasone suppression test, corticotropin-releasing hormone test) to rule out other conditions.

- Hyperprolactinemia occurs in 5–30% of women with PCOS. Prolactin levels are usually elevated by no more than 50% above the upper normal limit (30 ng/mL).

- 17-hydroxyprogesterone (17-OHP) should be tested in the early morning on an empty stomach during the first phase of the menstrual cycle.

- 17-OHP levels below 6 nmol/L generally rule out adrenal disorders, such as 21-hydroxylase deficiency.

- If 17-OHP is elevated, an ACTH stimulation test is required.

- Hormonal contraceptives and glucocorticoids affect 17-OHP levels, potentially leading to misinterpretation of results.

4.1.7. Modern Approaches to PCOS Treatment

Treatment for polycystic ovary syndrome is not a one-size-fits-all approach. It begins with a fundamental question: does the woman intend to conceive? For those planning pregnancy, ovulation induction is crucial, while others may prioritize menstrual cycle regulation. This individualized approach ensures that each woman's unique needs and goals are considered.

Weight normalization is the first-line treatment for PCOS. Even a modest weight loss of 5 kg can significantly improve menstrual regularity, providing hope and motivation for those managing the condition.

If pregnancy is not a goal, women may use low-dose oral contraceptives to regulate cycles. However, progestins have not been proven effective in PCOS treatment. Hirsutism treatment includes hormonal and non-hormonal therapies, as well as mechanical hair removal methods. Medications require 6–9 months of consistent use to show results.

In cases where pregnancy is desired, ovulation suppression treatments (hormonal contraceptives, progestins) should be avoided. Instead, reproductive technologies should be initiated immediately, including ovulation induction, using medications such as clomiphene, gonadotropins, aromatase inhibitors, or thiazolidinediones.

Surgical treatment (ovarian drilling, ovarian capsule incisions, or ovarian resection) is rarely performed. IVF (in vitro fertilization) may be recommended for the couple if all else fails.

4.1.8. Use of Progesterone in PCOS

Progesterone is frequently prescribed for women with PCOS, yet not all physicians fully understand which form and administration route should be preferred, considering its absorption characteristics and effects on both reproductive and non-reproductive organs.

Progesterone is used in PCOS for the following purposes:

- To induce withdrawal bleeding.

- To suppress LH production and regulate the menstrual cycle.

- To support ovulation induction in women resistant to clomiphene citrate.

- To maintain the luteal phase following assisted reproductive technologies (ART).

Women with PCOS not only experience irregular cycles but also prolonged cycles lasting weeks or even months, sometimes with no menstruation for 2–3 months. When a woman visits a doctor, she often does not know when her next period will occur, making it challenging to conduct hormone testing "at the right time." To address this, doctors prescribe short courses of progesterone (typically no more than five days) to induce withdrawal bleeding, creating an artificial menstrual period. This is not just a diagnostic tool but also a therapeutic approach to managing the irregular cycles in PCOS.

Thus, progesterone in PCOS is primarily used to optimize menstrual cycle assessment rather than to treat the underlying condition.

4.1.9. Dietary Supplements and PCOS

PCOS remains somewhat of a mysterious condition — it has multiple underlying mechanisms, is challenging to diagnose and treat, and remains unpredictable in its course. These uncertainties make it an ideal target for myths, supplement marketing, and miracle cures. However, what does evidence-based medicine say about the effectiveness of various supplements? Clinical trials provide disappointing results for many.

- Calcium and vitamin D — ineffective.

- B vitamins — ineffective.

- Vitamin B8 (inositol) — conflicting results.

- Chromium — ineffective.

- Vitamin D — ineffective.

- Omega-3 fatty acids — ineffective.

- Green tea (Camellia sinensis) — ineffective.

- Black cohosh (Cimicifuga racemosa) — ineffective.

- Cinnamon — ineffective.

- Spearmint (Mentha spicata) — ineffective.

This is only a partial list of the many remedies humanity has tested and continues to test for PCOS treatment.

4.1.10. Choosing the Right Diet for PCOS

What about diet? Since weight loss is the first-line strategy, it seems logical to focus on dietary approaches. However, clinical studies confirm that diet alone is not enough. Women must combine healthy eating with at least three hours of weekly exercise. When followed with patience and consistency, this holistic approach can bring noticeable effects after three months or longer, empowering women in their PCOS management journey.

Among all dietary approaches, the most effective are low-calorie diets (yes, calorie counting matters!) and diets based on glycemic index principles (often used by diabetics). Completely useless approaches include:

- Low-protein and high-protein diets.

- Diets rich in polyunsaturated fats.

- Low-carbohydrate diets (not to be confused with glycemic index-based diets).

High-carbohydrate diets may reduce hirsutism but worsen metabolic imbalances. Ketogenic diets (high fat, high protein, low carbohydrate) do more harm than good and are not recommended for PCOS treatment.

PCOS is a vast and complex topic that cannot be fully explored within the scope of this book. However, it is not something to fear.

4.2. Uterine Fibroids

All tumors of the uterine smooth muscle can be classified as benign or malignant. Benign uterine tumors are the most common neoplasms of the female reproductive system, with leiomyomas (fibroids) detected in 40% of women over the age of 35. By age 50, nearly 70% of white women are diagnosed with uterine fibroids.

Leiomyosarcoma is a malignant tumor of the uterus, though it is a rare condition, occurring in only 1.3% of all uterine malignancies.

Another category of uterine smooth muscle tumors is tumors of uncertain malignant potential. These tumors pose a significant challenge because their progression is unpredictable, and diagnosis without surgical intervention is difficult.

4.2.1. Causes of Uterine Fibroids

The causes of myometrial tumors remain unknown despite multiple hypotheses and theories.

Leiomyomas are monoclonal tumors arising from a **single cell** undergoing repeated division. What exactly triggers this cell's proliferation remains unclear. It is hypothesized that cellular mutations may disrupt the regulation of local growth factors and steroid hormones.

For years, estrogen was solely attributed to fibroid growth. However, extensive observations of progesterone-based therapies have unveiled that progesterone and progestins also play a significant role in fibroid cell proliferation. The progesterone receptors in fibroid tissue further confirm that the tumor responds to this hormone, adding a layer of complexity to our understanding of hormonal influences.

Animal studies have demonstrated that progesterone is equally significant as estradiol in fibroid growth.

It is incorrect to oversimplify the roles of estrogen and progesterone in fibroid development or other hormone-dependent conditions such as endometrial cancer, breast cancer, or endometriosis. This false dichotomy, portraying estrogen as a "bad hormone" and progesterone as a "good hormone", leads to misconceptions. Many of these conditions are associated with relative hypoestrogenism, where estrogen levels are lower than expected.

Progesterone plays a crucial role in regulating how cells utilize estrogen. If progesterone levels are insufficient or cells lose sensitivity to progesterone due to defective progesterone receptors, even small amounts of estrogen can trigger the growth of abnormal cells. This understanding of progesterone's regulatory role enlightens our knowledge of fibroid development.

Women with leiomyomas fall into two distinct age groups. Fibroids are uncommon among younger women (ages 20–35) and are typically linked to genetic predisposition. Researchers have identified two genes, HMGIC and HMGI(Y), associated with leiomyoma development. These women often have multiple small fibroid nodules that do not significantly affect fertility. Importantly, hormone levels in this age group are usually within normal ranges, which contradicts the "hyperestrogenism-hypoprogesteronemia" theory of fibroid growth.

Interestingly, pregnancy, a period of high progesterone levels, often causes fibroids to enlarge, but they may partially regress postpartum.

It's important to note that hormonal treatments, while beneficial in many cases, can sometimes stimulate fibroid growth. This cautionary information is crucial for medical professionals and patients, enhancing their awareness of potential treatment outcomes.

The second age group consists of perimenopausal women. This period is characterized by gradual declines in estrogen and progesterone levels and hormonal surges — sudden, short-term spikes in hormone levels. These fluctuations, particularly estrogen surges, disrupt hormonal balance and promote fibroid growth. However, with the onset of menopause, fibroids typically stop growing and gradually regress.

Fibroid growth is also influenced by various growth factors, including Platelet-Derived Growth Factor (PDGF), Heparin-Binding Epidermal Growth Factor (HB-EGF), Hepatocyte Growth Factor (HGF), Basic Fibroblast Growth Factor (bFGF or FGF-2), and Transforming Growth Factor-Beta (TGF-β).

4.2.2. Types of Fibroids

Fibroids can vary significantly in their microscopic structure, presence of necrosis (tissue death), atypical cells, mitotic (dividing) cells, and other characteristics. Because of these differences, their behavior can range from harmless incidental findings to potential threats that require medical or surgical treatment. Even among benign fibroids, there are three types that, under microscopic examination, may resemble malignant processes, making diagnosis challenging. These include atypical, mitotically active, and cellular leiomyomas. For this reason, whether specific markers exist to distinguish between benign and malignant uterine tumors has long been of interest to physicians. Accurate diagnosis is essential for predicting the course of the disease and selecting the most appropriate treatment.

One promising prognostic marker for distinguishing fibroid types is progesterone receptors' quantity and distribution pattern. Studying this pattern allows for the classification of leiomyomas. Research has also shown that most malignant smooth muscle tumors of the uterus lack progesterone receptors. However, despite its potential, determining progesterone receptor levels in leiomyoma nodules is not yet widely used in medical practice and remains under clinical investigation.

4.2.3. Treatment of Fibroids

Treatment for leiomyomas should be individualized based on symptoms, tumor size, growth rate, location, a woman's desire for pregnancy, and other factors. In most cases, uterine fibroids are asymptomatic and do not affect bodily functions, making treatment unnecessary.

Whenever possible, fibroid treatment should begin with conservative (medical) approaches. Traditionally, hormonal contraceptives have been used for fibroid management. Modern hormonal contraceptives, which contain low doses of synthetic estrogens and progestins, do not stimulate fibroid growth. While low-dose oral contraceptives do not shrink fibroids, they help regulate menstrual cycles, reduce bleeding duration, and decrease overall blood loss.

The use of progesterone and progestins in fibroid treatment remains controversial. Supporters argue that these hormones suppress fibroid growth, while opponents cite compelling evidence that progestins can accelerate fibroid growth, including with the widely used Mirena IUD with progestin. The effect of progestins on fibroids is highly individual and unpredictable. However, because progestins can reduce menstrual bleeding and blood loss, they are often prescribed to women with fibroids for this purpose.

Other hormonal therapies can temporarily shrink fibroids, but their effects are short-lived—fibroid growth resumes once the treatment is discontinued. For example, gonadotropin-releasing hormone (GnRH) agonists can reduce fibroid size by 50% within three months of therapy. Danazol, a synthetic androgen, can minimize fibroid size by up to 25%. These medications are not suitable for women planning pregnancy but are helpful in preoperative preparation when laparoscopic or hysteroscopic fibroid removal is planned.

Modern treatment strategies also focus on blocking growth factors with specialized drugs. RG13577 (a heparin-like compound) and halofuginone can inhibit DNA synthesis in muscle and fibroid cells without toxic effects on the body. Pirfenidone, a drug used to suppress fibrotic tissue growth, is currently being tested for fibroid treatment. Alpha-interferon (α-interferon), which may inhibit growth factors, is also under investigation. The development of these and other targeted treatments holds great promise and could significantly reduce the need for surgical interventions, including fibroid removal, hysterectomy, or uterine artery embolization (a procedure that blocks blood supply to the fibroids).

4.3. Endometrial Hyperplasia

Anovulatory (ovulation-free) cycles are prevalent in adolescents and young women. Typically, after age 21–22, the menstrual cycle becomes more stable, though anovulation may occur 1–2 times yearly. If factors suppressing the maturation of reproductive cells (e.g., stress) are present, anovulation may be more frequent. Cycle irregularities may persist in women with low or excessive body weight.

Anovulatory cycles are characterized by estrogen dominance. Progesterone levels remain insufficient since the corpus luteum does not form without ovulation. However, this is a relative progesterone deficiency, only compared to estrogen levels, not in absolute terms. In most women with anovulatory cycles, progesterone levels are within the normal range, though there is no peak production. Without the counterbalancing effect of progesterone, estrogen-driven endometrial growth intensifies, a process often referred to as endometrial hyperplasia.

It's crucial to dispel the common misconception that endometrial hyperplasia can be diagnosed based on ultrasound measurements of endometrial thickness. A physician or ultrasound technician may measure the endometrium and deem it abnormal simply because it does not align with their expectations, either falling outside the 'normal' range or not meeting their perception of what is expected. Accurate diagnosis requires a more thorough approach.

Measuring the actual thickness of the endometrium via ultrasound is not straightforward. Echogenicity, an ultrasound term describing tissues and organs' acoustic properties, adds a layer of complexity. Each ultrasound machine has a grayscale monitor that should be used to assess echogenicity objectively. However, in practice, many clinicians determine echogenicity 'by eye,' making it highly subjective. Image brightness and contrast settings also influence the appearance of structures, further complicating accurate assessment. This complexity challenges us to be more engaged in our diagnostic processes.

Endometrial thickness varies throughout the menstrual cycle:

- Menstrual phase (days 1–4): 1–4 mm

- Follicular phase (days 6–14): 5–7 mm

- Preovulatory phase: Two distinct layers are visible—an echogenic basal layer and a hypo-echoic functional layer, with a total thickness of 9–11 mm.

- Postovulatory phase (luteal/secretory phase): Within 48 hours after ovulation, the endometrium loses its layered appearance, making it harder to distinguish on ultrasound.

- Secretory phase: Endometrial growth halts due to the suppressive effect of progesterone. The glands and stroma undergo secretory changes, and the endometrium may appear slightly thicker (7–14 mm) due to cellular edema. However, measuring thickness at this stage is challenging, as both the endometrial layers and the stroma become hyper-echoic. As a result, the expanded endometrial glands in this phase are often mistakenly interpreted as focal adenomyosis (which will be discussed later).

Endometrial thickness is not a critical parameter for ovulating women of reproductive age, as it usually ranges from 5 to 15 mm. Consequently, thickness measurement in healthy women is rarely performed. It is most accurately assessed in the preovulatory phase.

In women with ovulatory dysfunction and irregular cycles, the endometrium may be expected to be thick but of poor quality. Physiological endometrial hyperplasia often results from prolonged estrogen exposure.

Endometrial thickness is primarily assessed in postmenopausal women with spotting or abnormal bleeding. Usually, postmenopausal endometrial thickness should not exceed 5 mm. However, is it genuinely problematic or necessary to perform a diagnostic curettage if ultrasound consistently detects an endometrial thickness of 6–7 mm in an asymptomatic woman? Each case requires an individualized approach that is empathetic and considerate of the patient's unique circumstances.

The term *"endometrial hyperplasia"* is histological, referring to cellular and tissue-level changes in the endometrium. It is not defined by its ultrasound thickness measurement, which is often inaccurate. Endometrial hyperplasia cannot be diagnosed "by eye" — it requires microscopic examination of a biopsy sample.

Endometrial hyperplasia is not a disease, pathology, or diagnosis — it is merely a descriptive characteristic of the uterine lining, reflecting a woman's hormonal status. It indicates estrogen dominance, whether from endogenous production or external hormone therapy. Hyperplasia is not due to a lack of progesterone per se but rather a failure in the hormonal shift

271

from estrogen to progesterone dominance, caused by anovulation or excessive estrogen exposure.

Anovulation can result from numerous conditions and situations, including overwork, nervous exhaustion, or emotional trauma.

Endometrial hyperplasia often presents with breakthrough bleeding, frequently mistaken for menstruation. These episodes may be mild (spotting), prolonged, or heavy, causing significant concern for affected women. Anovulatory cycles tend to be irregular, though they may occasionally alternate with ovulatory cycles.

4.3.1. Classification of Endometrial Hyperplasia

Despite the widespread practice of diagnosing endometrial hyperplasia based on ultrasound measurements of endometrial thickness, the actual diagnostic criteria for this condition (which describes the state of the endometrium rather than a disease) rely on cellular and tissue changes that can only be identified through histological examination.

There is still no universally accepted classification of endometrial hyperplasia, but the WHO classification is commonly used. It distinguishes between:

- Typical hyperplasiaSimple (glandular) hyperplasia

- Complex (adenomatous) hyperplasia

- Atypical hyperplasiaSimple glandular hyperplasia with atypia

- Complex atypical adenomatous hyperplasia

However, it's important to note that there is a significant disagreement with the WHO classification. For instance, some specialists argue that simple glandular hyperplasia with atypia already exhibits complex cellular changes, making it functionally complex hyperplasia. This disagreement underscores the need for a more comprehensive system that accounts for the different clinical presentations and diagnostic variations of hyperplasia, which often occur under various conditions.

An increasingly preferred classification in clinical practice is the therapeutic classification, which categorizes endometrial hyperplasia into:

1. Simple hyperplasia

2. Complex hyperplasia

3. Atypical hyperplasia

The last two types are further divided based on whether they occur before menopause (perimenopausal period) or after menopause. This classification is more practical for guiding diagnostic and treatment decisions, reducing unnecessary interventions and misdiagnoses. Its practicality should instill confidence in your decision-making process.

Simple glandular hyperplasia, commonly observed in reproductive-age women, is often overtreated by older-generation physicians using curettage or hormonal contraceptives, even when no treatment is necessary, especially in the absence of symptoms. Significantly, this type of hyperplasia does not progress to cancer.

4.3.2. Which Type of Hyperplasia Can Lead to Cancer?

The term "atypia" often causes alarm, as many people associate it with cancer. However, atypical cells are present in all human tissues, which does not necessarily indicate malignancy. In medicine, "atypical cells" means cells that do not conform to standard diagnoses. This deviation may be normal or a minor abnormality but not necessarily a cause for immediate concern. When evaluating potential precancerous or cancerous changes, specialized terminology is used in histological and cytological studies.

The only atypical hyperplasias that warrant concern are those occurring in postmenopausal women. Patients in this group typically present with persistent spotting or bleeding, often after 1–2 years of amenorrhea (absence of menstruation).

These cases require a thorough evaluation, which may include diagnostic curettage, but only under strict indications. Given the potential for serious implications, this careful consideration and appropriate action are crucial in cases of atypical hyperplasia in postmenopausal women.

By contrast, simple glandular hyperplasia is primarily problematic due to breakthrough bleeding or spotting, which is usually not dangerous — it does not cause anemia or other serious complications. However, it can provoke significant anxiety in women.

Heavy, irregular periods are also common in adolescents, but many mothers react with panic, subjecting their daughters to unnecessary curettage or hormonal treatments. In most cases, these irregularities result from endometrial hyperplasia due to anovulation and are self-limiting.

Another crucial point is that focal areas of atypical hyperplasia can develop within an otherwise normal endometrium, including cases where the endometrial thickness remains within normal limits. Women may have no symptoms at all in such instances. Endometrial cancer is often diagnosed only after postmenopausal bleeding occurs, even when an ultrasound shows a normal endometrial thickness.

Early-stage endometrial cancer often presents as a localized thickening of a small section of the endometrium, which is difficult to detect via ultrasound. Thus, clinical suspicion should be guided not only by imaging findings but also by:

- Family history

- Past medical conditions

- Number of pregnancies and childbirths

All these factors must be carefully considered to establish an accurate diagnosis.

4.3.3. Endometrial Hyperplasia Treatment: Is It Necessary?

In most cases of simple glandular endometrial hyperplasia, treatment is not required — neither curettage nor hormonal contraception or progesterone therapy.

It is always crucial to identify the underlying cause of excessive endometrial growth. If hyperplasia occurs during:

275

- Adolescence,

- The postpartum lactation period,

- Menstrual cycle delays due to significant weight fluctuations,

- Recovery from illness,

It is typically a physiological response that does not require treatment.

If a woman has persistent anovulatory cycles, the priority should be identifying the cause of anovulation rather than resorting to contraceptives to induce artificial menstrual cycles. Treating the primary disorder is essential if underlying systemic conditions, such as thyroid dysfunction, are present. Numerous conditions and diseases can lead to endometrial hyperplasia, and blindly suppressing endometrial growth is not the solution.

The endometrium is merely a target tissue that grows under the influence of estrogens. Instead of artificially suppressing this growth, it is necessary to determine the root cause of this estrogenic stimulation, whether it is due to true or relative hyperestrogenism.

Since progesterone suppresses endometrial growth, its use, including in the form of progestins, may help treat hyperplasia. Simple glandular hyperplasia is not inherently dangerous, but it may cause spotting or bleeding, which are often the primary reasons women seek treatment.

If a woman experiences three consecutive months without menstruation, progesterone may be used to induce withdrawal bleeding to prevent prolonged spotting or unexpected heavy bleeding. However, this artificially induced bleeding is typically shorter and lighter. If menstruation has been absent for less than 90 days, causing it is generally unnecessary.

It is disheartening to see women prescribed progesterone withdrawal therapy for a mere 1–2-week delay in menstruation under the false claim that severe hemorrhage due to endometrial hyperplasia could lead to dire consequences. This is simply untrue.

The mechanism of menstrual bleeding has been discussed in previous chapters. To artificially trigger withdrawal bleeding, progesterone is typically taken for 5 days, and bleeding occurs a few days after discontinuation.

If a woman has asymptomatic endometrial hyperplasia, progesterone therapy is not recommended. Withdrawal bleeding should only be induced after three months of amenorrhea, provided pregnancy is ruled out and the woman is not in menopause. However, it is crucial to be thorough and conduct further investigation to establish the correct diagnosis.

Even simple atypical hyperplasias often do not require treatment, mainly if curettage or hysteroscopy has already been performed.

Many women are prescribed progestins, including the levonorgestrel-releasing intrauterine system (Mirena), as a treatment option. Vaginal progesterone creams (containing synthetic progesterone) are less commonly used.

For complex atypical hyperplasia, hysterectomy (surgical removal of the uterus) is often recommended.

4.4. Endometriosis

Endometriosis, a complex condition, refers to visible endometrial tissue implants outside the uterus. Traditionally, this condition is considered estrogen-dependent, as the growth of endometrial tissue both inside and outside the uterus occurs under the influence of estrogens. When estrogen levels decrease, the growth of endometriotic lesions regresses, as observed in natural or induced menopause. This principle serves as the basis for existing medical treatments for endometriosis, which do not eliminate the disease but create a temporary effect of reducing the growth of endometriotic tissue and the endometrium by suppressing estrogen production. However, once treatment is discontinued, the symptoms of endometriosis return.

Surgical treatment of endometriosis has many limitations, offers only temporary relief, and is associated with a high risk of complications, so it is rarely performed.

Many modern doctors do not fully agree with the traditional definition of endometriosis, as it oversimplifies the understanding of this condition. Research shows that endometriotic lesions in different parts of the reproductive system and beyond can affect surrounding tissues differently, including their hormonal sensitivity. Additionally, it has been established that the reaction of the endometrium to progesterone in the mid-luteal phase differs between women with endometriosis and healthy women. In those with endometriosis, a condition known as "progesterone resistance" is observed, meaning that the endometrium does not correctly respond to progesterone.

Thus, endometriosis is not only an estrogen-sensitive condition but also a progesterone-resistant one, meaning it is a hormonal imbalance that manifests at the genetic level and disrupts the regulation of genes responsible for endometrial differentiation (17β-HSD-2, BCL-2, CALD1, CD14, CHRM3, CYP19, C1R, HOXA10, IL-6, KRAS, MMP3.7, MYH11, NF-KB, PGE2, PMAIP1, PTEN, RARRES1, RNASE1, THBS1, TIMP3, TGF-B, TNF-α).

Clinical studies show that endometriosis occurs 3–10 times more often among first-degree female relatives. Still, in many such cases, congenital anomalies of the reproductive organs are also present, leading to menstrual blood retention.

4.4.1. Mechanism of Endometriosis Development

The prevalence of endometriosis, a condition that has not been thoroughly studied, is a significant concern. Women most often seek medical help for lower abdominal pain and infertility during their reproductive years. It is believed that 5–10% of these women have endometriosis. Among those not planning pregnancy, 1–5% may have endometriosis. A hereditary link is found in 7% of cases. The highest prevalence of endometriosis is observed in women aged 35–44.

Why does endometriosis occur in some women who seem perfectly healthy while others who may have hormonal imbalances or reproductive system abnormalities never develop it? This question remains one of the great mysteries of endometriosis, which doctors, scientists, and researchers are working to unravel fully, providing hope for better understanding and treatment.

Despite being a common condition, endometriosis remains a mysterious disease, even under close medical scrutiny. Many theories and hypotheses attempt to explain its origins, but three are considered the most widely accepted.

According to the first **theory of retrograde menstruation**, endometrial tissue spreads with menstrual blood into the fallopian tubes or through open blood vessels and lymphatic pathways (implantation theory). It is known that during menstruation, 90% of women have blood in the abdominal cavity (particularly in Douglas' pouch).

The second theory, **coelomic metaplasia**, explains the development of endometriotic lesions due to changes in peritoneal lining cells influenced by adverse factors.

The third widely discussed theory attributes the development of endometriosis to the body's defense system's inability to destroy ectopic endometrial tissue and **abnormal differentiation of endometrial-like cells**. In this case, there is increased production of estrogens and progesterone, but at the same time, the tissues become resistant to progesterone.

Scientific data support these theories, yet none can fully explain the mechanisms behind the disease. In addition to these, there are other, less common theories.

Progesterone resistance in endometriotic lesions has also been observed in animals. It was logically assumed that this progesterone resistance could develop against the background of chronic inflammation in the pelvis since inflammatory reactions can suppress the activity of progesterone receptors through multiple mechanisms. For instance, some inflammatory mediators like interleukins and tumor necrosis factor can disrupt the function of other steroid hormone receptors, and certain inflammatory factors like prostaglandins can bind to progesterone receptors, blocking them. Additionally, oxidative stress and free radicals can interfere with the signaling pathways of progesterone receptors.

Interestingly, endometriosis is more common in women with chronic inflammatory bowel diseases than in healthy women. The presence of inflammatory foci in the pelvis may trigger the development of endometriosis, and conversely, endometriotic lesions may contribute to inflammatory processes in the intestines. The exact mechanism of this connection remains unknown.

4.4.2. Classification of Endometriosis

There are specific stages of endometrial cell implantation:

• Attachment and invasion (penetration);

• Vascular formation and growth;

• Inflammation;

• Formation of a lesion (tumor).

The clinical classification of endometriosis remains a complex and ongoing discussion. While doctors often differentiate between diffuse forms (small foci) and nodular forms (tumors), the lack of a clear classification system underscores the need for further research and understanding. Reproductive endometriosis affects the ovaries, fallopian tubes, and uterine ligaments, with lesions also found outside the reproductive system, including in the lungs.

Discussions about the staging of endometriosis continue due to the high degree of subjectivity involved in assessing the spread of endometrial lesions. However, determining the stage of the disease has no practical significance.

Among specialists performing laparoscopy, the most used diagnostic and treatment method for endometriosis, the American Society for Reproductive Medicine has proposed a laparoscopic classification that considers the color of the endometriotic lesion.

It is no secret that endometriosis is often discovered by chance during laparoscopy performed for non-gynecological reasons.

Modern recommendations state that **if a woman has no symptoms related to endometriosis, its lesions should not be removed**. Removing asymptomatic lesions may not improve the patient's quality of life and can lead to unnecessary surgical risks.

Inexperienced surgeons often mistake a slight purple or black lesion on the peritoneum for something dangerous and try to remove it. Dark-colored lesions are most frequently excised in the search for the cause of pain.

Endometriotic lesions vary in color — from clear to black (clear, white, pink, pink-red, red, blue-violet, black, yellow-brown), and may also appear as peritoneal damage. Studies have shown that pain levels depend on the type of lesion. The most painful lesions are red (84%), clear (76%), and white (44%), while black lesions cause pain in only 22% of cases.

Another feature of endometriosis is that **pain does not depend on the stage of the disease.** Pain is reported by:

- 40% of women at stage 1;

- 24% of women at stage 2;

- 24% of women at stage 3;

- 12% of women at stage 4.

It might seem logical that the more severe the endometriosis, the more it should affect a woman. However, paradoxically, even a barely visible lesion can cause more discomfort and suffering than a large endometriotic nodule in the abdominal cavity.

Endometriosis can also manifest as **endometriomas**, often referred to as *chocolate cysts*. These occur in 17–44% of women with endometriosis, and in 28% of cases, they are bilateral.

When choosing an observation or treatment strategy for endometriomas, three key factors are considered:

- Presence of symptoms;

- Size of the cyst;

- Ovarian reserve.

Chocolate cysts do not affect conception rates or pregnancy outcomes. They are monitored if smaller than 4–6 cm and do not cause pain or discomfort. If AMH (Anti-

Müllerian Hormone) levels are low, the cysts are also left untouched. **Medication does not treat chocolate cysts**.

When discussing endometriosis, it is crucial to mention **adenomyosis** — a condition in which endometrial lesions are found in the myometrial layer of the uterus. Adenomyosis is common in women over 35. In the past, such lesions were only discovered in removed uteri, typically after a hysterectomy performed for severe menstrual pain and heavy bleeding. Nowadays, adenomyosis is often overdiagnosed via ultrasound.

It is important to note that there is still no established:

• Classification of adenomyosis;

• Strict diagnostic criteria, including ultrasound criteria;

• Reliable data on its negative effect on fertility;

• Reliable data on its negative impact on pregnancy outcomes;

• Reliable evidence supporting treatment effectiveness.

The two most common symptoms of adenomyosis are heavy and painful menstruation. These symptoms typically appear after age 30, often following multiple pregnancies and childbirths, and tend to worsen with age.

Thus, adenomyosis is a benign condition of the uterus for most women, although it can be accompanied by painful and heavy periods.

4.4.3. Progesterone Resistance

At first glance, estrogen dependence and progesterone resistance are two names for the same phenomenon. However, they pertain to different menstrual cycle phases, where different hormones dominate.

The concept of "progesterone resistance" is based on studies showing that women with endometriosis exhibit dysregulated expression of more than 200 progesterone-dependent genes in both endometriotic lesions and the uterine endometrium. This phenomenon is thought to play a role in the development of tubal and ovarian dysfunction in women with endometriosis. Research has also demonstrated that this gene regulation disorder persists throughout the entire cycle, with the most significant deviations occurring in the early luteal phase. As a result, endometrial proliferation in these women is prolonged and not suppressed by progesterone.

At first, progesterone resistance might seem like an obvious explanation for infertility in some women with endometriosis. Logically, supplementing with exogenous progesterone should help facilitate pregnancy. However, the reality is more complex. The genes with disrupted hormonal regulation remain unresponsive to pharmaceutical progesterone. One study found that the expression of 245 genes in endometriotic tissue differed significantly from that of healthy women despite normal progesterone levels.

Unlike normal endometrial tissue, endometriotic tissue has lower sensitivity to progesterone, regardless of whether the lesions are outside the uterus (ectopic) or within the uterus (eutopic). It was also discovered that endometriotic lesions exhibit an imbalance of estrogen and progesterone receptors and a decreased ratio of progesterone receptor types A and B (PR-B/PR-A). This receptor imbalance may explain why these tissues are resistant to progesterone. Some researchers believe that a deficiency of PR-B receptors holds the key to understanding the development of endometriosis. Finding medications to activate these receptors could be the most effective treatment approach for the disease.

Progesterone resistance is also observed in other conditions, particularly in polycystic ovary syndrome (PCOS).

4.4.4. Modern Medical Treatment

Endometriosis, a complex and almost lifelong condition (until menopause) presents a significant challenge in the medical field. While it is practically incurable, medical intervention is necessary in cases of pain and/or infertility, requiring a multifaceted approach.

For pain management, preference is given to medical treatment, with drug selection based on minimizing side effects:

• Nonsteroidal anti-inflammatory drugs

• Hormonal contraceptives

• Progestins

• GnRH agonists

• Danazol

It is entirely irrational to induce artificial menopause without first trying gentler treatment methods. It is also unreasonable to treat endometriosis if it causes no symptoms. **The claim that untreated asymptomatic endometriosis leads to severe consequences is false.** Almost 25% of women with this condition experience no symptoms at all.

There are also excessive speculations about the advantages of different treatment methods for pain relief. A serious analysis of clinical studies (2017) revealed the following:

> • There is no difference in the effectiveness of surgical and medical treatment for pain relief in all stages of endometriosis

> • Pain reduction occurs after a certain period of treatment (12–24 months)

> • Long-term improvement or worsening of symptoms depends not on the type and duration of treatment but on lifestyle factors (diet, smoking, past trauma, abortions, alcohol abuse, bowel diseases, and other pelvic disorders).

Only a small number of studies on drug therapy for endometriosis report long-term treatment outcomes. Many women experience only limited or intermediate benefits from treatment:

> • 11–19% – no pain reduction

> • 5–59% – pain persisted

> • 17–34% – pain returned

- 5–16% – side effects led to treatment discontinuation

An individualized approach remains key in the treatment or monitoring of endometriosis.

Hormonal Therapy for Endometriosis

Progesterone's ability to suppress endometrial growth has been known for centuries. Although ancient healers and doctors had no concept of progesterone as a substance, they used ovarian extracts from animals to induce artificial menopause in women suffering from severe menstrual pain. Clinical descriptions from that time align closely with endometriosis cases.

Despite an understanding of progesterone resistance, **no adequate drug treatment has yet been found that both suppresses the growth of endometriotic lesions and restores normal tissue sensitivity to steroid hormones**. Along with the dysregulated expression of progesterone-dependent genes in endometriotic lesions, a structural defect in progesterone receptors also plays a role in progesterone resistance. As a result, supplementing with additional progesterone does not have a therapeutic effect.

The main goal of endometriosis treatment is to eliminate cyclic hormonal fluctuations, including ovulation. Thus, the use of *combined oral contraceptives* (COCs) and progestins, which suppress ovulation, can partially improve a woman's condition.

Doctors often prescribe COCs in a continuous regimen to avoid withdrawal bleeding during the 7-day hormone-free interval, as it is believed that even a small amount of menstrual blood entering the abdominal cavity during withdrawal bleeding could cause pelvic pain.

While progestins have a therapeutic effect, their pain relief is often short-term.

Dienogest can be combined with GnRH agonists, but recent studies have shown that it is effective even without them and causes fewer side effects. Since it has anti-estrogenic properties, the main side effects associated with its use are hypoestrogenic symptoms.

Depot progestin therapy is widely used for contraception. Medroxyprogesterone acetate (DMPA) depot injections are used for endometriosis treatment. This approach is gaining popularity among women as it is not only cost-effective (cheaper) but also eliminates the need for daily medication while providing contraceptive protection.

The most unpleasant side effect of depot progestin treatment is breakthrough bleeding, which can be heavy and prolonged. This method is not prescribed for women planning pregnancy, as these drugs can suppress the reproductive system for an extended period, disrupting ovulation and menstrual cycle regularity.

Long-term use of depot progestins requires additional calcium supplementation to prevent osteoporosis.

The intrauterine hormonal system (Mirena), which contains levonorgestrel, has anti-estrogenic effects, suppressing endometrial growth and often leading to amenorrhea (absence of menstruation), thus relieving pain in half of the women who have endometriosis. However, ovulation is not completely suppressed in all Mirena users.

The advantage of this treatment is that the levonorgestrel-releasing intrauterine system remains in the uterus for up to five years, providing therapeutic effects. However, the risk of endometriomas (chocolate cysts) may increase because ovulation is not entirely suppressed. In 5% of cases, the intrauterine system expels itself spontaneously.

Danazol is a derivative of male sex hormones and induces artificial menopause. It was widely used for endometriosis treatment about 20 years ago and is still used in some countries. This drug has side effects such as acne, hirsutism, weight gain, and breast atrophy. Some studies suggest that prolonged use of danazol may increase the risk of ovarian cancer.

GnRH agonists are a new class of drugs prescribed when other treatments fail or, in rare cases, in combination with other medications. These drugs should not be used without additional supportive (hormone replacement) therapy. Several GnRH agonists are available on the market, including buserelin, goserelin, leuprorelin, nafarelin, triptorelin, dienogest, and others.

Since these drugs have potent anti-estrogenic effects, their most serious side effect is estrogen deficiency (hypoestrogenism), which may cause hot flashes, vaginal dryness, insomnia, decreased libido, and reduced bone density with calcium loss (sometimes irreversible). To counteract these effects, hormone replacement therapy (a combination of estrogens and progesterone) is often prescribed, like treatments used for estrogen deficiency in menopausal women.

These medications induce prolonged amenorrhea, rarely leading to breakthrough bleeding. They should not be used by women planning pregnancy.

In several countries, clinical trials are underway for *aromatase inhibitors* as a potential treatment for endometriosis. These drugs work by inhibiting the aromatase enzyme, which endometriotic lesions use to produce estrogen. Aromatase inhibitors can be combined with other medications not only to manage endometriosis-related pain but also to prevent cyst formation following other treatments or after discontinuing previous therapies.

Surgical Treatment of Endometriosis

Doctors often overuse surgical treatment for endometriosis, particularly laparoscopy. Many women with chronic pelvic pain undergo this procedure, even though medical treatment, such as pain relief for *dysmenorrhea* (painful periods), can be initiated without surgery. If medication proves ineffective, laparoscopy may be performed for diagnostic purposes and as a surgical treatment method.

Modern recommendations for surgical treatment of endometriosis include only two groups of patients:

• **Patients with pelvic pain**:

A) who have not responded to medical treatment;

B) who have contraindications to medication;

C) who have refused medical treatment;

In emergency situations requiring urgent care, such as ovarian cyst rupture or torsion, surgery is a necessary and reassuring option for women with endometriosis.

D) who suffer from invasive endometriosis affecting the intestines, bladder, ureters, or pelvic nerves.

• **Patients with ovarian endometriomas**:

A) when an ovarian tumor of uncertain nature is detected;

B) who suffer from infertility and chronic pelvic pain.

Women whose endometriotic lesions are incidentally discovered during surgery (for example, during an appendectomy) do not require treatment for endometriosis.

Research shows that removing endometriotic lesions in women with infertility does not improve fertility rates. Therefore, laparoscopy is generally not recommended for women planning pregnancy.

4.4.5. Endometriosis and Infertility

Endometriosis has become a commercial diagnosis in some countries, a term used to describe the overdiagnosis and overtreatment of the condition. This is often driven by a woman's fear of infertility or future severe pain, leading to unnecessary medical procedures and prolonged treatment.

A strong negative psycho-emotional background accompanies infertility. It is precisely in the group of women struggling with conception that extensive examinations are conducted, leading to more frequent detection of endometriosis compared to reproductively healthy women.

Most infertile women have no idea that they have endometriosis. Only a tiny subset experiences pain severe enough to interfere with a regular sex life.

Due to the many speculations surrounding endometriosis and fertility, numerous serious clinical studies have been conducted. To this day, no proven link between endometriosis and infertility exists despite early publications claiming that endometriosis causes infertility. However, as research quality improves, more reliable data emerge. Here is what evidence-based medicine says about the widespread claims regarding the impact of endometriosis on fertility:

• The stage of endometriosis does not affect pregnancy progression or outcomes.

• Endometriosis does not affect egg quality.

• Luteal phase deficiency levels are not increased.

• The luteinized unruptured follicle syndrome does not occur more frequently in women with endometriosis.

• Endometrial quality is not impaired.

• Anti-endometrial antibodies may be elevated in some women with endometriosis, but they are also found in infertile women without endometriosis.

• Sperm transport through the fallopian tubes is not disrupted by endometriosis.

• The toxic effect of endometriosis on embryos is not confirmed.

• Endometrial receptors in the uterus are not damaged, only in endometriotic lesions.

• Endometriosis does not increase the risk of biochemical pregnancies.

• Endometriosis does not increase the rate of miscarriages or missed pregnancies.

• Treatment of stage 1–2 endometriosis does not improve conception rates.

• Progestins, GnRH agonists, and danazol do not increase conception rates; on the contrary, they reduce them by inducing anovulation.

• Surgical treatment of early-stage endometriosis does not improve conception or pregnancy rates.

• Surgical treatment of advanced endometriosis may improve conception rates by relieving pain and discomfort, thereby enhancing quality of life, including sexual health.

• IVF is less successful in later stages of endometriosis, though not due to egg quality.

These facts empower us to debunk the myths surrounding this condition, giving us a more precise understanding and control over our health.

Endometriosis is not as frightening as it is often portrayed. Understanding that asymptomatic cases require no hormonal or other treatment can bring relief. **There are no preventive treatment courses for endometriosis after removal of chocolate cysts, laparoscopy, pregnancy planning, or miscarriage.**

The problem for some women, especially those trying to conceive, is that they become fixated on a popular, trendy diagnosis, often imposed by an ill-informed doctor. As a result, they spend years trapped in a mental cage, wasting their time, money, and health on endless examinations and treatments.

If you feel trapped in a cycle of endless examinations and treatments, it's time to take control. Reassess your perspective, reason about the money and time spent, and take charge of your health. A lack of knowledge about one's own body and its processes creates fertile ground for fears, which in turn begin to control a woman's life, making her chronically unhappy.

If your doctor cannot relieve your suffering after a year, then this is not the right doctor for you. The problem is not the disease but the doctor's inability to diagnose and prescribe the proper treatment. And if you want a child, but your doctor is suppressing ovarian function without considering your wishes, change your doctor immediately.

Chapter 5. Hormonal Contraception

Hormonal contraception, a topic of enduring relevance and historical significance, has been a subject of societal discourse for the past sixty years. Its evolution and impact deserve a comprehensive exploration, so it merits a dedicated book to delve into its most critical aspects.

Approximately 70% of women of reproductive age are sexually active but do not plan pregnancy. Notably, about 40–50 years ago, 80% of unplanned pregnancies ended in abortion. The introduction of various contraceptive methods, including hormonal contraceptives, has significantly reduced abortion rates in all developed countries. While abortion rates remain high (25–50%), the role of hormonal contraception in preventing unplanned pregnancies is reassuring. However, global access to contraception remains a challenge, with around 60 million abortions performed worldwide each year, primarily in countries with low socio-economic conditions.

Approximately 18% of people using contraception rely on hormonal methods. In European countries, the United States, and Canada, up to 30% of women use hormonal contraception.

Despite this, many doctors and their patients in some countries still perceive hormonal contraception as something harmful, focusing on the potential serious side effects that occur in some women. However, history and medical practice show that in countries with low levels of hormonal contraception use, abortion rates, including illegal abortions, are incredibly high. The number of complications from pregnancy termination far exceeds the complications associated with hormonal contraception. Therefore, among the available options, hormonal contraception remains the most effective method of preventing pregnancy.

5.1. A Brief History of Hormonal Contraception

Historically, scientists and doctors have been interested in steroid hormones not so much for therapeutic purposes as for contraception. The search for hormones was so intense that within two decades at the beginning of the 20th century, hundreds of articles were published on ovarian hormones, particularly the corpus luteum. Not all these studies were printed in prestigious scientific and medical journals, making them difficult to access today. Nevertheless, the immense interest of researchers in female endocrinology remains striking. In other words, knowledge about ovarian hormones existed long before progesterone was isolated in its pure form.

Although computers and the Internet were not available in the 1930s and 1940s, information exchange among scientists was slow but still present. They were engaged in a fierce competition to find the ultimate contraceptive: progesterone. This was no mistake; the contents of the corpus luteum interested scientists solely from the perspective of pregnancy prevention.

The corpus luteum of certain animals was an easily accessible and inexpensive biological material. Doctors observed that pregnant women (as well as female mammals and other species) could not conceive again. Moreover, menstruation ceased during pregnancy. The same effect was noted when female animals and women were given corpus luteum extracts: false pregnancy occurred, menstruation stopped, and these females and women lost the ability to conceive. The corpus luteum extract, which was used to treat painful menstruation, often led to the cessation of menstrual cycles, effectively inducing artificial menopause. However, the most important discovery was that menstrual cycles resumed after treatment cessation, and women could conceive again, meaning the effect was temporary rather than permanent.

Further research led to the idea that pregnancy involves the release of a substance, also present in the corpus luteum, with strong contraceptive properties. That substance was progesterone. **The development of synthetic progesterone marked the beginning of hormonal contraception, and its principles remain unchanged to this day.**

The primary contraceptive component in all hormonal contraceptives is progestin — a synthetic form of progesterone.

The demand for hormonal contraception grew in the 1920s and 1930s, coinciding with the rise of the feminist movement advocating for women's emancipation, including their right to control conception and childbirth, as well as sexual freedom. The number of abortions began to rise dramatically, even though they were banned in many countries (and remain so in some today), and doctors performing abortions faced persecution and punishment. This increasing demand for a substance that could block the reproductive system accelerated the search for synthetic progesterone.

Progesterone was already known but under different names, and its contraceptive properties were recognized. The challenge was to produce it in a convenient and highly absorbable form.

In the 1930s, scientists obtained progesterone identical to the natural hormone. This breakthrough initially sparked enthusiasm, but it was soon followed by disappointment among doctors and chemists who discovered that in its pure form, progesterone did not provide the desired therapeutic effect.

It was found that progesterone metabolizes in the human body within minutes, making it rapidly eliminated. Administering large doses of progesterone via daily injections (sometimes multiple times per day) to achieve a contraceptive effect was impractical. Moreover, oral progesterone was utterly ineffective.

Thus, the discovery of progesterone led to many disappointments, unlike its synthetic analogs, it remained without practical application for years.

By the end of 1938, German chemists developed the first oral (tablet form) synthetic progesterone — *ethisterone*, which became the precursor of oral hormonal contraceptives. This form of progestin was well absorbed and maintained its contraceptive action after being ingested. Ethisterone is still used in some countries today.

In 1952, the first hormonal progestin contraceptive, *norethynodrel* (NET), was introduced in the United States. In 1960–1961, the first combined oral contraceptive, *Enovid*, was licensed in the U.S. and England. This pill contained both synthetic progesterone and synthetic estrogen. Enovid remained on the market until 1988 when it was discontinued due to its high estrogen content.

In 1940, Russell Marker extracted progesterone with a molecular structure identical to human progesterone from *diosgenin*, a compound found in yams (sweet potatoes). This method, known as semisynthesis, allowed to produce steroid hormones from plant-based raw materials. Thanks to the work of Percy Julian, other steroid hormones were soon synthesized from plant sources as well.

It was not until 1971 that progesterone was fully synthesized in a laboratory without using plant or animal sources. This development led to the production of relatively inexpensive hormonal contraceptives and the worldwide expansion of hormonal contraception.

Until 1973, the government regulated progesterone synthesis in the U.S., which amounted to just over 60 kg per year. However, by 1975, 13 types of hormonal drugs containing estrogens and progestins had appeared on the U.S. market, and by 1979, progesterone production had reached nearly 12 tons per year.

Synthetic progesterone substitutes appeared simultaneously with the discovery of natural progesterone. **Over the nearly one hundred years of the "progesterone era," hundreds of derivatives of progesterone and other steroid hormones have been synthesized, though not all have been used in practical medicine.**

Modern progestins are derivatives of progesterone, testosterone, and other steroids. All synthetic progesterones belong to the class of steroid hormones with 19 or 21 carbon atoms (C). Differences in molecular structure determine the varying effects of synthetic progesterones on the female body.

Progestins act on human cells and tissues by binding to progesterone receptors. Still, their unique feature is that they may bind more quickly or strongly to other steroid receptors, influencing their activity and effects.

Today, the global market offers over 500 types and formulations of synthetic progesterone — progestins. However, despite their availability, progesterone and progestins have not been widely used in obstetrics, except in countries where the myth of progesterone's benefit in maintaining pregnancy still prevails.

5.2. How Hormonal Contraception Works

I have already mentioned in this book that progesterone and progestins affect the endometrium and suppress oocyte maturation, which is the basis of progesterone action. If progesterone is taken at the beginning of the menstrual cycle, ovulation will not occur.

Over the past century, various terms have been used to refer to progesterone and its substitutes, meaning substances with progesterone-like and other properties.

In 1930, the German gynecologist Karl Klauberg, a professor at Königsberg University, created a classification of synthetic progesterone substitutes, introducing the terms "progestins," "progestagens," and "gestagens," along with a scale of their biological activity, based on studies of rabbit endometrium.

Progestagens is the group that includes progesterone and other hormones with similar properties. They are often referred to as *gestagens* in abbreviated form. The term "gestagen" means "progestational agent," indicating its connection with pregnancy (gestation). This group includes natural progesterone, bioidentical forms, and synthetic progesterone. However, in some sources, only synthetic forms are called progestagens, which is incorrect.

Progestins refer specifically to synthetic forms of progesterone.

There are four mechanisms by which progestins act as contraceptives:

1. **Inhibition of ovulation by suppressing LH and FSH in the middle of the cycle**. It is essential to know that in all hormonal contraceptive pills and other formulations, the main contraceptive effect is provided by the progestagen component. Estrogens are added to regulate withdrawal bleeding (by promoting better endometrial growth) and to prevent mid-cycle bleeding. Estrogens can also suppress ovulation by influencing LH and FSH production by the pituitary gland, but only in high doses.

2. **Thickening of cervical mucus**, which prevents sperm from entering the uterine cavity. This effect resembles the cervical mucus plug formed by progesterone during pregnancy.

3. **Endometrial quality is disrupted**, making it unsuitable for implantation. This effect is achieved by suppressing progesterone receptor activation, stimulating stromal cell growth, and reducing the number of secretory glands in the endometrium. Additionally, endometrial tissue swelling is observed.

4. **Reduction of fallopian tube mobility and slower movement of cilia**. This explains the increased risk of ectopic pregnancy when progestins are used for therapeutic purposes, especially in the second half of the cycle (risk of 5–6%).

Although many different progestins exist, all of them have the exact fundamental contraceptive mechanisms. However, each progestin may also have specific effects due to variations in the strength of these mechanisms. In other words, some progestins suppress ovulation more strongly, while others do so less effectively. Some significantly impact endometrial quality, while others are less so. These variations in effects can have implications for the effectiveness and side effects of hormonal contraception. For instance, some progestins may be more effective at preventing pregnancy, but they may also have more pronounced side effects. Some progestins exhibit strong anti-androgenic effects, while others have androgenic properties, and so on.

Progestins' biological properties can be weak, strong (positive), or absent (negative). The strength of their effects depends on their activity about different receptors.

PROGESTIN NAME	PROGESTOGENIC PROPERTIES	ESTROGENIC PROPERTIES	ANTI-ESTROGENIC PROPERTIES	ANDROGENIC PROPERTIES	ANTI-ANDROGENIC PROPERTIES	GLUCOCORTICOID PROPERTIES	ANTI-MINERALOCORTICO	ANTI-GONADOTROPIC	DAILY DOSE FOR OVULATION
Progesterone	+	-	+	-	+	+	+	+	300
Pregnanes									
Dydrogesterone	+	-	+	-	+	-	+	-	30

									- 35
Medrogesterone	+	-	+	-	+	-	-	+	10
Chlormadinone acetate	+	-	+	-	+	+	-	+	1.5 -2
Cyproterone acetate	+	-	+	-	+	+	-	+	1
Megestrol acetate	+	-	+	+	+	+	-	+	10
Medroxyprogesterone acetate	+	-	+	+	-	+	-	+	10
19-Norpregnanes									
Nomegestrol acetate	+	-	+	-	+	-	-	+	5
Promegestone	+	-	+	-	-	-	-	+	0.5
Trimegestone	+	-	+	-	+	-	+	+	0.5
Estranes									
Norethisterone	+	+	+	+	-	-	-	+	0.5
Lynestrenol	+	+	+	+	-	-	-	+	2
Noretynodrel	+	+	+	+	-	-	-	+	5
Gonanes									
Levonorgestrel	+	-	+	+	-	-	-	+	0. 05
Desogestrel	+	-	+	+	-	-	-	+	0. 06
Norgestimate	+	-	+	+	-	-	-	+	0. 2
Gestodene	+	-	+	+	-	+	+	+	0. 03
Dienogest	+	+	+	-	+	-	-	+	1
Drospirenone	+	-	+	-	+	-	+	+	2

Legend:

- "+" - Positive effect
- "-" - Negative effect
- "+/-" - Weak positive effect

(Compiled from comparative pharmacology and potency data in Kühl (2011), Goldstuck (2011), Sitruk-Ware (2006), and pharmacodynamic profiles of gestodene, drospirenone, and cyproterone acetate)

The effect of natural progesterone on progesterone receptors is considered 100%, and the comparative analysis of different progestins is expressed in numerical values, indicating how much stronger their effect on these receptors is compared to progesterone. For example, levonorgestrel is 150 times more potent, 3-keto-desogestrel is 150 times stronger, nomegestrol is 125 times, promegestone is 100 times, and gestodene is 90 times more potent than progesterone, and so on.

It is essential to understand that these comparative biological impact values are relative, as determining the exact effect of hormones in laboratory conditions or within the animal and human body is extremely difficult.

Considering these indicators, it becomes clear why the dosages of progestins used for therapeutic and contraceptive purposes vary so much. For example, while the daily dose of progesterone required to suppress ovulation is 300 mg, the daily dose of various progestins is minimal, ranging from 0.03 mg (10,000 times less than the progesterone dose!) to 30–35 mg. This is why excessive use of progestins and sometimes incorrect combinations of different progestagens by doctors can lead to serious adverse effects.

The same applies to the impact of progestins on other steroid receptors. The strength of synthetic hormones' effects on various receptors has been determined using comparative methods, analyzing their influence alongside other steroid hormones such as testosterone, estradiol, cortisol, and others. This also explains the potential side effects of hormones on different organs and body systems.

5.3. Types of Hormonal Contraception

The modern market offers a wide variety of different forms of progestins. They are often classified by generation. There are four generations of progestins, but this classification is not widely used in everyday medical practice.

The first generation of progestins, including norethisterone, the second — norgestrel, levonorgestrel, the third — desogestrel, gestodene, norgestimate, and the fourth — drospirenone (a derivative of spironolactone), each have specific properties. For instance, the third generation has a weaker effect on blood lipid levels than others and has lower androgenic properties. The fourth generation of progestins is characterized by a mineralocorticoid effect similar to spironolactone (a diuretic and competitor of adrenal hormones, influencing water-salt balance). Understanding these properties is crucial in selecting the most suitable progestin for therapeutic or contraceptive purposes.

Even before World War II, *noretynodrel*, a derivative of testosterone, was synthesized. Thanks to this first synthetic contraceptive, oral (tablet) contraceptives were developed in combination with synthetic estrogen. Two types of synthetic estrogens are used in combined hormonal contraceptives, but the composition most often includes *ethinylestradiol* (EE).

Some progestins can bind to progesterone receptors, others — to androgenic receptors, and others — to estrogenic receptors. Additionally, progestins can bind to mineralocorticoid and glucocorticoid receptors. Depending on the type of binding, progestins can exhibit *progesterone-like, estrogenic, anti-estrogenic, androgenic, anti-androgenic, glucocorticoid, and anti-mineralocorticoid properties.* Progestins can also affect the pituitary gland and suppress the production of gonadotropins, exerting an *anti-gonadotropic effect.*

These different properties of hormones are essential to consider when selecting a progestin for therapeutic or contraceptive purposes. The choice of hormonal drugs, including hormonal contraceptives, should always be individualized.

Modern women are fortunate to have a wide range of hormonal contraception options. Expanding this range, including pure progestin formulations and combinations with synthetic estrogen, empowers women to choose the method that best suits their needs. The technique of hormone administration further diversifies the options, categorizing all contraceptives into distinct groups.

Combined:

- *Oral* (through the mouth and gastrointestinal tract): Tablet contraceptives, including combined oral contraceptives (COCs) and progestins (mini-pills). The hormone package contains 21 to 28 tablets, which are taken daily.

- *Transdermal* – Contraceptive patch. Applied to the skin once a week for three weeks with a one-week break. It is a combined formulation containing estrogens and progestins.

- *Vaginal* – Vaginal ring, a combined hormonal contraceptive. Used for three weeks with a one-week break. A new type of ring is available on the market that can be used continuously for a year.

- *Subcutaneous* – Implants.

Progestin-Only:

- *Intramuscular* – Injections are usually required every three months.

- *Intrauterine* – The intrauterine hormonal system (IUD) contains progestin. Used for five years.

A separate category is **emergency contraception**, which can be carried out by several methods, including taking hormonal medications.

The introduction of such a variety of hormonal contraceptive forms to the market allows for better consideration of women's preferences. For example, some women do not tolerate tablet forms well or forget to take pills on time so that they may opt for a vaginal ring or patch. The intrauterine system containing progestin is successfully used not only for contraception but also to improve the quality of menstruation in women suffering from uterine bleeding.

Combined oral contraceptives contain synthetic doses of estrogen and progesterone. Depending on the estrogen dose, they are classified as *micro-dosed, low-dosed, medium-dosed, and high-dosed.*

- Microdosed and low-dosed COCs are usually used by young women, teenagers, and perimenopausal women.

- Medium-dosed COCs are popular among middle-aged women, especially those who have given birth.

- High-dosed COCs are primarily used for therapeutic purposes and less frequently for contraception.

Depending on the combination and dose of hormones, COCs are classified as *monophasic, biphasic,* and *triphasic.*

- Monophasic COCs were among the first developed; they contained high estrogen doses, which remained constant throughout the cycle.

- Biphasic contraceptives contain two different progestin doses.

- Triphasic contraceptives have varying doses of both estrogen and progestin.

The wide variety of types, doses, and forms of hormonal contraceptives may seem overwhelming when it comes to selecting the right drug. However, it's important to remember that in most countries of the world, hormonal contraceptives are chosen by a doctor. This professional guidance ensures that many factors and necessary contraindications are considered, providing reassurance in the selection process.

5.4. Effectiveness of Hormonal Contraceptives

Hormonal contraceptives are considered highly effective birth control methods due to their multiple mechanisms of action. In medical literature, effectiveness rates are often presented in ways that people may not easily understand without a medical background. Most individuals want to know their actual chances of accidentally getting pregnant. However, there are no calculations of effectiveness for just one month of hormone use. **The efficacy of all hormonal contraceptives is measured based on one year of use.**

The effectiveness of contraceptive methods is determined by the number of women who become pregnant within a year while using a particular contraceptive correctly.

Additionally, there is a distinction between *perfect use* and *typical use* of contraceptives. Perfect use refers to taking contraceptives under ideal conditions, ensuring maximum effectiveness. However, in reality, numerous factors influence the absorption and metabolism of hormones, including body weight, diet, metabolic rate, pre-existing health conditions, interactions with other medications, tolerance to contraceptives, adherence to dosing schedules, and more.

There is no contraceptive method with 100% effectiveness except for abstinence from sexual activity.

For those using any form of contraception, it is crucial to understand the effectiveness of the method under typical use, as achieving perfect use is extremely difficult. However, following instructions as closely as possible is important to maintain optimal contraceptive effectiveness.

TYPE OF HORMONAL CONTRACEPTIVE	EFFECTIVENESS WITH PERFECT USE	EFFECTIVENESS WITH TYPICAL USE	PERCENTAGE OF WOMEN CONTINUING USE FOR ONE YEAR
COCs (Combined Oral Contraceptives)	98–99%	91–95%	50–85% after 6 months, 60% after 1 year

Mini-pills	99%	91%	60–85%
Transdermal patch	99%	91%	50–67%
Intrauterine system (IUD)	99%	99%	88–93%
Injections	99%	94%	56–58%
Vaginal ring	99%	91%	50–67%
Implants	99%	99%	83–85%

Why do IUDs and implants maintain such high effectiveness? Because they eliminate the human factor — the hormonal drug is inside the body, and its action occurs automatically. Therefore, long-acting contraceptives are the most effective.

It is important to remember that 90% of pregnancies occurring while using hormonal contraceptives result from incorrect or inconsistent use.

5.5. When and How to Start Taking Hormonal Contraceptives

Hormonal contraceptives can be started on any day of the menstrual cycle, if pregnancy is ruled out. Contraceptives that include a 7-day break (or placebo pills) establish an artificial cycle that mimics the natural one. This break is designed to allow for withdrawal bleeding, which reassures the user that pregnancy has not occurred. These cycles are almost always 28 days long, even though natural menstrual cycles can range from 21 to 35 days and may vary by up to 7 days in either direction. A perfect natural 28-day cycle is rare among women.

For optimal effectiveness, especially with oral contraceptives, it is recommended to start taking them:

- On the first day of the cycle (the first day of menstruation);

- Between the 1st and 6th day of the menstrual cycle;

- On the first Sunday or Monday of the menstrual cycle.

Starting within this timeframe eliminates the need for additional contraception while the hormones take effect. If hormonal contraception is initiated after the 6th day of the cycle, additional contraceptive measures are required for the next 7–10 days. This is because the contraceptive hormones take some time to build up to adequate levels in the body, and during this period, there is a higher risk of pregnancy.

Progestin-only contraceptives are best started on the first day of the menstrual cycle, with additional contraceptive methods recommended for one month.

The vaginal hormonal ring is inserted between the 1st and 5th day of the menstrual cycle.

Hormonal injections are administered within the first five days of the cycle and are typically repeated every three months (12 weeks). A single injection provides contraceptive protection for up to 14 weeks.

Implants are placed under the skin within the first 7 days of the menstrual cycle and are usually removed after five years. The same applies to intrauterine hormonal systems.

It is important to understand that the need for additional contraception at the start of hormonal contraceptive use varies depending on the hormone dosage, the method of administration, and the timing of the cycle.

Hormonal contraception can be used immediately after an abortion and six weeks after childbirth.

5.6. Contraceptive Regimens

Dr. Gregory Pincus introduced the 28-day progestin-based contraceptive regimen in the 1950s. He proposed taking hormonal pills for 21 days, followed by 7 days of placebo pills to induce withdrawal bleeding, mimicking the natural menstrual cycle. Until 1960, only synthetic progestins were used as contraceptives.

Interestingly, this regimen was chosen to align with the lunar cycle, making hormonal contraception more socially and morally acceptable not only to women and doctors but also to the Catholic Church. Many clinical trials of hormonal contraceptives were conducted in countries where Catholicism was the predominant religion. To this day, 15% of Catholics consider hormonal contraception unacceptable.

This approach mimics a natural menstrual cycle and has proven convenient and reassuring. The 28-day cycle, with its artificially induced withdrawal bleeding, is often perceived as a natural period. This serves as a comforting reassurance that pregnancy has not occurred, providing a sense of security and confidence in the effectiveness of the contraceptive.

Until the late 1970s, no medical publications questioned the "classic" contraceptive regimen. However, in 1977, data emerged supporting the continuous use of active hormonal contraceptive pills for 84 days to reduce the frequency of menstrual bleeding.

Modern medical debates continue over whether women need monthly periods and, if so, how often. Proponents of "infrequent menstruation" argue that women in economically disadvantaged countries experience about 160 fewer menstrual cycles over their lifetime (equivalent to over 10 years without menstruation) compared to women in developed nations. This is attributed to demographic factors—later onset of menstruation, earlier and more frequent pregnancies, and extended breastfeeding. While these women have a shorter life expectancy, they are less likely to suffer from hormonally dependent conditions such as breast and endometrial cancer.

Supporters of 'classic menstruation' argue that maintaining regular 28-day artificial cycles is preferable. It reassures women that their contraception is working and reduces anxiety about unintended pregnancy. They also claim that this regimen minimizes adverse effects on the body. However, no evidence has been found that taking contraceptives continuously for three months causes harm. While extended-cycle regimens may not be suitable for all healthy women, they can significantly improve the quality of life for those with certain medical conditions, offering hope and optimism for those seeking relief from menstrual disorders.

Menstrual disorders that may benefit from cycle manipulation include painful periods (dysmenorrhea), excessive or frequent bleeding, and irregular uterine bleeding. Although premenstrual syndrome (PMS) is not classified as a disease, some women experience severe symptoms. Endometriosis is also entirely dependent on hormonal fluctuations and menstrual cycles. Additionally, some women suffer from menstrual migraines, where attacks occur just before their period. Sometimes, it may be necessary to postpone menstruation due to life events such as weddings, vacations, or exams.

Thus, adjusting the contraceptive regimen allows for menstrual cycle modification, known as menstrual manipulation or suppression.

Recent studies indicate that about 35% of women prefer to have monthly withdrawal bleeding, while around 50% would instead eliminate menstruation. As times change, so do preferences.

Modern contraceptives can induce artificial menopause or significantly reduce the frequency and volume of menstrual bleeding (as with implants, intrauterine systems, and injections). This is especially beneficial for women who struggle with taking oral contraceptives consistently.

5.7. How to Choose the Right Contraceptive Method

One of the most common questions women ask is: "How do I choose the right contraceptive method?" Given the wide variety of available contraceptives, both hormonal and non-hormonal, the selection process depends on numerous factors. This is why it is often the responsibility of a healthcare provider, who plays a crucial role in guiding and advising women on their contraceptive choices.

- **Age** – A key factor in assessing fertility potential.

- **Frequency of sexual activity** – Determines whether long-term contraception is necessary.

- **Number of sexual partners** – This is important for evaluating the need for protection against sexually transmitted infections.

- **Personal preferences** – The woman's understanding of why a particular method suits her.

- **Consistency of use** – Whether she prefers a daily contraceptive (e.g., oral pills) or a long-acting method (e.g., injections, implants, intrauterine systems).

- **Duration of contraceptive need** – Whether she requires protection for a few days, months, or years. Hormonal contraceptives are generally intended for women who do not plan to conceive for at least a year.

- **Medical history** – Presence of systemic or other health conditions.

- **Weight** – A critical factor in determining the suitability of hormonal contraception.

- **Additional medical indications** – Some women may use hormonal contraceptives for reasons beyond pregnancy prevention, such as regulating menstrual cycles or managing certain health conditions.

- **Contraindications** – Any medical conditions that may prevent the use of hormonal contraception.

These details are gathered through a consultation rather than a physical examination or testing. The conversation is the most important step in determining which contraceptive method best suits a woman's needs and preferences. This individualized approach ensures that each woman feels understood and cared for when selecting contraception.

There is no universal contraceptive method that suits all women.

The next step in contraceptive selection is assessing the woman's physical health and reproductive system, if necessary. A gynecological examination is not always required, especially if the woman has no complaints or concerning medical history and has had a routine check-up within the past 6–12 months. The doctor may recommend additional tests, such as an ultrasound or laboratory evaluation. Still, the primary goal is to rule out any conditions that could be contraindications for specific contraceptive methods.

In many countries, screening for serious health risks, such as breast, ovarian, and cervical cancer, as well as sexually transmitted infections, including HIV, is recommended. However, these tests are not mandatory, and women can decline them.

Before prescribing contraception, the following medical assessments may be conducted:

- Gynecological examination (speculum and manual examination) – Required for intrauterine devices (hormonal or non-hormonal), diaphragms, cervical caps, and vaginal rings.

- Blood pressure measurement – Necessary before prescribing combined oral contraceptives (COCs).

Laboratory tests are not mandatory but may be recommended when necessary. These may include blood sugar, lipid profile, liver enzymes, hemoglobin levels, and blood coagulation assessments. A woman's weight is always considered, especially in cases of obesity.

Once a contraceptive method is selected, the doctor must discuss it with the woman, highlighting both its benefits and potential side effects. Many healthcare providers focus on the advantages while neglecting to mention possible complications.

It's important to note that hormonal contraceptives carry the highest risk of side effects and complications (including serious ones) because they contain steroid hormones. These risks should be carefully considered and discussed with your healthcare provider when choosing a contraceptive method.

It is crucial to exclude pregnancy before starting contraception, especially in the second half of the cycle or if there is a delayed period. If there is any uncertainty, a pregnancy test or a blood test for hCG should be performed.

Most women can begin using contraception, including hormonal methods, immediately after a doctor's visit. While it is generally recommended to start hormonal contraception at the beginning of the menstrual cycle, in urgent cases, when pregnancy is ruled out, contraception can be initiated right away. In such instances, a follow-up pregnancy test may be advised after four weeks.

Choosing contraception is more than just a medical science — it is an art that requires balancing effective pregnancy prevention with minimal impact on a woman's health and well-being.

5.8. How Long Can Hormonal Contraceptives Be Used?

As women's reproductive years have extended and menopause now occurs at an older age, many wonder how long hormonal contraception can be used, especially after the age of 40. Understanding when hormone use should be discontinued is empowering. One of the main concerns is that hormonal contraception can make it difficult to determine whether ovarian function has declined, and natural menopause has occurred.

Current recommendations suggest that women over 40 are generally better suited to progestin-only contraceptives, which do not contain estrogen. These can be used up to 55 when most women naturally reach menopause. Low-dose combined oral contraceptives (COCs) may also be an option.

To monitor the transition to menopause while using hormonal contraception, it is recommended that women over 45 have their FSH levels checked every six months. This regular monitoring provides reassurance and care. Family history, specifically, when a woman's mother entered menopause, may offer some insight, though it is not a precise predictor.

Approaching 55 years of age, FSH levels should be monitored more frequently. If two FSH measurements taken at least one month apart are above 30 IU/L, this indicates ovarian insufficiency and suggests that menopause has begun. In such cases, a woman may continue progestin-only contraception for another year (or up to two years if she is under 50). Often, progestin contraception is supplemented with hormone replacement therapy (HRT), or the woman transitions entirely to HRT if needed, discontinuing progestin use.

5.9. The "Hidden Pitfalls" of Hormonal Contraceptives

Hormonal contraceptives are designed for pregnancy prevention — this is evident from their name. However, because they contain steroid hormones, they are classified as pharmaceutical drugs.

As mentioned earlier, progestins in hormonal contraceptives not only mimic progesterone but also interact with various receptors in the body, producing additional effects. In some cases, this provides therapeutic benefits.

Hormones such as estrogen, testosterone, and progesterone have been used as medications almost since their discovery, though their applications were initially limited due to an incomplete understanding of their functions. Today, synthetic hormone analogs are widely used in many other areas of medicine, including gynecology and endocrinology.

Hormonal contraceptives were also introduced for therapeutic purposes, primarily for women who required contraception as well.

Do hormonal contraceptives offer benefits beyond birth control? Yes, they have been shown to:

- Regulate the menstrual cycle (though not in all cases);

- Reduce menstrual flow (by up to 50%);

- Decrease menstrual pain;

- Improve acne;

- Reduce hirsutism (excess hair growth);

- Lower the risk of anemia;

- Alleviate premenopausal symptoms;

- Increase bone density;

- Decrease the risk of endometrial cancer;

- Lower the risk of ovarian cancer;

- Reduce inflammation in the reproductive organs;

- Slow the growth of fibroids;

- Relieve pain associated with endometriosis;

- Eliminate ovulatory syndrome;

- Decrease the risk of rheumatoid arthritis.

These positive effects may persist for up to 15 years after discontinuation, particularly after long-term use (over five years).

However, alongside these benefits, hormonal contraception also has drawbacks, which are more numerous and often more pronounced. Many women stop taking hormonal contraceptives due to side effects.

Hormonal contraceptive pills are among the most widely sold pharmaceutical products in modern medicine. Over the past 20–25 years, their sales have surged, mainly due to shifting attitudes among doctors. While physicians once viewed COCs as serious steroid medications and were cautious about prescribing them, today, many doctors actively promote these contraceptives. Some are directly affiliated with pharmaceutical companies that manufacture hormonal contraceptives and receive financial incentives for prescribing them. This dynamic has raised questions about the influence of profit motives on medical practice and patient care.

The desire for pregnancy control among women and the profit motives of pharmaceutical companies have played a key role in the widespread adoption of hormonal contraceptives.

When hormonal contraception is recommended, women typically hear only positive aspects. Much of the information is misleading or outright false. Marketing claims about "ovarian rejuvenation," "wrinkle prevention," and "preservation of ovarian reserve" have contributed to the perception of hormonal pills as harmless, everyday products.

Interestingly, many women avoid eating sweets daily because they are "bad for health." Yet, they take steroid hormone drugs daily without hesitation — to prevent pregnancy or for other reasons.

If you search for "hormonal contraception" online, you will find thousands of glowing articles and videos, often repeating the same promotional messages word for word. But ask yourself:

- How many women read the package insert before taking hormonal contraceptives?

- How thoroughly do doctors explain the side effects and risks rather than just highlighting the benefits?

322

- Why does the list of contraindications include so many common health conditions affecting women of reproductive age?

Reliable data on how many women stop using hormonal contraceptives due to side effects and never return to them is nearly impossible to find, even in professional medical literature.

In the section above, I presented data on the percentage of women using hormonal contraception for a year. It turns out that a significant number of women stop taking hormonal contraceptives within a year.

Supporters of hormonal contraception argue that the high cost of these medications is the main reason women discontinue them. However, statistical analyses in countries with the highest rates of hormonal contraceptive use indicate that financial factors are not the primary cause.

The main reason women stop taking hormonal contraception is the high number of side effects.

Data on the number of women who discontinue hormonal contraception remains unclear and inconsistent. The manufacturers themselves heavily fund clinical studies evaluating the effectiveness of contraceptives. But who funds research on the complications of hormonal contraception or investigates why women stop using it?

For example, U.S. studies report that after six months of using combined oral contraceptives (COCs), only 15–85% of women continue. The range between 15% and 85% is enormous! Other sources suggest that about 60% of women discontinue COCs within a year. These conflicting numbers highlight how critical yet unreliable this information is for patients and doctors.

One crucial but often overlooked factor is body weight. Almost all hormonal contraceptive doses are designed for women weighing 70 kg. Some formulations are ineffective in women over 90 kg, while underweight women experience more side effects. Obese women, in turn, have an increased risk of metabolic syndrome, which can lead to impaired lipid and glucose metabolism and rapid weight gain.

The significant risks of hormonal contraception arise from its side effects, some of which can develop into serious, life-threatening complications. These include:

- *Venous thromboembolism* – Risk increases 3–4 times with low-dose COCs and doubles with progestins.

- *Arterial thrombosis* – The risk of heart attack or stroke increases 2–3 times, especially with high estrogen doses, smoking, hypertension, and other cardiovascular risk factors.

- *Breast cancer* – The risk increases 1.5 times for women who start taking hormonal contraceptives at a young age. This elevated risk persists for 10 years after discontinuation.

- *Cervical cancer* – Risk increases 1.5 times with five or more years of hormonal contraceptive use and is compounded by other risk factors.

- *Gallstone disease* – Risk increases 1.5 times within the first five years of using oral contraceptives.

Hormonal contraception can also exacerbate or trigger conditions such as hypertension, diabetes, liver disease, migraines, systemic lupus erythematosus, depression, and candidiasis.

The most frequently reported side effects of hormonal contraception include:

- Irregular bleeding – Occurs in 10–30% of COC users, 35–45% with progestins, 7–8% with vaginal rings, and 18% with contraceptive patches.

- Absence of menstruation (amenorrhea) – Reported in 2–3% of COC users.

- Breast pain and swelling – Up to 30% for oral contraceptives, 3% for vaginal rings.

- Weight gain – Reported by 35% of COC users.

- Mood changes – Up to 30% of COC users.

- Skin changes (chloasma).

- Nausea – 4.5% for vaginal rings.

- Headaches – 12% for vaginal rings.

- Reduced libido – Up to 40% for COC users.

- Acne.

- Local skin reactions – 20% for contraceptive patches.

- Vaginitis – 13.7% for vaginal rings.

- Vision disturbances – 27% for COC users.

Data on the adverse effects of hormonal contraception is highly fragmented because there are many different formulations worldwide, and side effects are rarely systematically recorded. Similarly, there is no reliable data on the number of women who stop using hormonal contraception due to side effects.

Hormonal contraceptives do not reduce fertility, but ovulatory cycles may take 3–12 months to restore in one-third of women after discontinuation fully. In recent years, a growing number of women, especially young women, have been diagnosed with hypersuppression of gonadotropin function. This is an iatrogenic condition linked to:

- High-dose COCs

- Long-term use of hormonal contraceptives

- Early initiation of hormonal contraception (before complete maturation of menstrual cycle regulation)

A typical scenario is that mothers take their teenage daughters to a gynecologist due to irregular cycles, usually normal during adolescence. Many doctors prescribe COCs to "regulate" the cycle, but this often leads to pituitary suppression, preventing natural gonadotropin production.

Once this condition develops, it isn't easy to treat. Many young women experience long-term amenorrhea, yet they are repeatedly prescribed COCs to "regulate" their cycle — further reinforcing pituitary suppression. The same syndrome is observed after prolonged use of COCs for contraceptive purposes.

The most significant risk associated with hormonal contraception is contraindications, which both doctors and patients must carefully consider. Due to the high risk of complications, particularly thrombosis, and the extensive list of contraindications, some countries are proposing that doctors obtain written informed consent before prescribing any form of hormonal contraception. Women must be fully aware that they are taking steroid medications with a long list of side effects and contraindications.

Hormonal contraception is strictly contraindicated in the following cases:

- Conditions associated with an increased risk of thrombosis, especially in an active state.

- Unexplained vaginal bleeding.

- Acute or chronic liver failure.

- Acute or chronic kidney failure.

- Existing or suspected breast cancer.

- Existing or suspected pregnancy.

Hormonal contraception is also not recommended in many other cases:

- Smoking (more than 15 cigarettes per day) combined with age over 35.

- Hypertension (may be used with antihypertensive medications).

- Cardiovascular diseases (heart disease, history of heart attacks or strokes).

- Diabetes (low-dose COCs may be used if blood sugar and lipid levels are well-controlled).

- Dyslipidemia and hyperlipidemia (hormonal contraceptives that do not affect lipid metabolism may be used).

- Epilepsy (anticonvulsants reduce the effectiveness of COCs, requiring high-dose formulations).

- Gallstone disease.

- Hepatitis cirrhosis (absolute contraindications in the acute phase; may be used if liver function tests are normal).

- Inflammatory bowel diseases (ulcerative colitis, Crohn's disease) – episodes of diarrhea can significantly reduce contraceptive effectiveness.

- Migraine – use of high-dose COCs is hazardous.

- Systemic lupus erythematosus – only progestin-only contraceptives are considered safe.

Not long ago, breastfeeding during the first six weeks postpartum was considered an absolute contraindication for COCs. However, with the introduction of low-dose hormonal contraceptives, women can now use them while lactating. Typically, hormonal contraception is started six weeks after childbirth, as ovulation may resume by that time.

In several countries, commercial testing for thrombophilias is increasing, especially among pregnant women or those planning pregnancy. Many of these women are prescribed heparin therapy. However, postpartum thrombosis monitoring is often neglected. The most paradoxical aspect is the recommendation of hormonal contraception both before pregnancy and after childbirth, despite the well-known risks of thrombosis in these periods.

5.10. What Else Should Women Know About Hormonal Contraception

Since this book covers more than contraception, much information will remain beyond its pages. However, before concluding the topic of hormonal contraception, it is important to address some of the myths surrounding it. There are many misconceptions, which will be debunked in another book. For now, here are some facts about hormonal contraception:

- Women taking COCs may experience withdrawal bleeding, breakthrough bleeding, or no menstruation at all — all of which are considered normal.

- Neither COCs nor other hormonal contraceptives reduce a woman's ability to conceive in the future.

- It's important to note that hormonal contraceptives do not cause congenital disabilities in newborns if a woman becomes pregnant while taking them. This fact should provide reassurance and confidence to women considering or using hormonal contraception. Women over 35 can use hormonal contraception if they have no contraindications.

- There is no need to take breaks from hormonal contraceptives if they continue to meet a woman's needs.

- There are no specific discontinuation protocols for hormonal contraceptives, including progestins and progesterone.

- If side effects occur within the first three months, switching to another hormonal contraceptive is not recommended. The choice is either to continue taking the same medication or discontinue it entirely, depending on the situation.

- Switching contraceptives due to concerns about the body "getting used to" a specific medication is unnecessary unless symptoms arise.

- A woman can use hormonal contraception until menopause if she does not smoke and has no contraindications.

- Ovaries do not "rest" or "rejuvenate" when taking COCs.

- COCs do not reduce the risk of functional ovarian cysts and do not treat them.

- Vaginal rings, patches, injections, hormonal IUDs, and implants belong to the same category as COCs and therefore share the same side effects and risks.

- The contraceptive patch will not detach due to physical activity or sweating.

- Wearing the patch does not prevent showering, bathing, using saunas, or swimming.

- While the vaginal ring can be removed for up to three hours, frequent removal reduces contraceptive effectiveness.

- Taking hormonal contraceptives before planning a pregnancy does not increase fertility.

- Modern hormonal contraceptives do not increase the likelihood of multiple pregnancies after discontinuation.

- To achieve contraceptive effectiveness, there is no need to combine multiple hormonal contraceptives, nor is additional contraception required if the medication is taken as directed.

- No form of hormonal contraception is superior to another — they are simply different delivery methods. Each has its drawbacks, but when used correctly, all hormonal contraceptives are 99% effective.

With this, we conclude the discussion on hormonal contraception and move on to an equally fascinating topic: the role of hormones in pregnancy.

Chapter 6. Pregnancy and Hormones

It is impossible to imagine pregnancy without hormones, especially progesterone. Often referred to as the "progestational hormone," progesterone is critical in supporting gestation. Pregnancy is, in many ways, a state dominated by progesterone. However, its role in conception and pregnancy is frequently misrepresented, leading to unnecessary medical interventions involving this hormone.

Previous chapters have already mentioned pregnancy, including the role of certain hormones in ensuring a successful pregnancy. This chapter will further explore the hormonal mechanisms of pregnancy, including the roles of estrogen, hCG, and other hormones in addition to progesterone.

6.1. How Hormones Affect Conception

Pregnancy occurs when a female reproductive cell (egg) is fertilized by a male reproductive cell (sperm). However, fertilization alone does not guarantee pregnancy. For pregnancy to occur, the fertilized egg must successfully implant and develop within the uterus. **Many fertilized eggs fail to implant, and approximately 70–80% of conceptions do not result in birth.**

Conception is an intricate, multi-step process that demands the precise interaction of male and female reproductive systems. Even a minor disruption can lead to failed fertilization or infertility, underscoring the need for caution and respect for the process.

After ejaculation, sperm entering the vagina must undergo a series of biochemical changes to become capable of fertilization. Even in healthy semen, only 10% of sperm acquire fertilizing potential, while most remain inactive. Fertilization occurs in the ampullary region of the fallopian tube, where a single sperm penetrates the egg's protective layers.

While the fertilization process may sound straightforward, it is a complex interplay of precise molecular signaling and hormonal interactions. The hormone progesterone is a key guiding factor for sperm movement, underscoring its crucial role in the process.

Sperm movement is activated only when ovulation has occurred, and a mature egg is present in the fallopian tube. Just before ovulation, the dominant follicle releases high concentrations of progesterone, significantly higher than the levels in the bloodstream. When the follicle ruptures, it releases the egg and follicular fluid rich in progesterone.

The fallopian tubes contain finger-like fimbriae, which help capture the egg and follicular fluid after ovulation. This results in a much higher progesterone concentration in one fallopian tube, guiding sperm toward the egg.

Progesterone directly affects sperm motility by stimulating calcium channels in the sperm tail, causing a rapid calcium influx. This enhances sperm movement and helps it navigate toward the egg. Unlike other hormonal processes, this activation is independent of genetic regulation, as mature sperm lack complete chromosomal sets.

Sperm do not all respond to progesterone equally. Their reaction depends on the number of progesterone receptors on the sperm membrane. A specialized structure called the *acrosome* covers the sperm head. It functions like a cap containing digestive enzymes, and this *acrosome reaction* is essential for sperm penetrating the egg's outer layer.

Upon contact with the egg, the sperm attaches to it, and the acrosome breaks down, releasing enzymes that help dissolve the egg's protective barrier. Progesterone, estradiol, and other signaling molecules regulate this process.

Successful conception is not just about the presence of sperm and egg. It requires the precise timing and coordination of sperm movement, quantity, and quality, underscoring the significance of these factors in the process.

Once fertilization occurs, the *zygote* begins its journey toward the uterus, undergoing sequential cell divisions. This process takes 4–6 days. Approximately 30 hours after fertilization, the first cell division occurs, setting the stage for embryonic development.

As division continues, the embryo reaches the 16-cell stage, at which point cell differentiation begins. At this stage, the developing embryo is called a *morula*. The morula enters the uterine cavity, where it continues dividing. Once fluid accumulates inside the morula, it becomes a *blastocyst*.

The blastocyst contains primitive *chorionic villi*, which help it implant into the uterine lining. This is when the pregnancy hormone - human chorionic gonadotropin (hCG), a hormone that supports the continued production of progesterone and estrogen, begins to be produced, ensuring the continued hormonal support of pregnancy.

6.2. What Is Needed for a Healthy Pregnancy

Every woman planning or carrying a pregnancy hopes for a healthy child. As mentioned earlier, the loss rates of fertilized eggs are remarkably high. **Most embryonic losses occur before clinical pregnancy is even detected, meaning before rising hCG levels and ultrasound confirmation**.

It's important to remember that early pregnancy losses are not unique to humans — they occur across the animal kingdom and are a natural part of reproduction. **This process is beyond our control, and while it may seem harsh, it's simply a biological reality.**

Reproductive studies in agriculture have advanced decades ahead of human reproductive medicine. For example, it is well-documented that over 60% of early pregnancies in cattle fail, with up to 80% of these losses occurring within the first days of embryonic development and implantation (between days 8 and 16 after fertilization). Nearly identical rates have been observed in humans.

What causes embryo loss? The key factors include genetic, physiological, endogenous (internal), and external (environmental) influences. Genetic factors play the most critical role — when errors occur at the genetic or chromosomal level, the development of healthy, viable offspring becomes impossible. All species, including humans, have high genetic and chromosomal abnormality rates.

**The laws of nature apply to all living beings —
anything unfit for survival is naturally eliminated**. It
is a mistake to place humans above other species regarding
reproductive success. Humans have far more reproductive
limitations than animals. Fertility is lower, multiple
pregnancies are considered a pathology, and due to human
brain size and skull expansion, childbirth has become a
complex and high-risk process.

Age is fertility's greatest adversary. It's a well-
established fact that fertility decreases with age, which is why
marriages were traditionally arranged at a young age, often
right after puberty. In 1895, American physician Dr. Duncan
published a study on fertility, infertility, and their
relationship to a woman's age, further solidifying this
understanding.

In the past 50 years, the average age for first-time
pregnancy has risen to 30–37 years in many countries. By
this time, signs of ovarian aging appear, with a declining
ovarian reserve and a significant drop in egg quality. This
affects conception and the early stages of embryonic
development, including cell division and implantation.

Hormones play an essential role in pregnancy,
particularly sex hormones and progesterone. Their impact
depends on the stage of pregnancy, which ultimately
determines pregnancy outcomes.

Studies have shown that removal of the ovaries during
the early days or weeks of pregnancy leads to slowed embryo
transport through the fallopian tubes, embryonic loss, and
failed implantation. However, research has revealed that
estradiol plays a far more significant role in guiding the
fertilized egg through the fallopian tubes than progesterone.

When estradiol is administered after ovary removal, it restores regular embryo transport, but does not improve embryo survival in the uterus, even when progesterone is supplemented.

Progesterone does play a role in moving the embryo through the fallopian tubes. When estrogen is absent, progesterone helps the embryo reach the uterus and supports blastocyst differentiation. However, neither estradiol nor progesterone alone is enough to ensure a healthy pregnancy. Their interaction is crucial — without a proper balance between these two hormones, pregnancy cannot be established or sustained.

The interplay between estrogen and progesterone is fundamental for pregnancy progression. Both hormones affect the embryo and the reproductive organs, and any imbalance, whether excess or deficiency, can prevent pregnancy from occurring or lead to early pregnancy loss.

No doctor, scientist, or researcher has determined the "ideal" ratio of estrogen to progesterone needed for pregnancy success.

Hormone levels measured in blood tests do not reflect the actual hormonal balance within the body. These tests only show hormone concentrations, which can fluctuate hourly, following natural biological rhythms that remain unknown to medicine. What is considered a "hormonal balance" in nature does not always align with medical definitions, and what doctors define as "normal" hormone levels may, in reality, be an anomaly for a particular woman or pregnancy.

Over 70 years of research on animals and humans has debunked many outdated medical theories about the role of sex hormones and progesterone in pregnancy. However, many doctors rely on these disproven theories in clinical practice.

Many factors influence pregnancy maintenance, which I discuss in detail in my book "9 Months of Happiness: A Practical Guide for Pregnant Women." If you are particularly interested in this topic, I recommend reading my book on pregnancy.

6.3. How Hormonal Levels Change During Pregnancy

Studying the intricate hormonal processes in the female body, particularly in pregnancy, I once humorously remarked that human life begins in a 'hormonal brine.' The egg matures in a follicle brimming with high concentrations of hormones — progesterone, testosterone, and estrogens. Later, the placenta churns out copious amounts of hormones at levels that would be unbearable for a non-pregnant woman if they entered her bloodstream directly. The fetal bloodstream is also a hub of hormones received from the placenta, adding another layer of complexity to this fascinating process.

6.3.1. Progesterone during Pregnancy

This book has repeatedly underscored the pivotal role of progesterone in various functions of the female body. In a non-pregnant woman, progesterone is produced by the corpus luteum, which forms after ovulation from the ruptured follicle. This type of progesterone is aptly named *luteal progesterone*, highlighting its origin. During pregnancy, the placenta takes over progesterone production, ensuring a steady supply of this crucial hormone for both the pregnancy and the developing fetus.

The corpus luteum of pregnancy is simply the ovarian corpus luteum that forms after ovulation. Before implantation, progesterone is produced independently of whether fertilization has occurred. However, once the first signals of pregnancy are received through various biochemical pathways, the corpus luteum continues functioning; it remains active until the luteal-placental shift occurs, meaning the placenta begins producing its progesterone.

For over 60 years, progesterone has been known to be the primary hormone produced by the ovaries. However, the function of the corpus luteum was not fully understood for many years.

Early progesterone extraction was primarily conducted using animal ovarian tissue, ranging from small rodents to cattle. In pregnant cows, the corpus luteum is large and cystic (luteomas), and this was the primary source for obtaining solid progesterone. At that time, scientists did not realize that progesterone production varies significantly among pregnant animals. Pregnancy relies entirely on corpus luteum progesterone in some species, while the placenta and fetus contribute considerably in others.

For example, cows depend entirely on corpus luteum progesterone. At the same time, pigs rely on both the corpus luteum and the placenta, and sheep transition from corpus luteum progesterone to placental progesterone by mid-pregnancy. **Each mammalian species has different progesterone sources and different roles for this hormone —attempts to model human pregnancy after cattle pregnancies led to incorrect conclusions.**

In the 1920s and 1930s, early experiments on animals showed that removing the ovaries in early pregnancy caused pregnancy loss. Scientists then hypothesized that corpus luteum secretions were essential for pregnancy maintenance.

Research on corpus luteum function in pregnancy began over 70 years ago in animals and 50 years ago in humans during the early days of reproductive medicine. The results of these early studies formed the basis for four decades of progesterone use in IVF and other assisted reproductive technologies (ART). However, the optimal duration of progesterone supplementation remained debated among doctors.

Studies from the 1970s–1980s showed that removing the corpus luteum before 7 weeks of pregnancy led to a progesterone drop and pregnancy loss. However, after 8 weeks, removal did not affect progesterone levels or pregnancy continuation. These findings confirmed that luteal progesterone is only essential until 7–8 weeks of pregnancy.

Further research in reproductive medicine later revealed that corpus luteum progesterone supports pregnancy only until 4- to 5 weeks (the first three weeks after conception). By 7–8 weeks, the placenta becomes the primary progesterone source, marking a natural and reassuring progression of hormonal changes during pregnancy.

As progesterone levels increase during pregnancy, so do the levels of its derivatives, particularly sex hormones.

Progesterone stimulates growth hormone production in both the maternal and fetal pituitary glands. Fetal growth depends on sufficient levels of this hormone. Two other hormones — prolactin in the mother and placental lactogen in the placenta, structurally similar to growth hormone and contribute to tissue development. Their levels rise significantly during pregnancy.

The breasts begin to grow and enlarge, preparing for not only childbirth but also breastfeeding in the baby's first year of life. Progesterone and prolactin, like siblings, work together to stimulate breast development.

The increase in progesterone levels also raises concentrations of many other essential pregnancy hormones, ensuring normal fetal growth. There is no need to fear these hormonal changes, nor should they be medically altered unless clinically necessary.

Interfering with the natural hormonal processes of pregnancy can increase the risk of pregnancy loss.

Progesterone and Pregnancy Outcome Prediction

How do doctors predict pregnancy outcomes? This question is most relevant in reproductive medicine, particularly after IVF and other assisted reproductive technologies (ART), where success rates are crucial due to high costs and emotional investment. Many protocols exist to monitor pregnancy progression, yet none offer a clear advantage or high enough sensitivity to be universally recommended.

One of the earliest methods for predicting pregnancy outcomes was measuring progesterone levels before pregnancy (during the luteal phase) and between 4–8 weeks of pregnancy. However, this method proved to be unreliable for several reasons:

- Progesterone levels fluctuate throughout the menstrual cycle, making single measurements inaccurate.

- Luteal progesterone can be low even in regular menstrual cycles without affecting conception or implantation.

- Healthy menstrual cycles can present with varying progesterone levels—from low to high—without predicting pregnancy failure.

- The corpus luteum's progesterone production is regulated by pregnancy-related factors and signals from the embryo. If the embryo is abnormal, supplementing progesterone does not improve pregnancy outcomes.

- By 7–8 weeks of pregnancy, the luteo-placental shift occurs: corpus luteum progesterone decreases while placental progesterone rises.

- Placental progesterone production is independent of the mother's body—it functions autonomously, regardless of fetal health.

- Administering external (exogenous) progesterone does not affect placental progesterone levels and is not utilized by the placenta or fetus.

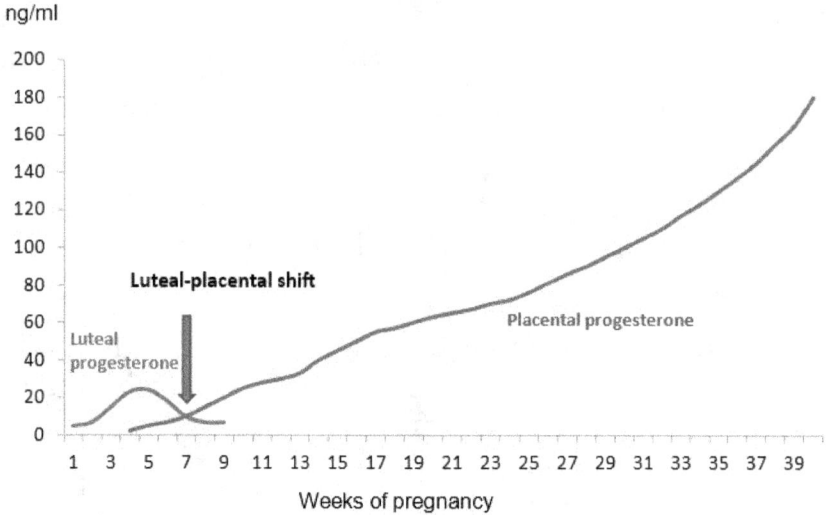

ng/ml

Weeks of pregnancy

Thus, measuring progesterone levels before and after pregnancy onset has little predictive value and is not used in modern obstetrics. If implantation is compromised, corpus luteum and placental progesterone levels naturally decrease. However, implantation failure is not caused by progesterone deficiency but rather by an unhealthy embryo.

For multiple pregnancies, early progesterone measurement is also ineffective in predicting pregnancy outcomes. Until 7–8 weeks, luteal progesterone dominates in the mother's bloodstream, and the number of embryos does not influence progesterone synthesis. Until 10 weeks, there is no difference in luteal or placental progesterone levels between singleton and multiple pregnancies. After 10 weeks, progesterone levels vary significantly between women, making measurements impractical. Most spontaneous pregnancy losses (including twin pregnancies) occur before 8 weeks, rendering progesterone measurements useless for prediction.

Progesterone and Pregnancy Outcomes in Cases of Vaginal Bleeding

If progesterone levels cannot reliably predict pregnancy outcomes in asymptomatic women, could they be beneficial for women experiencing vaginal bleeding, often diagnosed as threatened miscarriage? Can progesterone levels help detect ectopic pregnancy?

Doctors commonly consider progesterone levels between 3.2 and 11 ng/mL (10 and 35 nmol/L) normal before 14 weeks. Some define the minimum normal threshold as 5 ng/mL (16 nmol/L).

Clinical studies indicate that:

- If progesterone levels in women with bleeding, pain, and inconclusive ultrasounds are below 3.2 ng/mL, the probability of a non-viable pregnancy is 99%.

- If progesterone is above 6 ng/mL, the risk of pregnancy loss is 44%.

- When progesterone is below 6 ng/mL, the risk of a missed miscarriage is about 74–75%.

- However, progesterone testing is unreliable for diagnosing ectopic pregnancy.

Among women with bleeding or pain whose ultrasound confirmed an intrauterine pregnancy, the average minimum normal progesterone level was 10 ng/mL. Nearly 97% of women with progesterone below this level had a missed miscarriage, while 37% of those with progesterone above 10 ng/mL also had non-viable pregnancies.

The higher the progesterone level, the harder it is to predict whether the pregnancy will continue or fail. Conversely, the lower the progesterone, the harder it is to measure accurately, though very low levels strongly suggest pregnancy loss.

Although various graphs and models have been developed to correlate progesterone levels with pregnancy outcomes, they have not been adopted in clinical practice. The main reasons are measurement inconsistencies, including differences between total, free, and bound progesterone levels in plasma and serum.

A single progesterone measurement is only helpful in diagnosing missed miscarriage in cases of vaginal bleeding, abdominal pain, and unclear ultrasound findings. However, it is entirely unreliable for diagnosing ectopic pregnancy, normal pregnancy viability, or spontaneous miscarriage.

For women with symptoms but no ultrasound findings, progesterone testing is not a reliable method for confirming a viable pregnancy and is not recommended by most doctors.

Important Additional Information About Progesterone

Entire books could be written about progesterone; every time one is published, new research and updated recommendations emerge from professional organizations. I strive to share these latest findings on my official website and social media with as many people as possible. There is overwhelming information, so that I will highlight some of the most common misconceptions regarding progesterone.

- There is no such thing as "pregnancy-preserving therapy," which is why progesterone is not prescribed in the first trimester for bleeding, hematomas, or lower abdominal pain.

- Progesterone is not prescribed for non-viable pregnancies, such as blighted ovum or missed miscarriage.

- In modern obstetrics, progesterone medications are not combined in different forms.

- Excessively high doses of administered progesterone can block progesterone receptors, disrupting the body's natural progesterone production and utilization potentially leading to pregnancy complications.

- Although progesterone is sometimes prescribed for recurrent pregnancy loss (three or more early miscarriages), its effectiveness is low.

- Vaginal progesterone is prescribed after IVF and sometimes in other reproductive technologies as part of supportive therapy. The duration of progesterone use is 15 days, or rarely until 6–8 weeks of pregnancy.

- There is no withdrawal protocol for progesterone. A woman can stop taking it immediately, which will not affect a normal pregnancy's progression.

- Vaginal progesterone is used in women with a short cervix (less than 2.5 cm) who have had previous pregnancy losses, typically from 16 to 32–34 weeks. The recommended dosage remains a subject of debate.

- Vaginal progesterone may be used to prevent preterm birth in women who previously delivered prematurely due to cervical insufficiency.

- Progesterone is not used after 34 weeks of pregnancy in any form.

- Oral progesterone is poorly absorbed in pregnant women, which is why vaginal formulations are preferred.

- Due to its low effectiveness, progesterone is no longer used to stop preterm labor (as a tocolytic).

6.3.2. Male Sex Hormones During Pregnancy

Pregnancy is a unique physiological state that triggers massive changes in the female body, including significant hormonal fluctuations. In recent decades, some doctors have begun treating pregnancy as if it were a disease, requiring frequent testing and "corrections" simply because laboratory values often fall outside the normal range for non-pregnant women. The problem is that many laboratories do not provide reference values for different trimesters, leading to unnecessary concerns.

Pregnancy is not a disease. Many biological markers in the blood change over nine months, including male sex hormones (androgens). Due to rising estrogen levels, the concentration of sex hormone-binding globulin (SHBG) increases, which binds testosterone, leading to a rapid rise in total testosterone levels, detectable as early as two weeks after conception. The ovaries, specifically the corpus luteum of pregnancy, are the primary source of this early testosterone increase.

During pregnancy, total testosterone rises due to an increase in the bound testosterone fraction, while free testosterone remains unchanged until the third trimester (week 28), after which it doubles. The source of this late pregnancy testosterone increase remains unknown but likely involves both maternal and fetal contributions. Women carrying male fetuses tend to have slightly higher testosterone levels than those carrying female fetuses.

In the third trimester, androstenedione levels rise, and DHEA-S levels increase early in pregnancy, thought to originate from the fetus. However, DHEA-S levels decline significantly by the second half of pregnancy, influenced by the placenta. Despite these changes, free testosterone levels remain stable until the third trimester, and even then, its increase does not significantly affect target tissues.

Androgen concentrations in maternal blood are three to four times higher than in the fetus's umbilical cord blood.

Despite increased maternal total and free testosterone levels, most women and fetuses are protected from androgenic effects and do not develop hyperandrogenic symptoms. Several robust mechanisms ensure this protection:

- SHBG levels increase, reducing free testosterone activity.

- Progesterone suppresses androgen receptor sensitivity and inhibits the conversion of testosterone precursors into active testosterone.

- The placenta converts testosterone into estrogens (estrone and estradiol).

- The placental barrier prevents significant maternal testosterone from reaching the fetal bloodstream.

Elevated maternal androgens do not affect male fetuses. Hyperandrogenism can only impact female fetuses, particularly between weeks 7 and 12, when external genital development occurs. This is the most critical period during which excess androgens may cause clitoromegaly. After week 12, the risk of genital abnormalities decreases, and labial fusion does not occur.

It's important to note that hyperandrogenism during pregnancy does not lead to pregnancy loss or miscarriage, providing reassurance about the safety of the pregnancy despite hormonal changes.

The most common cause of androgen elevation in pregnant women is *luteomas* — benign ovarian growths caused by the massive proliferation of luteinized cells. These false tumors develop only during pregnancy and disappear spontaneously after childbirth. Luteomas can grow from 1 to 25 cm, with an average size of 6–10 cm. In half of cases, both ovaries are affected. Ultrasound may reveal hemorrhagic areas within the tumor, but no treatment is required, pregnant women are monitored. Surgical removal is rare and performed only in exceptional cases.

Theca-lutein cysts are another source of elevated androgens in pregnancy. They are most seen in multiple pregnancies, gestational trophoblastic disease (hydatidiform mole, choriocarcinoma), and mothers with diabetes. Women with polycystic ovary syndrome (PCOS) may also develop theca-lutein cysts during pregnancy. Unlike luteomas, cysts are not tumors—they are fluid-filled reservoirs.

A third cause of increased androgens in pregnant women is the *use of synthetic hormones*, including progestins and androgens.

True hyperandrogenism in pregnancy is an infrequent occurrence, reinforcing the robustness of the body's regulatory mechanisms.

6.3.3. Female Sex Hormones and Pregnancy

Estrogens are essential for fetal development. They increase blood flow in blood vessels, particularly in the uterine arteries, which enhances the delivery of oxygen and nutrients to the growing fetus.

For the first 5–6 weeks of pregnancy, the corpus luteum is the exclusive producer of estrogens, particularly 17β-estradiol, for the developing embryo. By the end of the first trimester, the fetus and placenta take over estrogen production, leading to a 300-fold increase in maternal estrogen levels by the end of pregnancy (from 0.1 ng/mL to 30 ng/mL).

17β-estradiol acts as a blood flow stimulator, while other estrogens are less active. Estrogens also regulate placental progesterone production, stimulate breast growth (together with progesterone), and influence the development and function of the fetal adrenal glands.

Placental estriol (E3) appears in maternal blood by week 9 of pregnancy. This hormone's levels increase even more dramatically than estradiol levels, from 0.01 ng/mL in non-pregnant women to 30 ng/mL before labor — a nearly 3000-fold rise. Between weeks 35 and 40, estriol levels increase sharply, signaling hormonal changes in preparation for labor.

Estrone (E1), like estradiol, is produced in the first 4–6 weeks by the ovaries, adrenal glands and partly by maternal fat tissue. Later, the placenta becomes the primary source of circulating estrone. By the end of pregnancy, estrone levels increase 100-fold (from 0.3 ng/mL to 30 ng/mL).

Estrogen levels vary among pregnant women, fluctuating between 2–30 ng/mL. These fluctuations are due to the changing needs of the developing fetus and the mother's body. Estrogen levels significantly rise before labor, signaling the body's preparation for childbirth.

Measuring estrogen levels in pregnancy has no clinical application. However, one specific type of estrogen — unconjugated estriol (uE3) — is used in prenatal genetic screening tests.

6.3.4. Placental Lactogen

Placental lactogen, also known as chorionic somatotropin or chorionic growth hormone, is closely related to human growth hormone (hGH), although it is 100 times weaker in its cellular effects.

The term "lactogen" highlights its similarity to prolactin — another hormone that stimulates mammary gland development in preparation for breastfeeding.

Placental lactogen, like a silent guardian, influences maternal blood sugar levels. During pregnancy, especially under stress, maternal blood becomes more 'sugar-loaded,' ensuring that the growing fetus receives sufficient energy and nutrients.

In the past, placental lactogen levels were thought to be a crystal ball for predicting pregnancy outcomes, especially in complications. However, like many others, this method proved to be a mirage and is no longer used in clinical obstetrics.

6.3.5. Prolactin and Pregnancy

There is a close relationship between prolactin, the endometrium, and pregnancy. The activity of endometrial prolactin and prolactin receptors plays a crucial role in signal transmission during *endometrial decidualization* and *implantation*. A deficiency of endometrial prolactin during implantation has been observed in women who have infertility and recurrent spontaneous miscarriages. Similar findings have been reported in studies investigating the role of endometrial prolactin in animal models.

Women with endometriosis also exhibit impaired prolactin absorption. However, there is no conclusive evidence that endometriosis increases the risk of spontaneous abortion.

The rise in prolactin levels during pregnancy contributes to the growth of mammary glands and their preparation for lactation. The highest prolactin levels are observed before childbirth, at the end of the third trimester. It is hypothesized that prolactin may be involved in the mechanism triggering labor.

6.3.6. Human Chorionic Gonadotropin (hCG)

Pregnancy hormones, particularly human chorionic gonadotropin (hCG), are integral. This hormone is present only during pregnancy. As the name suggests, hCG is a derivative of the chorion, the part of the fertilized egg that later develops into the placenta. "gonadotropin" indicates its chemical relationship with pituitary gonadotropins (FSH and LH). Chorionic or placental gonadotropin is found in some primates but is absent in other mammals.

The practical significance of determining hCG levels in early pregnancy cannot be overstated. It confirms the presence of pregnancy and provides crucial information about its progression. In most cases, hCG testing is used to diagnose ectopic pregnancy, a practical application of our research findings.

Human chorionic gonadotropin (hCG) is produced by the cells of the fertilized egg, meaning it is not a maternal (female) hormone. However, it can be detected in very small amounts in the blood outside of pregnancy. Even in cases of an anembryonic pregnancy (blighted ovum), hCG levels may still be elevated. Additionally, certain ovarian and, in some cases, other tumors can produce hCG.

A unique feature of hCG is that it consists of two subunits — alpha and beta:

- The α-hCG subunit has the same structure as the corresponding subunits of other female hormones: luteinizing, follicle-stimulating, and thyroid-stimulating hormones.

- The β-hCG subunit has a unique structure specific to pregnancy-related hCG. Therefore, β-hCG is most measured in blood serum.

This hormone must reach a specific concentration to be detected in blood serum, where it appears 7–8 days after conception (i.e., days 21–23 of the menstrual cycle) and in urine 8–9 days after conception. hCG levels increase until weeks 10–12, and their growth slows down, followed by a secondary rise after 22 weeks.

hCG levels below 5 mIU/mL are considered negative for pregnancy, while levels above 25 mIU/mL are considered positive.

Many doctors have adopted the standard that hCG levels should double every two days as an indicator of a developing pregnancy. However, research has shown that doubling may occur more slowly, and an increase of 1.4 times every two days is also a normal parameter. Moreover, such a pattern of hormonal growth is observed only in the first 4–5 weeks of pregnancy.

In 85% of pregnant women, hCG levels double every 48–72 hours. After reaching peak levels at 9–10 weeks, hCG production declines and, after 16 weeks, stabilizes at levels similar to those observed at 6–7 weeks of pregnancy. In the second half of pregnancy, hCG levels constitute only 10% of their peak at 10 weeks.

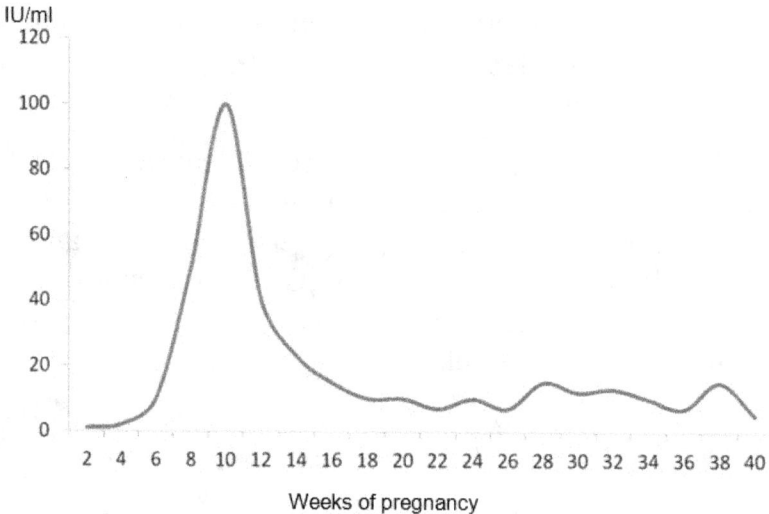

hCG levels vary so widely that determining the exact gestational age based on them is impossible. For example, at 4 weeks, hCG levels can range from 23 to 4,653 mIU/mL, and at 5 weeks, from 114 to 45,800 mIU/mL. The same woman may have completely different hCG levels in separate pregnancies. Additionally, certain pregnancy conditions and multiple pregnancies may be associated with elevated hCG levels. From a practical standpoint, the exact gestational age should be known before measuring hCG levels.

While measuring β-hCG can help diagnose spontaneous miscarriages and ectopic pregnancy, it is important to note its limitations. It is unreliable for predicting pregnancy outcomes when a live embryo is present in the uterine cavity. This underscores the need for further research and the development of more reliable prognostic methods in reproductive health.

Despite its inaccuracy in predicting pregnancy outcomes, measuring progesterone, hCG, or both is still widely used in clinical practice due to the absence of more reliable prognostic methods.

In all publications, especially older ones, textbooks, and even my previous publications, it is stated that hCG supports the function of the corpus luteum during pregnancy. This belief is a medical dogma accepted by doctors and their patients, with rare exceptions. It has become a habitual assumption, reinforced by adopting research findings from half a century ago. But how reliable is this assertion?

No causal link has been established or proven between hCG production and progesterone production, nor has any evidence demonstrated that progesterone synthesis depends on hCG production.

The peak function of the corpus luteum, as I previously mentioned, is observed at 4–5 weeks, and by 7–8 weeks, this function ceases. Placental progesterone production begins with the onset of implantation, just like hCG in general. The peak of hCG occurs around 9–10 weeks, after which its level rapidly declines and, upon reaching

356

values similar to those at 6 weeks, remains stable, except for short fluctuations in the second half of pregnancy. At the same time, placental progesterone production increases significantly despite the decline in hCG levels.

Could the rising hCG levels suppress progesterone production by the corpus luteum? If hCG truly stimulated luteal progesterone synthesis, then additional administration of hCG would help sustain pregnancies by supporting implantation and stimulating the corpus luteum. However, numerous experimental studies have shown that this does not happen.

When carefully tracking corpus luteum progesterone production, the peak occurs precisely during implantation — between 3 and 5 weeks of pregnancy. From week 5 onward, luteal progesterone begins to decline while hCG rises intensively, nearly doubling from weeks 4 to 5.

Thus, hCG does not play a key role in stimulating the corpus luteum. Then what does? It appears that the embryo itself while traveling through the fallopian tube into the uterine cavity and awaiting the implantation signal (a process that typically takes 7 days), secretes certain substances that support corpus luteum function and luteal progesterone production. This could be tau-interferon, chaperonin 10, early pregnancy factor, or another specific protein—possibly an as-yet-undiscovered substance. However, hCG levels do not rise significantly until the chorion develops. In the first week after conception, hCG remains very low, while corpus luteum function remains unchanged. Conversely, as soon as hCG starts rising rapidly, luteal progesterone production declines, and by week 7, its levels drop significantly while placental progesterone production increases.

Despite the parallel rise of hCG and placental progesterone, these are two independent processes. This discovery, which challenges previous assumptions, significantly advances our understanding of early pregnancy. **No direct link has been found between hCG levels and placental progesterone production.** After reaching its peak, hCG declines to very low levels while placental progesterone production continues steadily.

As a result, many physicians, me included, are increasingly questioning the long-held belief that hCG stimulates corpus luteum function, which is likely incorrect.

In obstetrics, studying the effects of hCG on pregnancy has largely been overlooked, as hCG has not found a practical role as a medication. In reproductive medicine, it is still sometimes used to stimulate ovulation, though other gonadotropins are now more commonly prescribed. However, with the evolving understanding of hCG's role, its potential applications in reproductive medicine could also change.

I would also like to mention the recent trend of testing pregnant women for hCG antibodies, especially among those who have experienced pregnancy loss. Such testing has no practical application in obstetrics. Any attempts to detect or 'eliminate' these antibodies from the body should be regarded as medical malpractice rather than sound clinical practice, as they can lead to unnecessary treatments and potential harm to the patient.

6.4. Gestational Diabetes

Since we are discussing pregnancy hormones, it is impossible not to mention gestational diabetes, a relatively new diagnosis in disease classification. Many people are aware of the dangers of diabetes. Worldwide, complications from diabetes lead to up to 3 million deaths annually, and approximately 180 million people suffer from this condition. However, gestational diabetes is not caused by excessive consumption of sweets and baked goods.

In all pregnant women, two key processes occur that have a profound effect on glucose metabolism. The first process is **accelerated fasting**, closely related to the natural drop in blood sugar levels overnight. Since women do not consume food during sleep, it is logical that blood sugar levels decrease significantly.

Morning blood sugar measurement is commonly used to diagnose diabetes and monitor its treatment. However, pregnant women experience an even more significant drop in glucose levels due to their body's response to overnight fasting (which explains why many women wake up hungry and need to eat at night). In addition to low blood sugar, fatty acid levels in the blood increase, accelerating the formation of ketones (ketone bodies are frequently detected in the urine of pregnant women and are considered normal).

Low blood sugar levels in the first trimester are also associated with gradual plasma volume expansion. However, the growing fetus uses a significant amount of glucose as energy as pregnancy progresses.

The liver increases glucose production by 30%, automatically stimulating insulin secretion from the pancreas. However, certain placental hormones reduce cellular sensitivity to insulin. Poor dietary habits (such as skipping breakfast) can lead to rapid metabolic disturbances and intensify accelerated fasting.

The second process observed in pregnant women is the **increased breakdown of nutrients**, primarily to ensure a rapid supply to the fetus. Changes in maternal insulin sensitivity affect carbohydrate metabolism and protein and fat metabolism. As a result, a pregnant woman's blood becomes rich in energy-producing substances — fatty acids and triglycerides, which also play a role in hormone production by the placenta and the fetus.

Despite experiencing accelerated fasting and enhanced nutrient breakdown, pregnant women often gain weight quickly, a pattern also seen in type 2 diabetes. Weight gain is linked to self-preservation mechanisms that store energy for successful fetal development since pregnancy significantly strains the female body. Oxidative processes are intensified in pregnancy, which is why pregnancy is sometimes referred to as a state of oxidative stress, potentially leading to oxygen deficiency in various organs.

It has been established that most women who develop gestational diabetes (but have normal blood sugar levels before and after pregnancy) are at increased risk of developing diabetes later in life.

Measuring blood glucose levels alone is insufficient for diagnosing diabetes, as these levels fluctuate throughout the day and are influenced by various factors. What matters is not just glucose levels but how the body processes and utilizes energy derived from glucose metabolism and how it responds to excess sugar and other carbohydrates in the diet.

For this reason, the glucose tolerance test (GTT) was introduced in the early 1980s. This test provides a more accurate prediction of diabetes risk and is now widely used by doctors worldwide.

Pregnant women are generally a young population group, far from the typical demographic at risk for diabetes. However, GTT results show that many pregnant women have abnormal glucose metabolism. In 10–15% of cases (depending on the country or region), gestational diabetes is diagnosed. Furthermore, studies have shown that women with abnormal GTT results have a higher incidence of pregnancy complications (e.g., large-for-gestational-age babies, stillbirth, and complications during delivery). Approximately 25–30% of women with gestational diabetes give birth to babies weighing over 4 kg.

Diagnosing gestational diabetes remains challenging, as I have discussed in many of my publications on pregnancy, including my book "9 *Months of Happiness*." Gestational diabetes screening is recommended between 24–28 weeks of pregnancy.

Gestational diabetes is a field in obstetrics that still requires extensive research to establish optimal guidelines for both pregnant women and healthcare providers.

Chapter 7. Menopause and Hormones

As you've journeyed through this book, you've become familiar with menopause and its challenging symptoms. This knowledge empowers you to navigate this phase with confidence and control. With increasing life expectancy, a significant portion of a woman's life is now spent in menopause, a phase that is as inevitable as it is manageable.

Some women mistakenly believe that they lose their femininity once menstruation stops. The unpleasant symptoms of menopause are linked not only to hormonal changes but also to psycho-emotional factors. In many women, psychosomatic responses dominate, amplifying other contributing factors.

Modern women, whose social and professional activity is much greater than previous generations, are concerned with maintaining a youthful and healthy appearance. They explore ways to slow aging or even reverse it. At the same time, as they enter menopause, many look for ways to counteract declining hormone levels, often viewing menopausal hormone therapy as the optimal solution.

7.1. Can Aging Be Slowed Down?

Aging is a normal physiological process for all living beings. Cells, tissues, and organisms age over time. I often hear pregnant women say that some doctors frighten them with the term "placental aging," insisting on urgent hospitalization and rejuvenation treatments. In such cases, I recommend reminding the doctor that over nine months of pregnancy, not only does the placenta age, but so do the fetus, the pregnant woman, and the doctor.

It's important to remember that aging is a natural part of life, not something to be feared. Old age often brings various bodily dysfunctions, chronic illnesses, and limitations in mobility, but these are all part of the human experience. With the proper care and support, these challenges can be managed, allowing us to embrace the fullness of life.

However, the fear of aging has given rise to numerous myths, fueling a market for "anti-aging" solutions. Throughout history, people have sought "elixirs of youth," "elixirs of life," and "elixirs of beauty." Yet, ironically, none of the creators of these "miraculous antidotes" have become younger or lived longer than their peers.

Today, thanks to the internet, the advertising and sale of countless "anti-aging" and "rejuvenation" products have skyrocketed. There is immense psychological pressure from mass media, dictating beauty and youth standards to society.

Men, too, struggle with aging, as 60% of men over 40 experience erectile dysfunction. While they do not go through menopause, they still age, even though sperm production can continue into old age. However, sperm quality significantly declines after 55–60 years.

I will not discuss skin rejuvenation, supplements, hormone treatments, or plastic surgery. Instead, let's focus on the so-called "rejuvenation" of the ovaries using hormonal contraceptives.

Since women now postpone childbirth until later in life, the question of preserving ovarian reserve (the limited number of eggs a woman has from birth) has become increasingly relevant. A lack of knowledge about reproductive function often leaves women struggling with infertility later on. This has led to the development of technologies aimed at preserving eggs, much like sperm banking. Although significant limitations remain, egg and ovarian tissue freezing is now used in medical practice.

Since the timing of menopause largely depends on ovarian reserve, what reduces it? This is a genetically predetermined process beyond a woman's conscious control. However, several external factors can accelerate ovarian depletion, including:

- Surgical interventions involving the ovaries or pelvic organs (e.g., laparoscopies) that disrupt ovarian blood supply.

- Medication use or overuse, particularly drugs that stimulate egg maturation or impair microcirculation in the pelvis.

- Radiation therapy and chemotherapy.

- Any disruption of blood supply or nerve function in the ovaries and pelvic organs.

- Harmful habits, mainly smoking, damage microcirculation in ovarian tissues.

Genetic mutations (e.g., in the FMR1 gene) can also accelerate follicular depletion. These mutations may be inherited or occur spontaneously.

Thus, if a woman has even one of these risk factors, menopause may occur significantly earlier.

Once ovarian reserve is lost, it cannot be restored. No drug or medical method can slow or stop egg depletion.

Hormonal contraceptives do not halt ovarian depletion, even though they suppress ovulation. Some doctors claim that contraceptives "put the ovaries at rest" and "rejuvenate" them, but this is misleading, whether due to ignorance or commercial interest. It is important to acknowledge two key facts:

- Women who have taken hormonal contraceptives for 10–15 years have not remained younger nor preserved their youth. They age at the same rate as women who never used contraceptives. The external signs of aging are identical in both groups.

- Women who delayed childbearing and used hormonal contraceptives for 10–15 years face fertility challenges just as frequently, if not more so, than those who never used them. They often experience more difficulties since ovulation may take several months to resume after discontinuation.

Hormonal contraceptives suppress ovarian function by inhibiting the hypothalamic-pituitary system. This is a forced intervention in hormonal regulation, replacing natural hormone production with synthetic substitutes. Calling this process "ovarian rest" is simply wordplay designed for specific agendas — in reality, it is the manipulation of women's health.

Menopausal hormone therapy (previously known as hormone replacement therapy) consists of essentially the same synthetic hormones as contraceptives, only in lower doses. However, this therapy does not have rejuvenating effects — it merely suppresses ovarian function and replaces natural hormones.

What slows aging? The answer is surprisingly simple: a healthy lifestyle! This includes:

- A balanced, nutrient-rich diet.

- Regular physical activity.

- Positive cognition (the ability to interpret and respond to life and people positively).

Life is a unique, strange, and complex journey that includes youth, maturity, and old age. Each phase is irreplaceable. Life always moves toward death, yet many people remain trapped in past suffering and future fears, failing to live in the present or appreciate what they have. Old age is not a sentence — it is normal.

Fearing old age is like burying yourself alive in the past. No "rejuvenation" has ever made a person younger or happier.

7.2. Menopausal Hormone Replacement Therapy

Hormone therapy (HT), a significant medical intervention used in menopause to treat climacteric syndrome and various gynecological conditions, holds a rich historical significance. It was once more popular than hormonal contraceptives and predates them by several decades.

The rise in HT usage was primarily driven by the baby boomer generation, born between 1946 and 1964. As they entered retirement while striving to maintain their social and professional activities, the need for HT became more pronounced. This connection to a specific generation makes the topic more relatable.

7.2.1. A Brief History of Hormone Therapy

After the discovery of estrogens in 1923, research into hormone-based treatments progressed rapidly, with the first estrogen-containing drugs hitting the market by 1926. These drugs, initially used to treat climacteric syndrome, became a global health trend, especially among wealthier white women in the U.S. and Europe. However, access to these medications was limited for most women worldwide.

Until the late 1940s, estrogens were prescribed for menopause symptoms based more on theoretical assumptions than on proven effectiveness. The first suggestion that estrogen therapy could prevent climacteric syndrome came from Drs. Geist and Spielman in 1932. Shortly after, Dr. Reifenstein proposed a connection between osteoporosis (bone loss) and menopause, suggesting hormone therapy as a treatment.

Robert Wilson conducted the most in-depth research on this topic. In the 1950s, he described the direct relationship between ovarian function decline, the onset of climacteric symptoms, and multiple aging-related changes in the female body. To counteract these effects, he advocated the use of estrogen therapy.

In 1966, Wilson published a book in the UK titled "Feminine Forever," which became enormously popular, not just among doctors but especially among women in Europe and the U.S. In this book, he introduced the concept of "estrogen deficiency syndrome," proposing estrogen therapy as the treatment.

In 1969, the International Health Foundation, responding to public debates about hormone therapy for menopause, conducted a survey of women in five European countries (400 women per country). The study revealed that women's knowledge about menopause and its treatment was directly influenced by media coverage — the more widely the topic was discussed, the more informed women were about hormone therapy. German women were the most knowledgeable about estrogen therapy, and Germany had the highest readership of Wilson's book.

Following these discussions, the rationale for prescribing hormone therapy was widely debated. By this time, several synthetic forms of progesterone had been developed, and the first hormonal contraceptives had entered the market. It was proposed to combine progesterone with estrogen in HT to counteract the potential adverse effects of estrogen on the uterine lining, which could increase the risk of endometrial cancer. This combination was believed to provide the benefits of estrogen therapy while minimizing its risks.

Many women and even some doctors mistakenly viewed hormone therapy (and some still do) as a rejuvenation treatment, a panacea for reversing menopause and restoring premenopausal youth. Dr. Robert Norman, a prominent figure in the field, opposed this view, emphasizing that **the primary goal of HT is to help women manage menopause symptoms at the hormonal (endocrine) level, not to reverse aging.**

European countries were the first to embrace HT as a standard treatment for climacteric syndrome, and soon, it was widely prescribed. including to women who had undergone hysterectomies or oophorectomies. Moreover, hormone therapy was sometimes offered to asymptomatic women in perimenopause simply as a preventative measure to delay ovarian aging, even though ovaries age regardless of hormone use. Some doctors even advocated lifelong HT for all women over 45.

The UK was an exception among European countries, approaching HT more skeptically and cautiously. The British medical community adopted HT approximately eight years later than Germany and other European nations. The growth of HT use in the UK can largely be credited to Wendy Cooper, whose 1975 book, "No Change: Biological Revolution for Women," actively promoted hormone therapy.

Interestingly, many myths about medications, and their widespread use, originate from "sensational" books, often written by non-medical authors with media connections rather than scientific expertise.

In the U.S., the situation was quite different. Until the early 1990s, American doctors were mainly resistant to HT — only a small number of physicians prescribed hormone therapy to menopausal women. However, the publication of books by Dr. Lee, a retired family physician, sparked a surge in progesterone prescriptions among menopausal women, often at their request.

7.2.2. How Hormone Therapy Can Be Beneficial

Perimenopause and menopause are accompanied by a range of symptoms, many of which I have already discussed in previous chapters. To better understand when hormone therapy (HT) is effective and when it is not, let's categorize the most common symptoms into three groups:

- **Vasomotor symptoms**: hot flashes, excessive sweating, chills.

- **Urogenital system changes**: vaginal dryness, vaginal inflammation, painful urination, urinary incontinence.

- **Psycho-emotional issues**: mood disorders, anxiety, insomnia, depression.

In addition to these symptoms, there are long-term health risks that remain unnoticed for a certain period:

- Loss of bone density (osteoporosis).

- Increased risk of cardiovascular disease.

Each woman experiences a unique combination of symptoms and risks. The doctor's role (and it must be a doctor's role) is to determine:

1. To what extent do these symptoms affect a woman's quality of life?

2. Whether non-hormonal treatments can alleviate the symptoms.

3. If hormone therapy is required, which medication and form should be preferred?

For many older women, hormone therapy offers a ray of hope amid menopausal symptoms, particularly hot flashes. To mitigate the potential side effects of estrogen, women often combine it with progesterone. The most prescribed hormones for managing menopause symptoms are estrogens, progesterones, and, in some cases, androgens.

While hormone therapy can alleviate symptoms and prevent bone loss, it's important to note that it can also affect breast tissue. Studies have shown that HT can increase breast tissue density, especially when estrogen and progesterone are combined. Additionally, using 'natural' estrogen has been linked to more abnormalities than synthetic progesterone, which can complicate the detection of breast cancer.

Since estrogen is often mistakenly considered a "bad hormone" and progesterone a "good hormone," women have increasingly turned to different forms of progesterone. Numerous clinical studies have compared the effects of micronized progesterone (MP) and medroxyprogesterone acetate (MPA), a synthetic form of progesterone. However, many of these studies contain biases and inconsistencies. No significant difference has been observed in symptom relief or breakthrough bleeding between different forms of progesterone. MP and MPA have similar effects on the breasts, cardiovascular system, and other organs.

Endocrinology societies in some countries warn against the claims that micronized progesterone is safer or superior, stating that such claims are unproven, premature, and lack scientific evidence. Most professional obstetrics and gynecology associations strongly discourage the combination of different forms of progesterone or switching from one form to another.

Progesterone is a form of hormone therapy regardless of its formulation, and both doctors and patients must recognize a simple fact: a hormone is a hormone, regardless of how it is administered.

7.2.3. Concerning Facts About Hormone Therapy

In 2002, the results of the American clinical study Women's Health Initiative (WHI) were published, examining the use of estrogens and progestin (MPA) in hormone replacement therapy for menopausal women. The study revealed a 26% increase in breast cancer risk, along with a higher incidence of cardiovascular diseases, strokes, blood clots, and thromboembolism compared to the control group of women who took a placebo. The study included 16,608 women aged 50–79 from 40 U.S. clinical centers and was conducted between 1993 and 1998.

The results shocked not only doctors but also millions of women who were either undergoing hormone therapy or planning to start it in search of a safer treatment option combining estrogens and progesterone. Following the publication, the prescription rate for estrogen-progesterone therapy dropped by 63% within just three months. This meant that millions of women were suddenly left without treatment. In response, around 70 books critically analyzing hormone therapy were published in English, with many more in other languages in a very short period.

Another large-scale study in the United Kingdom, conducted between 1996 and 2001, examined the impact of hormone therapy on breast cancer risk in 1,084,110 women aged 50–64. The findings confirmed that HT significantly increased the incidence of breast cancer, especially when estrogen and progesterone were used together, much more so than with estrogen alone.

Some of my Canadian colleagues, who were trained in medical school during the 1990s, recall that prescribing hormone therapy to all postmenopausal women was not just a recommendation — it was a dogma. Young doctors believed in it so strongly that few ever questioned whether the data supporting the benefits of HT could be inaccurate or even misleading.

By 1999, more than 90 million women worldwide were taking hormones after menopause. The results of the WHI study and the UK study shocked the medical community, particularly gynecologists and family doctors, who were the primary prescribers of hormone therapy. Many abandoned the practice due to concerns about severe side effects and the ethical questions it raised. How could they continue to recommend a treatment that had been proven to have serious risks? How can patients trust doctors if their recommendations, and the scientific knowledge behind them, are false?

However, to the credit of American and European physicians, as soon as new data emerged, they openly and courageously began warning women about the potential risks of HT. Despite the controversy it may have stirred, this proactive approach reassured women that their doctors were committed to their well-being.

By 2005, follow-up studies, though smaller in scale, indicated that most menopausal women were now aware of the serious risks associated with hormone therapy, and they had received this information primarily from their doctors.

Yet, the publication of new findings on the dangers of HT led to another unintended consequence: the search for alternative treatments for menopausal symptoms. At first glance, this is a positive shift. However, the reality was that many doctors and patients quickly turned to "natural" progesterone as a replacement for synthetic forms despite these products being sold without regulation or quality control.

The problem was that many so-called "natural" progesterone products contained little or no actual progesterone, and the dosages were not clinically validated. None of the available "natural" progesterone formulations had undergone rigorous clinical trials for safety and efficacy.

The media further fueled the controversy. While some headlines painted doctors as the villains, accusing them of only prescribing 'approved pharmaceuticals' while ignoring alternative treatments, it's important to note that this was not the universal view. When serious clinical studies failed to support 'natural' hormone therapies, some media outlets blamed doctors for not recommending these unverified alternatives, suggesting that women should take matters into their own hands. However, other media sources provided balanced coverage, highlighting the need for evidence-based medicine and the potential risks of unregulated 'natural' hormone therapies.

Such misleading arguments were actively promoted, and not without financial incentive, by pharmaceutical companies selling "natural" hormones, eager to increase their sales.

A review of 130 studies on alternative treatments for menopausal symptoms, including "natural" progesterone creams, found that their effects were no greater than placebo. This does not diminish the potential value of alternative medicine, but it confirms a crucial psychological factor: woman's mindset profoundly influences her experience of menopause and its symptoms. If she believes a treatment will help, it likely will. No conventional or alternative treatment will make a difference if she does not.

7.2.4. The Modern Approach to Prescribing Hormone Therapy

The history of hormone therapy outlined earlier shows that it began with estrogen. Today, women have a much wider range of options, including:

- Estrogens

- Combined estrogen-progestin therapy

- Selective estrogen receptor modulators (SERMs)

- Gonadomimetics (containing estrogens, progesterone, and androgens)

Hormones can be administered in various forms, like hormonal contraception. This variety of options, including tablets, rings, patches, injections, and implants, allows patients to choose the method that best suits their needs. Creams and gels are also available for localized use.

What are the modern indications for hormone therapy? You may be surprised to learn that they remain contradictory. While hormone therapy was once widely prescribed, today, there is a noticeable gap between understanding its necessity and its actual use. The fear of cancer, blood clots, and the responsibility for potential severe complications from steroid hormones make both doctors and patients cautious.

There is also debate over whether hormone therapy should be used preventatively. When it is prescribed for symptom relief, the goal is clear:

- To reduce vasomotor symptoms (hot flashes).

- To alleviate urogenital symptoms.

These are currently the primary indications for hormone therapy.

Hot flashes can occur before menopause, but their frequency increases as menopause approaches. They are typically most intense during the first one to three years of menopause and then subside. However, a small percentage of women experience them for a more extended period (up to 10 years). In such cases, hormone therapy for 1–3 years can provide relief from frequent and severe hot flashes.

Urogenital symptoms tend to worsen with age, making long-term hormone therapy necessary in some cases.

Hormone replacement therapy may also be used to prevent or slow the progression of osteoporosis, but it is not a standalone indication for hormone use. In other words, hormone therapy should not be prescribed solely for osteoporosis prevention, especially in women with natural menopause.

For early menopause, hormone therapy remains a controversial recommendation. On one hand, these women may experience hot flashes, which can justify treatment. On the other hand, their symptoms may be mild, leading to the question of whether osteoporosis prevention alone warrants hormone therapy. **Currently, there are no clear guidelines on using hormone therapy solely for osteoporosis prevention in women with early menopause**. If a woman does not want to take hormones, a calcium-rich diet and regular physical activity can be just as beneficial as hormone therapy.

Beyond these indications, there are no additional reasons to prescribe hormone therapy. This may seem surprising given the widespread use of hormones in Europe, the U.S., and Canada just a few decades ago.

What about hormone therapy in reproductive-age women? There has been considerable overuse in this group as well. The justification often sounds simple: hormone therapy "supplements" ovarian hormone production, which is supposedly insufficient. This claim, however, is false. Hormone therapy suppresses ovarian function and, in most cases, prevents ovulation, acting as a contraceptive. Women planning pregnancy should not take hormone therapy.

There is no solid evidence in modern gynecology supporting the use of hormone therapy to treat diseases or support various health conditions, except in cases of functional ovarian insufficiency (early menopause, artificial menopause, or natural menopause).

It is essential to understand that menopausal hormone therapy is neither safer nor better than hormonal contraceptives. These are still estrogens and progestins — steroid hormones. Therefore, the contraindications for hormone therapy are nearly identical to those for contraceptives. However, because hormone therapy has been in use much longer than general hormonal treatment, and many of its early prescriptions predate evidence-based medicine, its guidelines remain contradictory and inconsistent. The field remains unclear and full of conflicting information.

The main contraindications for hormone therapy include:

- History of breast cancer
- History of endometrial cancer
- Acute liver disease
- High levels of fatty acids
- Blood clotting disorders and thrombosis
- Unexplained vaginal bleeding

These are not the only contraindications. For some medications, endometriosis and fibroids are also considered contraindications.

Interestingly, medical guidelines do not consistently list contraindications and side effects. Many drug package inserts also lack complete and accurate information. Many outdated recommendations have become dogma, and some doctors still adhere to them. This is why it is essential to ask questions:

- Is hormone therapy necessary in your case?
- Are there alternatives? (There almost always are.)
- What are the potential risks?

A well-informed approach is key to making the right decision.

7.3. Myths About Phytohormones

Understanding the nature of phytoestrogens and phytoprogesterones is crucial when considering their use in treating various gynecological conditions. It's also important to clarify the concept of 'non-hormonal hormones' of plant origin, a term often used by doctors. Let's delve into the facts about phytohormones to gain a comprehensive understanding.

Steroids structurally similar to sex hormones and progesterone have been found in 60–80% of plant species studied over the past few decades.

Interest in the biochemical structure of plants dates back nearly a century, coinciding with the development of organic chemistry. However, the study of plant-derived compounds peaked in the 1950s and 1960s, when researchers were fervently searching for anticancer drugs. This period saw the study of hundreds of thousands of natural and synthetic compounds, some of which were named due to their applications in both alternative and conventional medicine.

Research on plant steroids is a dynamic field that continues to evolve. The discovery of new steroidal compounds underscores the increasingly close connection between the plant and animal kingdoms. While some steroids are unique to plants, their study is instrumental in developing new pharmaceuticals.

The animal kingdom is also rich in steroid compounds, including sex hormones and metabolites. All mammalian species produce progesterone. Interestingly, the role and application of progesterone in animals, particularly those raised in agriculture, have been studied in far greater detail than in humans.

7.3.1. Phytosterols

Virtually all plants contain organic sterol compounds, commonly referred to as phytosterols. Fungi contain ergosterol, while animals have only one type of sterol— zoosterol, or cholesterol. These sterols are essential for the survival of both plants and animals, playing a role in numerous biochemical reactions and serving as building blocks for hormone production.

Phytosterols, the plant-based sterols used in progesterone synthesis, differ structurally from human progesterone molecules. As a result, they cannot be converted into progesterone or estrogens inside the human body.

Progesterone from Wild Yam

The conversion of phytosterols into progesterone or estrogens occurs only in laboratory settings and never in nature. This is because the sterol molecule must be modified to resemble human cholesterol. For example, stigmasterol undergoes 11 chemical reactions before transforming into progesterone.

Cholesterol is a natural precursor of progesterone, so one might assume that producing progesterone from cholesterol would be the most efficient approach. However, this process is costly and economically unviable. Therefore, progesterone is synthesized from plant sources such as soybeans (Glycine max), various species of yam (Dioscorea composita, floribunda, mexicana, villosa, deltoidea, nipponica), agave, fenugreek, calabar beans (Physostigma venenosum), certain lilies, yucca, nightshade plants, and corn. The most used phytosterols for progesterone production are *stigmasterol, diosgenin, beta-sitosterol, campesterol, hecogenin, sarsasapogenin,* and *solasodine.*

Many promotional materials for progesterone-based supplements claim they contain "natural progesterone derived from wild yam" or "natural progesterone from diosgenin." But is modern "diosgenin-based" progesterone genuinely natural, or is it a synthetic derivative of wild yam?

Wild yam is considered a medicinal plant in several countries. Indigenous peoples of South and North America have long used it to treat diabetes, gastrointestinal disorders, arthritis, and tumors.

Scientists have known since the 1930s that Mexican wild yam contains diosgenin. In 1940, American chemist Russell Marker patented a method for synthesizing progesterone from diosgenin, a process that became known as "Marker degradation" in his honor.

It's a common misconception that progesterone derived from wild yam is natural. It's a semi-synthetic, bioidentical progesterone. This method uses diosgenin and was widely used for nearly 40 years until American chemist William Summer Johnson successfully synthesized progesterone in 1971.

Marker's groundbreaking discovery sparked a global search for yam species capable of producing larger quantities of progesterone, underscoring the collaborative nature of scientific research.

Wild yam is cultivated as a food crop in many countries. The most common edible species include white yam (Dioscorea rotundata) and yellow yam (Dioscorea cayenensis), which have over 200 subspecies and are primarily grown in Africa. Purple, or water yam (Dioscorea alata), is popular in South Asia and some parts of Africa. Japanese mountain yam, or Chinese yam (Dioscorea opposita), is commonly known as sweet potato in Europe and is widely used in Chinese and Japanese cuisine. Unlike wild yam, cultivated edible yam species do not contain diosgenin.

In the 1950s, the annual collection of approximately 5,500 tons of dried wild yams for steroid hormone production was a significant economic endeavor. The cost of producing 1 gram of progesterone had dropped from $200 in 1940 to 30 cents by 1956, a testament to the advancements in progesterone synthesis. Mexico's monopoly on diosgenin production for over 20 years further underscores the economic implications of this field.

As wild yams became increasingly difficult to harvest, the cost of transporting raw materials from remote jungles to processing centers made production even more expensive. This led to a global search for alternative yam suppliers capable of producing diosgenin identical to the Mexican variety.

Today, China is the primary supplier of diosgenin extracted from soybean oil. With the introduction of soy-based diosgenin in 1980, yam-derived progesterone production was almost entirely phased out. The use of soybeans significantly reduced the cost of progesterone production, and within the last 10 years, most pharmaceutical companies producing progesterone have switched to soy-based sources.

Diosgenin is also found in fenugreek seeds (Trigonella foenum-graecum), which were used early in ancient Egypt to induce labor. Hippocrates mentioned fenugreek in his writings, and it was commonly used in Europe to treat gynecological conditions.

Due to its structural similarity to cholesterol and other steroids, diosgenin has been used to synthesize various steroid hormones. Other commonly used saponins in pharmaceutical production include hecogenin and tigogenin.

Progesterone obtained via semi-synthesis from diosgenin and other saponins is structurally identical to human progesterone produced by the ovaries. This means it can be absorbed by the body's cells and tissues with minimal resistance, making it more bioavailable than fully synthetic progestins. Additionally, this progesterone can synthesize other hormones once in the body rather than always acting as pure progesterone in target tissues. This does not occur with synthetic progestins.

Many so-called "natural progesterone" products are labeled as containing diosgenin or being derived from diosgenin, leading many women to assume that all such products offer identical high-quality progesterone. The problem is further exacerbated by doctors recommending wild yam extracts containing diosgenin as so-called "natural homeopathic alternatives" for gynecological and obstetric conditions. But let's be honest — no one truly knows what inside dietary supplements, creams, and ointments is marketed as "natural progesterone."

When applied to the skin in cream form, diosgenin is not absorbed and does not affect tissues sensitive to estrogen and progesterone. No study has confirmed that diosgenin can be converted into progesterone inside the human body. This substance is not bioidentical to human hormones.

When considering the production of pharmaceuticals, 75% of medications used to treat infectious diseases and 60% of anticancer drugs available on the market since the 1980s are derived from natural sources. Other categories of drugs also contain a significant number of plant- and animal-derived ingredients. However, no one refers to these drugs as "natural."

If a product labeled "natural progesterone" contains an extract from soybeans, yam oils, agave, or other plants, it does not contain progesterone.

7.3.2. Phytoestrogens

As soon as hormone replacement therapy (HRT) was linked to an increased risk of cancer and various side effects, the search for estrogen substitutes and alternative treatments for menopausal symptoms began.

Since menopausal symptoms appear to be less frequent among Eastern women (Chinese, Korean, Japanese, and Vietnamese), it was hypothesized that the consumption of large amounts of soy products helps them tolerate menopause better. However, the situation turned out to be different. In Eastern cultures, menopause is perceived as a new stage of life dominated by wisdom, experience, and mastery. In other words, in most cases, unpleasant symptoms, especially hot flashes, are manifestations of psychosomatics.

The perception of menopause as a natural part of life prevents the occurrence of hot flashes. Multiple clinical studies have confirmed this.

Phytoestrogens are plant-derived compounds believed to have estrogen-like activity but not hormones. Why are phytoestrogens so popular? They fall into the category of dietary supplements, meaning they do not require oversight by regulatory bodies responsible for evaluating the quality, efficacy, and safety of pharmaceutical drugs. They do not require extensive clinical trials before being introduced to the market or used in medical practice. Unlike hormones, they can be sold without a prescription. However, it's important to note that their benefits remain unproven, and their risks are still poorly studied. This should make us more cautious and critical of unsubstantiated claims, as they have become an attractive commercial product, generating enormous profits for manufacturers.

Nonetheless, let's examine phytoestrogens from a scientific and medical standpoint. Until 1990, there were virtually no publications on this topic. Interest in phytoestrogens surged after studies linked HRT to an increased risk of cancer and thrombosis. The peak of such publications occurred between 1998 and 2000.

Estrogenic ingredients (but not estrogen itself) have been found in more than 300 plant species, but they are hardly absorbed in the human and animal body, with only a few exceptions.

Phytosterols, which were mentioned earlier, are not hormones. Among phytosterols often mistakenly attributed with estrogenic properties, β-sitosterol, campesterol, and stigmasterol do not bind to estrogen receptors in animals, including humans, and therefore do not exhibit hormonal activity.

The first discussions of phytoestrogens arose in agriculture. In the 1980s, scientists observed declining fertility among cows and sheep grazing on clover. Formononetin in clover also affects bird reproduction. This led to further studies of plants containing phytosterols and phytoestrogens.

The exact number of compounds in nature that can be conditionally classified as phytoestrogens is unknown. There may be several hundred. A little over 100 phytoestrogens have been described in detail, and some have been studied in animal models (mainly in agricultural research).

By chemical structure, phytoestrogens are classified into the following categories:

- Chalcones
- Flavonoids (flavones, flavonols, flavanones, isoflavonoids)
- Lignans
- Stilbenoids
- Other classes

Isoflavonoids have been studied more extensively than other classes. They include subclasses such as *isoflavones, isoflavanones, pterocarpans,* and *coumestans.* However, in popular literature, there is excessive confusion in the naming and classification of phytoestrogens.

Regarding their effects on humans, the best-studied phytoestrogens come from soy, red clover, chickpeas, hops, licorice, rhubarb (rheum), yam, and vitex. Phytoestrogenic isoflavonoids have also been found in beans, peas, kudzu root, sesame seeds, sunflower seeds, peanuts, oats, rye, strawberries, cranberries, blueberries, raspberries, red cabbage, broccoli, zucchini, carrots, beets, black and green tea. The list of phytoestrogen-containing foods could go on.

The sheer number of plants, including fruits and vegetables that supposedly contain beneficial "hormones" has led to an explosion of various dietary supplements in the modern market, whose quality and efficacy have never been scientifically proven. Most importantly, **no established dosage for their use exists, meaning that any manufacturer can set their dosage recommendations**.

Sometimes, people ask: why not simply consume all these vegetables and fruits to "restore hormonal balance" instead of spending money on questionable supplements? This is not a question for experts but for anyone with common sense.

Almost all isoflavones in plants exist in a unique glycosylated form, meaning they are bound to carbohydrates, and the absorption of these forms varies among different animal species. As a result, no reliable animal models could be used to study the effects of phytoestrogens on humans.

Moreover, data from animal studies is often misinterpreted and exaggerated, leading to misleading claims about their actual significance in human health.

Gut bacteria can break down certain flavonoids into forms that the human body can absorb. The interaction with intestinal microbiota plays a key role in determining how phytoestrogens are metabolized and their potential biological effects on the body. Despite many phytoestrogens, only enterodiol and enterolactone, formed from genistein and daidzein in soy, have been studied in humans. Interestingly, one-third of people are unable to absorb these compounds.

After changing in the intestine, some phytoestrogens may bind to estrogen beta-receptors. Theoretically, they could exert effects similar to estrogen, as estrogen receptors exist in various tissues and organs. However, no conclusive evidence exists that this occurs in the human body. In other words, the estrogenic effect of phytoestrogens in the human body remains purely theoretical despite numerous laboratory experiments. In reality, we do not fully understand whether phytoestrogens act through hormonal or non-hormonal mechanisms due to a lack of research on these substances.

The vast number of publications on the potential benefits of phytoestrogens for the reproductive, skeletal, immune, and nervous systems, as well as for skin health and other organs, suggests that the topic is popular. However, the scientific evidence supporting these claims remains extremely weak. The amount of reliable data available allows only for speculation about the potential benefits of phytoestrogens without clearly understanding their actual effects or an effective dosage. More research is needed in this area.

Many scientists and doctors remain hopeful that phytoestrogens could lead to new, high-quality medications for treating various conditions, including cancer. However, just like true estrogens, phytoestrogens may also increase the risk of breast cancer and other reproductive system disorders.

The central conflict between scientific research and commercial pseudoscience lies in the fact that conducting large-scale clinical trials on phytoestrogens according to the principles of evidence-based medicine requires significant funding. Meanwhile, phytoestrogen supplements are already a profitable business that does not require scientific validation — only aggressive advertising with grandiose claims about their miraculous ability to solve all women's health problems.

Thus, the decision to take soy and clover supplements (the most marketed) ultimately falls on the individual woman and her belief in the effectiveness of phytoestrogens.

7.4. Myths About Bioidentical Hormone Therapy

After the decline of interest in hormone replacement therapy (HRT) due to the publication of serious side effects in the early 2000s, a vacuum emerged in the medical field regarding the treatment of menopausal conditions. The absence of an effective and simultaneously safe alternative led to the spread of various rumors, myths, and misinformation, which caused as much harm as hormone therapy itself. This is how the myth of the safety and benefits of bioidentical hormone therapy (BHT) arose, where the word "replacement" was swapped for "bioidentical," which many people perceived as "natural." As a result of this wordplay, bioidentical hormone therapy (BHT) was born.

The promotion and endorsement of this therapy were taken up by various individuals, including doctors and popular "elite celebrities." Suzanne Somers, an American actress, singer, and savvy businesswoman, became a vocal advocate for the same hormone replacement therapy but under the rebranded name of BHT. In 2006, she published the book *Ageless: The Naked Truth About Bioidentical Hormones*, where she confidently claimed that bioidentical hormones could help maintain a slim figure, shiny hair, wrinkle-free healthy skin, good brain function, and strong protection against cancer, heart attacks, and other diseases. Without medical education, the author confused several critical aspects of hormone classification and failed to provide clinical research data to support her claims.

Somers's book was artificially elevated to a sensation level due to her media connections, including television. Millions of American women purchased the book in hopes of gaining reliable information about hormone therapy, especially since Somers herself had been using hormones for years.

In 2009, Oprah Winfrey, a well-known television host, invited Somers onto her show, where the actress recommended using this therapy, dismissing doctors' warnings that bioidentical hormones were neither safe nor a genuine alternative to HRT. Interestingly, Somers was diagnosed with breast cancer in 2001, and in 2008, she underwent a hysterectomy due to precancerous endometrial changes, possibly even cancer.

Doctors had warned Suzanne that her health issues could be linked to years of hormone therapy use. According to one interview, Somers received daily injections of growth hormone, vitamin B, estrogen suppositories, and estrogen applications and took 60 different dietary supplements — all of which she believed were the foundation of youth and a way to prevent aging.

Suzanne Somers is one example of how celebrities and media figures can significantly influence public opinion. Their advice on health and medicine, often backed by financial ties to companies profiting from high product sales, can shape public perception. This underscores the importance of critical thinking and independent research regarding health decisions.

What exactly is a "bioidentical hormone"? Unfortunately, no standardized definition creates significant confusion among doctors and individuals using these hormones. This lack of clarity underscores the need for reliable and accurate information in the field of hormone therapy.

The term "bioidentical" can apply to both natural (not artificially created, even through semi-synthesis) substances and synthetic ones, as long as their structure and function match those of naturally occurring hormones in the human body. This is why most professional medical organizations define a bioidentical hormone as molecularly and chemically identical to a hormone produced by the human body.

It is crucial to understand that the term 'bioidentical' does not specify the source or method of obtaining the substance. In modern medicine, numerous pharmaceuticals are bioidentical yet synthetically produced. This underscores the need for informed decision-making in hormone therapy based on a clear understanding of sources and classifications. Modern medicine still does not have a genuinely natural progesterone.

All hormones used in contemporary gynecology can be classified as either bioidentical or non-bioidentical — meaning substances that do not exist in nature or within the human body. These include:

- Estrogens: synthetic conjugated estrogens, natural animal (non-human) conjugated estrogens, bioidentical plant-derived estrogens

- Progesterone: synthetic progestins, bioidentical progesterone

- Combination estrogen-progesterone therapies: combinations of synthetic conjugated estrogens, animal-derived conjugated estrogens, and progestins.

All combined forms of estrogen and progesterone are not bioidentical hormones, even though some estrogens are derived from the urine of pregnant animals, most commonly horses.

All bioidentical estrogen products have a chemical structure of 17-β-estradiol, derived from plant-based sources, and are available in various forms (tablets, capsules, creams, gels, patches, sprays, vaginal tablets). The production of these medications is strictly regulated and adheres to manufacturing standards in most developed countries. However, no large-scale studies have been conducted to compare the efficacy and safety of bioidentical versus synthetic estrogens due to the vast number of estrogen products available (several dozen), making it impossible to compare them all, especially since they come in different forms.

Currently, there is only one type of bioidentical progesterone on the market — micronized progesterone, although it is sold under different brand names and in various forms (tablets, vaginal tablets, creams, gels). Unlike bioidentical estrogen products and synthetic progesterone forms, bioidentical progesterone production is not regulated or standardized in most countries.

The topic of menopause and hormone therapy is vast. Even with the desire to cover as much as possible, there comes a point where one must stop, because there are still many interesting and important topics related to hormones and their impact on the human body. I will write a separate book about menopause. For now, let's turn to emotions and their connection to hormones.

Chapter 8. Hormones, Emotions, Mood, and Feelings

In recent years, the number of cases involving psychosomatic reactions has increased, especially among women. *Psychosomatics* refers to the influence of the psycho-emotional state on the appearance of symptoms resembling those of certain diseases. The most common psychosomatic reactions in women include lower abdominal pain (often mistaken for an inflammatory process), itching of the external genitalia, and menstrual cycle irregularities. Are hormones involved in psychosomatic reactions? We will discuss this next.

Delving into the late 18th century, we find that the ovaries were once believed to be part of the nervous system. Viennese gynecologist Chrobak's oophorectomies on women to treat hysteria, anorexia, and even nymphomania and Joseph Halban's transplantation of women's ovaries into guinea pigs were pivotal in demonstrating the connection between ovarian function and female behavior. These experiments significantly influenced the study of hormones and their use in treating various conditions, marking a significant milestone in our understanding of the subject.

8.1. Hormones and Cognition

When assessing people's reactions to life events and bodily changes, both external and internal factors, we often discuss cognition.

The term "cognition" (from the Latin *cognitio*, meaning "knowledge" or "learning," and the Greek *gnosis*, meaning "thought" or "reflection") is rarely found in popular literature. However, psychologists and psychiatrists frequently use it to describe human cognitive processes. In medicine and psychology, cognition refers to the mental (psychological, intellectual) processes involved in acquiring, processing, and assimilating information, such as perception, categorization, thinking, speech, and behavior. Cognition also includes self-awareness and the evaluation of oneself about the surrounding world, shaping behavior, attitudes toward people, external events, and one's own body.

Many hormones can influence cognition. Elevated thyroid hormone levels can lead to irritability and a negative perception of events and people. Conversely, low thyroid hormone levels are often associated with tearfulness, apathy, and melancholy.

Over the past few decades, it has been well-established that steroid hormones exert a profound influence on cognition and human behavior. Numerous clinical studies and experiments have examined this intricate relationship. Observing mood swings and emotional shifts in women throughout the menstrual cycle reveals a fascinating connection between hormonal fluctuations and cognitive function, underscoring the complexity of the human body.

Changes in estrogen, testosterone, and progesterone levels affect both short-term and long-term memory. In the first half of the follicular phase, when hormone levels are low, perception-based memory and spatial orientation improve. In the first half of the luteal phase, when hormone levels rise, verbal and visual memory and memory for routine, habitual actions improve.

Emotional memory is intricately linked to the influence of steroid hormones on the brain, particularly the limbic system. This part of the brain is a fascinating study area, with its key role in forming emotions and feelings related to reproduction, food-seeking, survival, environmental responses, and interactions with other living beings. It governs emotions such as fear, aggression, irritation, and anger, as well as those that drive sexual behavior — the search for a sexual partner and the experience of sexual satisfaction.

The amygdala, a structure within the limbic system, serves as a repository of memory — it stores and "filters" all experiences, retaining only those that provoke a strong emotional response, such as intense fear, overwhelming worry, or great pleasure.

The connection between stress hormones and emotions, particularly emotional memory, has been known for a long time. Fear and anxiety trigger increases in cortisol, adrenaline, and norepinephrine levels. A slight increase in cortisol can enhance memory, while prolonged or excessive elevation impairs it. Norepinephrine, which rises during the second half of the menstrual cycle, also influences women's emotional memory. However, the relationship between these hormones and cognition is more pronounced in men than women.

Sex hormones and progesterone, particularly their fluctuations and proportional balance, are considered central factors affecting a woman's behavior, cognition, memory, emotions, and feelings. Women are more likely than men to experience mood disorders, depression, and stress-related conditions.

8.2. The Influence of the Menstrual Cycle on Women's Behavior

Despite the thorough understanding of the physiological processes of the menstrual cycle, including the molecular-level changes in the ovaries and uterus, the influence of hormonal fluctuations, ovulation, and menstruation on female behavior and reactions remains a largely unexplored area in the medical literature. This lack of research underscores the urgency and importance of understanding how women respond to external and internal stimuli depending on their menstrual cycle.

In contrast, veterinary science and zoology have extensive data on how hormonal changes in the reproductive system influence animal behavior.

Although observations about women's states and behaviors depending on their menstrual cycle have been passed down for centuries, often in the form of jokes, songs, and amusing stories, medicine has primarily overlooked this subject. Only recently has it begun to receive more attention. The primary reason for this omission is the tendency of many specialists to assess women's health concerns without considering sex-specific differences. Even when statistics indicate that certain diseases are common in women compared to men, this information is typically viewed as an epidemiological fact rather than being analyzed concerning the distinct physiology of the female body, which includes unique periods such as menstruation, pregnancy, postpartum, and menopause.

Anxiety is always rooted in fear — a woman's fear of something or someone, which is fueled by negative thinking and emotions. In other words, it is the projection of internal mental content onto the physical body, often nothing more than self-suggestion. To some extent, analytical thinking can regulate anxiety and suppress fear. However, most people do not develop this type of reasoning to the level where they critically analyze information rather than unquestioningly accepting what they hear, see, or read, including their behavior as a response to information. Women are no exception, and for many, the limbic system of the brain dominates behavior, leading to chronic anxiety, irritability, blind conformity to group beliefs, and resistance to alternative perspectives on events and phenomena.

Medicine recognizes two key processes: pathophysiological and psychobiological. The first describes the body's pathological response to a stimulus, how diseases develop under the influence of risk factors. The second describes the individual's psycho-emotional reactions and behaviors, which can exacerbate or mitigate the pathophysiological process.

For example, some women experience heightened anxiety leading up to menstruation, which can trigger physical disturbances. Conversely, the onset of physical symptoms before menstruation may provoke an exaggerated psycho-emotional reaction. This creates a vicious cycle that many women fall into simply due to a lack of understanding of their physiology.

There are numerous examples of the disconnect between a woman's psychological and physical states, particularly among those who either desperately want to conceive or are terrified of pregnancy. Others, without actively planning for pregnancy, live in constant fear of ectopic pregnancy or miscarriage, ironically, heightening their risk of such outcomes. Some women engage in extreme behaviors, obsessing over every bodily sensation in the days leading up to their period, escalating their anxiety with excessive monitoring. Many take multiple pregnancy tests per day, rush to get ultrasounds, or repeatedly visit doctors without a clear medical need.

The effects of the menstrual cycle on cognition, memory, and behavior in reproductive-age women have only been superficially studied. Globally, only a handful of research studies have focused on this topic. At the same time, significantly more attention has been given to the impact of hormone therapy on cognition and memory in postmenopausal women.

One study utilized the Bem Sex Roles Inventory (BSRI), a psychological assessment tool consisting of 60 characteristics:

- 20 traits traditionally associated with masculinity (e.g., ambition, independence, aggressiveness)

- 20 traits associated with femininity (e.g., emotionality, sensitivity, expressiveness)

- 20 neutral characteristics and emotions (e.g., happiness, satisfaction, confidence).

The results indicated that a woman's sense of "femininity" remains relatively stable throughout her cycle — women remain women. However, the expression of traditionally "masculine" traits fluctuates depending on the cycle phase: during the pre-ovulatory phase, masculine traits decline, whereas during menstruation, when hormone levels are at their lowest, these traits increase. This understanding can help better manage women's health and behavior, especially when they might exhibit more 'masculine' traits.

Menstruation is characterized by heightened emotional sensitivity, irritability, and aggression. Women tend to be more talkative during the second half of their cycle, and this verbal expressiveness peaks during menstruation. Women generally employ a verbal-analytical problem-solving strategy, unlike men, who prefer a holistic approach. The verbal-analytical method emphasizes details and focuses on individual components of a problem, whereas the holistic approach prioritizes the broader picture rather than its smaller elements.

Research has also shown that around ovulation, women appear more attractive and draw increased attention from men. Their bodies release specific pheromones that enhance their appeal. During ovulation, women dress more stylishly and vividly, use makeup more frequently, and choose clothing that reveals more skin. Hormonal fluctuations do not solely dictate this behavior but are also influenced by evolutionary instincts related to reproduction and mate attraction, which persist in human behavior.

The impact of the menstrual cycle and hormonal fluctuations on women's cognitive states and behaviors is an area that demands further research. The existing findings confirm the existence of such influences and support many observations about female behavior passed down through generations. However, the potential for discovery and advancement in this field through further studies is vast and promising.

8.3. Hormones and Emotions

Emotional memory, negative emotions, fear, and anxiety in women, particularly those influenced by the menstrual cycle, have been the subject of significant research. Several studies have revealed that progesterone and its metabolites have a cumulative effect on brain hormones (neurotransmitters), particularly serotonin and norepinephrine, which regulate emotions. Notably, one study found that progesterone plays a more significant role in men's emotional stability than women's. While research on women primarily focuses on progesterone's role in reproductive function, studies on men emphasize its impact on brain function, particularly in cognitive enhancement. These findings shed light on the complex relationship between hormones and emotions, providing a deeper understanding of this intricate interplay.

The brain's limbic system contains specific receptors that respond to various substances derived from steroid hormones, particularly progesterone. A deficiency of these substances is associated with increased anxiety. In the late luteal phase of the menstrual cycle, progesterone levels drop significantly, triggering negative emotions in response to stress if such situations arise during this period.

Animal model studies have confirmed the link between low progesterone metabolites and behaviors dominated by fear and aggression. When progesterone was introduced into the amygdala of female rats that had undergone oophorectomy (and thus had low progesterone levels), the animals displayed significantly reduced anxiety, fear, and aggression. Conversely, when substances that inhibited progesterone production were administered, the animals exhibited heightened anxiety, sought shelter from others, and spent less time in open spaces. Their stress response was prolonged, often resulting in a "freeze" reaction, where they remained motionless in fear.

8.4. Hormones and Depression

Women experiencing periods of low mood, tearfulness, insomnia, and fatigue have been well-known long before the term "depression" was introduced. This understanding of women's mental health has been present in literature and culture for centuries, connecting us to the historical evolution of mental health understanding.

Despite advances in science and technology making modern life significantly more comfortable than our ancestors, humanity has gradually lost its survival instincts. This has led to an increased focus on introspection and a cultural trend of psychiatric self-diagnosis. The phrase "Oh, I have such depression!" has become a typical exaggeration among both men and women. Even young children learn to recognize their mothers' so-called "depressive episodes" and know when it's best not to ask unnecessary questions.

The widespread use of antidepressants has become another trend, heavily fueled by pharmaceutical companies. Experiencing depression is now an inherent part of modern life. However, if you tell someone they have a mental disorder (which depression technically is), you may be met with extreme defensiveness and even anger. "I suffer from a mental illness" carries a social stigma, whereas "I have depression" sounds trendy and relatable — even adolescents use the term liberally.

Nonetheless, depression is a clinical diagnosis and is classified as a psychiatric disorder. The first person to note a gender difference in depression prevalence was Charles Dickens, the famous English writer who himself suffered from depression. While studying hospital records from a well-known London psychiatric institution, he observed that women were disproportionately affected by depression, a fact he later mentioned in his writings. He also noted that depression was more prevalent among women from specific social classes. Dickens' observations remain consistent with those of modern physicians.

This high prevalence of depression among women led to the identification of "reproductive depression," which is linked to the menstrual cycle, postpartum period, and perimenopause. Depressive episodes in women most frequently occur during times of hormonal shifts after childbirth and in the years leading up to menopause. Research confirms that the highest rate of depression in women occurs in perimenopause, typically two to three years before menstruation ceases.

The triad of *premenstrual depression, postpartum depression,* and *menopausal depression* was officially classified as reproductive depression in 2009, recognizing its association with hormonal fluctuations regulated by the ovaries. Establishing reproductive depression as a distinct diagnosis helps reframe the condition, not merely as a psychiatric disorder but as a complex physiological response occurring during different life stages. It also underscores the crucial role of sex hormones and other steroid hormones in shaping women's mental health, validating the experiences of many women who have struggled with these conditions.

Since estrogen and progesterone receptors are present in brain tissue, the impact of these hormones on brain function is undeniable.

8.4.1. Premenstrual Depression

As previously mentioned, approximately 10% of women experience premenstrual dysphoric disorder (PMDD). This condition causes significant discomfort and impairs work capacity and daily life. Healthcare professionals must recognize the symptoms and provide timely diagnosis and treatment. Depression, mood swings, and emotional disturbances characterize PMDD.

Many gynecologists and psychiatrists disagree with the term "dysphoric," which equates severe PMS with a psychiatric disorder. Some doctors suggest renaming it "ovarian cyclic syndrome," emphasizing its dependence on ovarian function and the cyclical nature of symptoms.

The mechanism of premenstrual depression is unknown, although it is similar to PMS. A drop in progesterone levels in the second half of the menstrual cycle may trigger depressive symptoms.

Premenstrual depression is characterized by:

• Symptoms occur with every menstrual cycle

• Depression disappears during pregnancy

• Symptoms return in the postpartum period as postpartum depression

• After menstrual cycles resume postpartum, depression reappears before each period

• The condition worsens with age, especially in perimenopause

• Often accompanied by menstrual migraines, breast pain, bloating

• Symptom-free periods last 7–10 days per month, mainly in the first half of the cycle

We must engage in better mental health discussions to address the complexities of premenstrual depression. The fact that suppressing ovulation with a combination of estrogens and progesterone (or progestins) or hormonal contraceptives relieves symptoms confirms that premenstrual depression is linked to ovarian function. Many doctors believe that antidepressants are not appropriate for treating premenstrual depression. Progesterone is rarely used, although some attempts have been made.

8.4.2. Postpartum Depression

This type of depression often goes undiagnosed because, after childbirth, many women become socially isolated and fully immersed in caring for their newborns. The first months of breastfeeding, adaptation, and sleep deprivation demand physical and emotional energy.

Many symptoms of postpartum depression are mistaken for postpartum fatigue, sleep deprivation, concerns about breastfeeding, the baby's health, or thyroid dysfunction. These symptoms can include persistent feelings of sadness, anxiety, or irritability, changes in appetite or sleep patterns, difficulty bonding with the baby, and thoughts of harming oneself or the baby.

Postpartum blues, unlike depression, appear within the first week after birth due to a sudden hormonal shift and do not always require antidepressants or treatment. Postpartum depression develops later and can last throughout the postpartum period, sometimes transitioning into premenstrual depression.

Obstetricians and gynecologists typically focus on reproductive health, and the first postpartum checkup often does not happen until 8–10 weeks after birth. Even during this visit, women rarely discuss mental health symptoms, and doctors frequently do not ask about them.

If a woman with postpartum depression seeks help from a psychiatrist or family doctor, the connection between postpartum depression and past premenstrual depression may be overlooked, leading to inappropriate antidepressant prescriptions.

Early intervention is crucial in the treatment of postpartum depression. Some modern publications suggest using progesterone or progestins to treat postpartum depression. However, most psychiatrists do not recognize these methods, recommending antidepressants instead. Obstetricians and gynecologists are not trained to diagnose or treat postpartum depression, making early intervention even more difficult.

Interestingly, some studies suggest that estrogens may improve mood and help treat postpartum depression, while certain types of progestins may worsen the condition.

Postpartum depression demands more attention from researchers and healthcare providers, as many critical questions about its causes, diagnosis, and treatment remain unanswered.

8.4.3. Climacteric Depression

The perimenopausal and menopausal periods are accompanied by numerous symptoms, which can, in themselves, trigger negative emotions and distress in women.

A defining characteristic of climacteric depression is that it develops against the background of premenstrual depression, with symptoms intensifying 2–3 years before menopause, especially if the woman has previously experienced postpartum depression.

Hormone replacement therapy (HRT) can help relieve many symptoms of this form of depression. However, most of these women end up categorized as psychiatric patients, where antidepressants become the primary treatment prescribed by psychiatrists.

Some gynecologists treat this type of depression with estrogens, but most psychiatrists reject this approach. Progestins are usually prescribed in combination with estrogens, but their effect on climacteric depression remains unstudied.

The term "reproductive depression" is a new diagnosis. Still, it will likely be vehemently opposed by psychiatrists, as it places too much emphasis on ovarian function, a subject they have only a superficial understanding of.

Gynecologists are also unlikely to diagnose it frequently, as the word "depression" still carries strong associations with psychiatric disorders.

How long will it take before women's health is viewed through the lens of reproductive function? No one knows. For now, many women will remain on antidepressants.

Chapter 9. Hormones and Cancer

Understanding the role of hormones in cancer is of paramount importance. While all hormones produced in the human body play vital roles in specific functions, it's crucial to recognize that many hormones can trigger malignant (cancerous) processes independently or in combination with other substances. The most harmful effects are associated with steroid hormones, particularly sex hormones and progesterone.

In the group of hormone-dependent tumors — ovarian, testicular, endometrial, prostate, breast, thyroid cancers, and osteosarcoma — the influence of both endogenous (naturally produced) and exogenous (medically administered) sex hormones and progesterone plays a crucial role in stimulating cancer cell growth.

9.1. What Are Carcinogens

Many people know that carcinogens are substances linked to the development of malignant processes, and extensive research confirms this.

Dr. Siddhartha Mukherjee's book *The Emperor of All Maladies: A Biography of Cancer* contains a wealth of unique information about how perspectives on malignant diseases have evolved since ancient times, the search for cancer causes, how society's attitude toward cancer has shifted, and how money has been made from human suffering. The book also traces improvements in diagnosing and treating various types of cancer. This monumental work contains significant information on hormone-dependent tumors, whose growth is influenced by hormones.

It's widely known that tobacco (specifically, various compounds in cigarette smoke) and alcohol are classified as carcinogens. However, it's important to remember that the first publications linking smoking and lung cancer appeared as early as the 1930s. Despite this, tobacco companies invested significant efforts into suppressing and falsifying the results instead of publicizing them. This underscores the need for awareness of the risks associated with smoking and alcohol.

Today, cigarette packaging includes warnings about the increased risk of lung cancer but achieving this took over 50 years of relentless struggle by courageous scientists, doctors, and activists. Many of these individuals lost their jobs, positions, reputations, families, and even their lives in the fight against smoking. It took nearly 30 years to pass laws banning smoking in public places, a testament to the courage and sacrifice of those who fought against this harmful habit.

Of course, doctors frequently warn that smoking while taking oral contraceptives (OCs) is strongly discouraged — to put it bluntly, it is incompatible with OCs. But many women still smoke occasionally, ignoring their doctors' warnings. Beyond smoking, the use of alcohol and drugs while on OCs also increases the risk of serious health conditions.

Alcohol is also a teratogen, meaning it contributes to congenital disabilities, which is well known among women, particularly those planning pregnancy. However, far fewer people are aware of the proven link between alcohol consumption and an increased risk of cancers of the throat, larynx, mouth, lips, esophagus, liver, breast, and colon. For example, daily consumption of

- Two bottles of beer (350 ml each)

- Two glasses of wine (300 ml total)

- Or about 100 ml of hard liquor

doubles the risk of breast cancer compared to non-drinkers (National Cancer Institute, USA). Yet, alcohol labels contain no warnings about these risks.

Natural estrogens and progesterone can also stimulate the growth of certain malignant tumors in both women and men — these are often referred to as hormone-dependent cancers.

In 1999, the World Health Organization (WHO) and the International Agency for Research on Cancer (IARC) published a monograph from the Program for the Study of Carcinogenic Risk, stating that estrogen and progesterone should be considered human carcinogens.

For nearly 15 years, the U.S. National Toxicology Program (Department of Health and Human Services, USA) has supported this conclusion in its reports on carcinogens.

9.2. A Few Words About Malignant Diseases

Many people have a superficial understanding of tumors. The word *"cancer"* refers only to a specific type of disease — *malignant growth* of epithelial cells forming the skin, mucous membranes, and glands.

Excess tissue appears when a cell begins dividing at a rate exceeding the normal speed of cell division. In medicine, we refer to this as *"plus tissue."* This formation is called a tumor. All Latin tumors (excluding cysts) have the suffix *"-*

oma": endometrioma, luteoma, carcinoma, sarcoma, choriocarcinoma, etc. Therefore, if a diagnosis contains a term ending in *"-oma,"* it indicates the presence of a tumor-like process. Some conditions are given general names describing the disease, such as leukemia.

Not all tumors are malignant, so we distinguish between benign and malignant processes. In other words, not every "plus tissue" formation is cancer. The term "neoplasm" is also commonly used.

Benign tumors do not spread throughout the body (do not metastasize), although their adverse effects can still be significant. Some conditions are not malignant but may affect the entire body, destroy cells, tissues, and organs, and require long-term treatment.

Having a benign condition does not necessarily mean it will become malignant. The term "precancerous condition" does not mean a person has a benign tumor. At the same time, any disease that does not lead to death is considered benign. However, when discussing benign tumors, the majority do not progress to cancer.

The most common types of benign tumors are adenomas, lipomas, fibroids, and hemangiomas.

Medicine also recognizes borderline tumors — those that can become malignant. However, the exact risk of malignancy for many borderline conditions remains unknown, and there are still no clear guidelines on how they should be monitored or treated.

A precancerous condition is a laboratory diagnosis that describes cellular changes that *may* develop into a malignancy. However, this transformation does not occur in

100% of cases. Examples of precancerous changes include hyperplasia, atypia, metaplasia, dysplasia, and carcinoma in situ ("cancer in place").

It is important to note that these cellular changes are also common in normal biological processes. For example, inflammation, tissue healing, and regeneration often involve metaplasia, atypia, and cellular proliferation. Dysplasia can also be a temporary transitional state. In most cases, these changes do not require treatment, except in cases of carcinoma in situ.

Multiple classifications of malignant tumors exist, including those based on the type of tissue they originate from: carcinomas, sarcomas, blastomas, and germ cell tumors. In clinical medicine, the focus is on the extent of tumor spread and organ involvement, which is why doctors use staging classifications that consider lymph node involvement and metastases (TNM classification).

There are hundreds of different diagnoses for benign and malignant tumors. For example, more than 30 types of ovarian cancer have been identified. However, in 98–99% of cases, ovarian tumors are benign.

The causes of many cancers remain unknown, making diagnosis and treatment challenging. However, modern medicine has made significant progress, and many cancers, when detected early, can be successfully treated.

Cancer is not a death sentence. As long as a person is alive, there is always hope for recovery.

Among my friends and relatives, many have faced malignant diseases. Some did not survive because they either sought treatment too late or refused treatment altogether.

However, others have overcome cancer and are now living full lives for 10–30 years post-diagnosis.

Although a cancer diagnosis is terrifying, advances in modern medicine now offer a wide range of high-quality and effective treatments.

9.3. Which Hormones Are Associated with Malignant Diseases

The role of steroid hormones in the development of various cancers has been known for a long time, and with each passing year, more research on this topic emerges. Estrogens receive particular attention, as they significantly increase the risk of breast and endometrial cancer and are also linked to ovarian cancer. Testosterone is associated with an increased risk of prostate cancer. Cortisol, the stress hormone, is considered a risk factor for the development of several malignant tumors. Anabolic steroids can provoke kidney, lung, and testicular cancer.

Other hormones that do not belong to the steroid class are also involved in carcinogenic processes. For example, elevated insulin levels have been linked to the development of cancers of the intestines, pancreas, kidneys, and uterus. Insulin-like growth factors (IGFs), or growth hormone, are involved in developing prostate, breast, and colorectal cancers.

The role of prolactin in breast cancer is a topic of heated debate among researchers. While its connection to breast cancer remains controversial, elevated prolactin levels are often found in cases of lung, kidney, rectal, and ovarian cancers. The potential impact of prolactin on cancer formation in other organs is a subject that demands further study.

In the past, estrogen was thought to stimulate the growth of precancerous breast cells. However, pregnancy-related breast cancer is often estrogen-insensitive (negative). Some researchers suggest that elevated prolactin levels may act as a trigger for breast cancer development. It is also known that prolactin levels naturally increase with age in women.

However, the highest prolactin levels are not observed postpartum or during lactation but instead in the third trimester of pregnancy, just before childbirth, reaching up to 200 ng/mL. After delivery, if a woman does not breastfeed, prolactin levels drop rapidly and return to pre-pregnancy levels within 8–10 weeks.

For breastfeeding mothers, prolactin production depends on the frequency and duration of nursing. Just 45 minutes after breastfeeding, prolactin levels double, initiating new milk production for the next feeding. However, despite these fluctuations, prolactin levels never reach pregnancy levels during lactation. Even in nursing mothers, prolactin gradually decreases.

- In the first 3–6 months of breastfeeding, prolactin levels usually do not exceed 100–110 ng/mL (for non-pregnant women, normal levels do not exceed 25–30 ng/mL).

- Once menstrual cycles resume, prolactin drops to 50–70 ng/mL.

- In the later months of lactation, prolactin rarely exceeds 50 ng/mL.

415

Thus, it is likely that a combination of high progesterone and prolactin levels during pregnancy may act as a trigger for breast cancer development.

Understanding how various hormones negatively impact cells and contribute to malignant transformations is a complex and ongoing challenge. To fully grasp this influence, a more comprehensive approach, particularly one that delves into genetic changes, is needed.

As science advances, we must maintain our optimism that a breakthrough in this field will lead to new, effective treatments for malignant tumors. The potential for progress is accurate, and we must not lose hope.

Chapter 10: Hormones and Sex

Did you know that the word "sex" has been one of the most frequently searched terms on the internet since the rise of personal computers and search engines? Regardless of moral or religious principles, sexuality remains an inseparable part of human life.

All physiological processes in the human body are ultimately aimed at ensuring reproduction. Whether or not people want children, their biological mechanisms function through the lens of reproduction and sexual maturity. Since humans reproduce only through sexual intercourse, sex plays an essential role in human life.

What role do hormones play in sexuality? They play the same role in puberty, reproductive system function, and fertility, primarily in the ovaries and testes. Hormone production and fluctuations are closely linked to human behavior and sexual activity.

Since the topic of sex is vast, we will focus on a few aspects of how hormones influence sexual relationships.

10.1. The Influence of Hormones on Sexual Desire

What determines sexual desire? Before answering this question, let's clarify what we mean by sexual attraction, sexual desire, and libido. In essence, there is no real difference between these terms, though some sexologists may argue otherwise. Sexual desire is simply another name for libido, which exists in both women and men. Some mistakenly believe that libido refers only to female sexuality, but this is incorrect.

Over the past 70-80 years, the meaning of the word "libido" has undergone a fascinating evolution, shedding light on our understanding of human desire.

In ancient times, Cicero (106–46 BC) used the Latin term "libido" to mean desire, longing, or even forbidden sexual craving. Saint Augustine (354–430 AD) expanded the definition to describe desire in all its forms.

During the Middle Ages and Renaissance, terms such as "animal spirit" and "anima" were used instead of libido to describe sexual impulses.

In the 19th century, German psychiatrist Albert Moll (1862–1939), known as the father of modern European sexology, introduced hypnosis into sexual disorder treatment. In his book "Studies on Sexual Libido," he described libido as a biological force that governs relationships, including sexual ones.

Swiss psychiatrist and founder of analytical psychology, Carl Jung, defined libido as a creative (psychic) force that fuels personal development and self-actualization. He did not view libido as purely sexual desire.

However, Sigmund Freud, the Austrian physician who was Jung's close associate for many years, redefined libido as an instinctive, subconscious energy — a force that drives sexual behavior. In his book "Three Essays on the Theory of Sexuality," Freud explicitly labeled libido as the sexual instinct.

Over time, the concept of "instinctive energy" was narrowed down to purely sexual attraction. According to Freud, if libido represents the energy of creation, its opposite is destrudo, which is often associated with aggression, including hostility toward the opposite sex.

It's important to differentiate between sexual desire (libido) and sexual arousal, as they represent distinct aspects of human sexuality:

- Sexual desire (libido): the interest in sex and sexual activity.

- Sexual arousal: the body's physiological response to sexual desire, including physical changes in the reproductive organs.

There is a connection between these concepts: if there is no desire, there is usually no arousal. However, arousal does not always occur, even in the presence of desire.

A decrease in sexual desire can occur in both men and women, but women are more often wrongly accused of being "frigid" or uninterested in sex.

Sexual desire and arousal tend to decrease in the presence of chronic illnesses, depression, pregnancy, and prolonged stress. Socioeconomic factors can also suppress libido, such as job changes or unemployment, financial difficulties, raising young children, or living with parents or other relatives in the same household. A strict upbringing, childhood psychological trauma, and excessive parental control can leave a lasting negative imprint on a woman's life, contributing to sexual dysfunction. Unpleasant situations or crises in intimate life may awaken deep-seated, unconscious fears and prohibitions, which in turn manifest as sexual problems.

I will not rewrite textbooks on sexology, leaving them for those who wish to explore the subject further. Instead, I will mention a well-known fact that many men are unaware of: female libido is influenced by the menstrual cycle. This applies to women who are not taking hormonal contraceptives.

During the first phase of the menstrual cycle, as estrogen and testosterone levels rise, sexual desire increases, peaking around ovulation. Physiological changes accompany this period — vaginal secretions alter in quantity and consistency, external genitalia and nipples become more sensitive, and the body releases pheromones, which have a specific scent that attracts the opposite sex. While a woman herself may not perceive this scent, it still affects a man's sense of smell.

In the pre-ovulatory phase, oxytocin levels surge, which can lead to uterine contractions and, in some cases, even orgasms, particularly during sleep. Women's behavior also changes — many become more uninhibited, use more makeup, and wear brighter clothing.

Conversely, in the days leading up to menstruation, sex hormone levels decline, leading to a decrease in libido. The effects of progesterone, such as tissue swelling, bloating, and breast tenderness, further contribute to reduced sexual desire.

Interestingly, during menstruation, sexual desire may increase due to heightened uterine sensitivity and contractions triggered by oxytocin. Many women experience erotic dreams and orgasms during their periods. However, embarrassment over menstrual discharge often suppresses the urge for sexual intimacy.

In menopause, many women experience a decline in libido due to hormonal changes and uncomfortable symptoms, particularly vaginal dryness and alterations in the skin of the external genitalia. Additionally, psychological factors play a role — fear of aging and loss of femininity after the cessation of menstruation can further diminish sexual interest.

Endocrine disorders frequently contribute to reduced sexual desire. Conditions affecting the pituitary gland, thyroid, and adrenal glands are particularly influential. These disorders impact sexual function through complex mechanisms, ranging from direct hormonal imbalances affecting the brain to disruptions in reproductive organ function. Even the awareness of having a chronic illness can suppress sexual desire.

When low libido is linked to hormonal deficiencies, small doses of testosterone or estrogen may sometimes be prescribed. The diagnosis of androgen deficiency, or low levels of male sex hormones, particularly in postmenopausal women, remains controversial. Many physicians question this diagnosis due to the lack of clear diagnostic criteria.

To this day, there is no universally established minimum level of testosterone required for female health. Each laboratory has its reference values for these hormones. However, studies have shown that even women with low testosterone levels can maintain regular sexual activity. As I previously mentioned in the chapter on sex hormones, male hormones serve as precursors to female hormones, meaning their levels fluctuate significantly, particularly with age. Additionally, various human cells can produce their testosterone from its precursor, progesterone. This locally produced testosterone may exert effects without entering the bloodstream, adding another layer of complexity to understanding its role in female sexuality.

Testosterone is most prescribed to women in menopause. However, the challenge of such treatment lies in the fact that, for women, including those in postmenopause, the absolute levels of male and female sex hormones matter less than their proper physiological ratio. In menopausal women, the ratio of testosterone to estrogen is naturally high, and adding testosterone can further disrupt this balance, leading to significant side effects. Conversely, estrogen therapy lowers the proportion of free testosterone, which can also affect sexual function. A combination of both hormones has been shown to improve libido in postmenopausal women, though this approach remains infrequent, particularly for younger women.

Synthetic estrogens are sometimes prescribed to menopausal women to enhance libido, often as part of hormone replacement therapy. Vaginal estrogen creams are also recommended, especially for women experiencing vaginal dryness or thinning of vulvar skin. However, there is insufficient evidence supporting their effectiveness in treating sexual dysfunction.

For premenopausal women, estrogen-based medications are not typically used to treat sexual dysfunction.

Beyond hormonal treatments, sexologists have begun exploring other pharmacological options. One such drug is tibolone, a steroid (anabolic) compound prescribed primarily to menopausal women for osteoporosis prevention. Studies suggest that tibolone may enhance sexual arousal, although these trials were conducted on healthy women without complaints of sexual dysfunction.

Several other medications claim to boost sexual desire, but most come with a range of adverse effects. To date, no actual "female Viagra" exists despite periodic market releases of products marketed as groundbreaking solutions for female sexual dysfunction.

10.2. Orgasm and Hormonal Surges

There are many myths and misconceptions about orgasms, especially regarding the so-called different types of female orgasms. There is only one — just an orgasm. However, some women become so focused on achieving a vaginal orgasm that they stop enjoying their sex life altogether.

Orgasms are often attributed to exaggerated positive effects on the body, including hormonal surges, energy bursts, and the release of various biochemical substances.

Every sexual act follows a sequence of phases, a normal and natural process. The first phase, arousal, begins before penetration. Whether a penis or another object is involved does not affect the sequence of sexual responses. During masturbation, a person experiences the same four phases as in intercourse. The sensations in each phase vary depending on the type of sexual activity and technique used, and orgasm is not always reached, though sexual pleasure can still be significant.

The second phase, the plateau, is a brief "calm before the storm" leading up to orgasm. Its duration varies from person to person, and it either transitions into orgasm or fades away. Many women become so afraid of not reaching orgasm that they remain stuck at the end of the first phase, never progressing further. Since the plateau phase often happens automatically, it isn't easy to control. Some sexual techniques allow for delaying orgasm, such as tantric sex, which teaches how to extend arousal for prolonged pleasure, though not everyone enjoys this approach.

The third phase is orgasm, often considered the highest point of pleasure. It isn't easy to describe, as each person experiences it differently. In both scientific and popular literature, orgasm is sometimes referred to as the "O-word." This individuality of experience should be respected and understood.

The fourth phase is resolution (satisfaction or post-orgasmic phase).

Without the first two phases, the third phase (orgasm) does not occur. Proper arousal and physiological preparation of the sexual organs are necessary for orgasm to happen.

Women typically progress through these phases more slowly than men. A man may experience all four stages in 4–5 minutes, while a woman often requires 10–20 minutes just for the first two phases. About 50% of women reach orgasm within 10–12 minutes, while others need more time. Early in a woman's sexual life, when sexual attraction and emotional connection with a partner are firm, 25% of women may reach orgasm within one minute of penetration.

Orgasms occur in both women and men. In men, ejaculation is the physiological equivalent of orgasm, accompanied by intense pleasure. However, with age, men experience orgasms less frequently due to increasing erection and ejaculation difficulties. In contrast, many women experience orgasms more often with age due to greater sexual experience, a better understanding of their bodies, and improved control over contraception. However, because sexual activity generally declines with age, orgasm frequency also decreases.

Why is female orgasm so often discussed? Likely because people have tried to categorize it into different types — vaginal, clitoral, anal, nipple, and even breast orgasms. Some even promote the idea of "mental orgasms," supposedly achieved through thought alone using techniques borrowed from yoga. Debates over female ejaculation continue as well.

Surveys on simultaneous orgasm show conflicting results, as men and women are usually questioned separately. 25% of men and 14% of women claim that simultaneous orgasm is an essential part of their relationship. Oral sex is also a significant source of pleasure — 10% of men and 18% of women report reaching orgasm through this type of sexual activity.

In the past, perceptions of female orgasm were often bizarre and even comical. Since orgasms were observed more frequently during ovulation, it was mistakenly believed that orgasm was a sign of ovulation and that conception (referred to as "insemination" at the time) was guaranteed.

In 1660s London, some men feared women who experienced orgasms, believing that orgasm itself could cause pregnancy. While some doctors and scientists criticized this idea, others mistakenly believed that orgasm allowed women to control sperm movement, influencing which partner would father their child. This led to the incorrect belief that a woman could have multiple partners but conceive only from the one with whom she had an orgasm.

Sexual arousal activates specific areas of the brain, sending impulses through the spinal cord, which increases blood flow to vaginal muscles by dilating arteries. This process is driven by the release of vasoactive intestinal peptide (VIP) and nitric oxide.

During orgasm, oxytocin, DHEA, and other hormones are released. However, the role of hormones in orgasm remains poorly understood, which has led to many myths about the health benefits of sex.

One widespread but questionable claim is that sex reduces pain, particularly in women. Some sources claim that oxytocin levels increase fivefold before orgasm, supposedly leading to pain relief for headaches, arthritis, and menstrual cramps. However, the actual impact of this hormonal surge on pain relief is a topic of ongoing research and debate.

However, a 1987 study by Carmichael and colleagues found that oxytocin levels rise slightly before orgasm in both men and women but remain elevated for only five minutes before returning to normal. Later studies showed that oxytocin levels increase only briefly — no longer than one minute.

Thus, even if oxytocin levels do rise before or during orgasm, the effect is too short-lived to provide significant pain relief. Furthermore, oxytocin in women is released in pulses, influenced by factors such as the menstrual cycle phase and pregnancy status. Its exact role in sexual function and pain relief remains unclear, fueling ongoing speculation.

Another claim suggests that the "hormonal surge" from orgasm prevents osteoporosis, a condition characterized by bone density loss and increased fracture risk, especially in postmenopausal women.

Some research suggests that artificially increasing testosterone levels in older women may improve libido and enhance sexual function. Since testosterone positively affects muscle and bone metabolism, it has been speculated that it could help prevent osteoporosis.

However, while testosterone levels may increase slightly before and during sex, this effect is brief. Canadian psychologist Sari van Anders, who has extensively studied testosterone fluctuations before and after sexual activity, argues that even if testosterone rises after sex, its impact on female health remains unknown. Thus, claims that sex and orgasm prevent or treat osteoporosis are purely speculative.

10.3. Frequency of Sexual Activity and Hormonal Balance

Supporters of frequent sex often argue that it benefits human health, while opponents highlight its potential negative consequences. However, amid this debate, one fundamental truth remains: if sexual activity occurs without mutual consent, it will never be beneficial. In such cases, neither the frequency of intercourse nor its type or position matters.

Among animals, sex is an essential part of reproduction and occurs mainly during mating seasons, which are often tied to seasonal cycles. In contrast, humans have transformed sex into a means of pleasure, making it acceptable at any time of the year, at any time of day, and any frequency.

There is no such thing as "too much sex" as long as it does not cause discomfort to those involved. Some couples engage in sex daily or even multiple times a day, while others have sex once a week, once a month, or even once a year. Any frequency of sexual activity is considered normal if it does not lead to negative consequences and is mutually satisfying for both partners. Likewise, "too little sex" is also a misleading concept, though partners may have differing needs regarding sexual frequency.

For men, regular sexual activity is physiologically more important than for women, not due to hormonal balance but because of the prostate. The prostate gland produces prostatic fluid, a key component of semen. If this fluid is not regularly released, its stagnation can lead to prostate dysfunction and other health issues. Therefore, regular ejaculation, either through intercourse or masturbation, is necessary for male health.

How the frequency of sexual activity affects hormonal levels in men and women remains unclear, as no in-depth studies have been conducted on this topic. However, some medical publications have explored the impact of sexual activity on ovulation.

Studies on animal models have yielded intriguing results. Rats, often used in research due to their physiological and behavioral similarities to humans, show notable differences in ovulation mechanisms. Unlike women, rats do not ovulate spontaneously, ovulation occurs only in response to mating. In female rats, the corpus luteum does not form on its own; signals from the vulva, vagina, and cervix must trigger its development during copulation in the mating period. Sexual activity in these animals stimulates corpus luteum function and progesterone production. This type of induced ovulation is also observed in mice, cats, camels, and llamas.

In women, the primary trigger for ovulation is not sexual intercourse itself but acute stress, which can arise from an unplanned sexual encounter or sexual assault.

A 2001 study published in medical circles claimed that the rate of spontaneous conception following rape was higher than after consensual intercourse — 8% compared to 3.1%.

While chronic stress suppresses ovulation, acute stress can trigger a surge in luteinizing hormone (LH) due to interactions between the adrenal glands and progesterone. In this process, progesterone, primarily sourced from the adrenal glands under acute stress, rises before LH levels increase. This effect occurs against the backdrop of high estrogen levels.

Numerous animal studies and clinical research on women have shown that acute stress, including the administration of stress hormones, affects ovulation and ovarian function differently depending on the phase of the menstrual cycle. During the mid-follicular, mid-luteal, and late luteal phases, acute stress has a stimulatory effect, raising the possibility of a second ovulation.

The size of the dominant follicle, compared to those undergoing atresia (gradual shrinkage and resorption), ranges from 10 to 17 mm (expanding further during the pre-ovulatory period). However, even in the second half of the cycle, the ovaries may still contain follicles larger than 15 mm, which began developing alongside the dominant follicle but stopped growing. Despite halting their growth, these follicles remain potential vesicles capable of ovulation.

Studies have found that 10% of healthy women experience a second surge in follicle-stimulating hormone (FSH) and LH levels. In 6% of women, three gonadotropin surges occur within a cycle, starting from the mid-follicular phase. While multiple ovulations remain extremely rare, they are possible.

Thus, an unplanned sexual encounter or rape may indeed stimulate ovulation, mainly if it occurs in the middle of the first or second phase of the cycle. However, whether regular sexual activity without stress induces ovulation in humans remains doubtful. Unlike in certain animal species, ovulation in humans appears to be largely independent of sexual intercourse. A more definitive answer would require further research.

Chapter 11. Hormones and the Skin

Throughout this book, the impact of certain hormones on the skin has been mentioned multiple times. A clear example of this influence can be seen in menstruating women who do not use hormonal contraceptives. Many notice that their skin becomes oily before menstruation, acne, and breakouts appear, and the skin becomes more sensitive to various irritants. However, after menstruation ends, the opposite occurs due to rising estrogen levels.

Pregnant women's skin also changes under the influence of increased hormone levels. Pigmentation spots, especially on the face (*chloasma*), appear but typically fade after childbirth. The skin of the nipples and areolas darkens, as well as the midline of the abdomen (*linea nigra*) and the area around the eyes — these are regular occurrences. Stretch marks (*striae gravidarum*) often develop on the abdomen, breasts, and thighs, though effective treatments are practically nonexistent. The activity of sweat glands increases, making pregnant women more prone to sweating. Additionally, the blood contains increased levels of relaxin, a unique protein that softens and loosens ligaments in preparation for childbirth.

Hair loss after discontinuing combined oral contraceptives or following childbirth, vaginal dryness during menopause, pigmentation changes, and various skin conditions during pregnancy — all these are direct examples of how hormones affect the skin.

In 2011, German dermatologist Dr. Jörg Reichrath published an article in a professional journal titled *"Hormones and Skin: An Endless Love Story!"* The title alone encapsulates the deep and fascinating connection between hormones and the skin. Much like a relationship between a loving couple, there are moments of harmony and conflict. This subject continues to captivate researchers and medical professionals worldwide.

I often refer to the skin as a mirror of the body's internal state, literally and figuratively. The skin's condition reflects any illness, especially those involving hormonal imbalances. Stress, emotional turmoil, lack of sleep, and intense emotional reactions also manifest as visible skin changes.

Traditional medical teachings have long emphasized the skin's role as a reflection of internal health, interpreting it as a projection of internal dysfunctions, much like a screen displaying the body's internal health. Unfortunately, many modern doctors no longer know how to 'read this documentary film' about a person's health through their skin.

11.1. Skin Condition and Hormones

The skin's multifunctionality is evident in its role as a protective covering for bones and muscles and as a thermoregulatory system. Sweating is one of the body's key cooling mechanisms.

Additionally, the skin plays a crucial role in absorbing thyroid, parathyroid, sex hormones, and certain steroid hormones. It also synthesizes various substances, including vitamin D. Given the vast surface area of the skin, it is the largest target organ for hormonal influence.

It is important to remember that the skin consists of multiple structural components. The primary tissue of the skin is keratinized stratified squamous epithelium. The skin has three layers:

- Epidermis

- Dermis

- Subcutaneous fat tissue (hypodermis)

I will not delve into the intricate anatomy of the skin. Still, it is worth emphasizing that healthy skin depends more on the condition of small blood vessels (capillaries) and the nutrients they deliver than on external sources of fats, vitamins, or minerals. Without proper nutrition, healthy skin is impossible.

Numerous external interventions — creams, gels, masks, and other cosmetic products — do not prevent skin aging and barely penetrate the skin. This is because multiple layers of dead epithelial cells create a protective barrier that prevents most substances from being absorbed.

Genetic factors also influence skin conditions, including pigmentation (determined by melanocyte count), fat distribution, collagen levels, and the rate of aging. Some people naturally appear younger than their biological age without using any special treatments, while others look older than their years. Unhealthy habits — smoking, alcohol consumption, drug use, and, of course, stress — further accelerate premature aging.

Pigmentation changes in the skin can also reflect hormonal fluctuations. For instance, some women develop pigmentation spots while taking hormonal contraceptives.

Conditions such as polycystic ovary syndrome (PCOS) and Cushing's syndrome are among the most common endocrine disorders that cause visible skin changes. Pregnancy, however, holds the leading position in producing various skin manifestations, from pigmentation and stretch marks to pregnancy-related dermatoses, including itching and rashes.

11.1.1. Skin and Aging

While many external factors, such as sun exposure, extreme temperatures, dryness, and chemical exposure, can negatively affect the skin, it's important to recognize that internal factors also play a significant role. Aging is the most influential of these internal factors.

With age, collagen, elastin, and hyaluronic acid — the three key components of skin tissue — gradually decline. These substances are often surrounded by speculation, particularly in the beauty industry. When menopause begins, the loss of these components accelerates each year. On average, the skin loses 2.1% more collagen annually after menopause.

It's crucial to understand that skin elasticity is entirely genetically determined. This means that no external treatments can fundamentally alter collagen and elastin levels in the skin. However, it's worth noting that sex hormones do have some influence on these substances.

While some studies suggest that hormone therapy (HT) can increase collagen levels in postmenopausal women, it's important to note that it does not 'rejuvenate' the ovaries. The effect is not strong enough to justify HT as an anti-aging treatment. Unfortunately, some doctors overprescribe

434

hormones without medical necessity, promoting the false belief that hormones slow down aging. While estrogens may play a role in collagen synthesis and hyaluronic acid regulation, scientific research has not consistently confirmed these claims.

There is also a widespread belief that women who have used hormonal contraceptives or hormone replacement therapy (HRT) for an extended period develop fewer and less pronounced wrinkles than those who have never taken hormones. However, serious studies have debunked this claim, showing that hormonal drugs do not reduce wrinkle formation in either premenopausal or postmenopausal women.

Genetically determined racial and ethnic factors also influence aging. While darker skin tones offer better protection against ultraviolet rays, they do not slow aging. Regardless of skin color, prolonged sun exposure leads to similar aging rates. Black women tend to develop fewer wrinkles, not because of melanin levels but due to structural differences in their skin composition.

As the skin ages, it also becomes drier. However, applying thick layers of cream does not effectively reduce skin dryness. Moisturizers fall into two categories:

- Water-based creams provide hydration.

- Oil-based creams soften the skin.

A proper skincare routine should incorporate both types of creams, applied based on the time of day, environmental conditions, and skin type. However, oil-based creams can clog pores and worsen skin conditions if overused.

435

To prevent skin dryness, women should stay hydrated and engage in physical activity, which improves blood circulation in the skin, delivers essential nutrients, and aids in waste removal through sweat.

Clinical research has not scientifically proven the effectiveness of collagen, hyaluronic acid, and other supplements, including injectable treatments, for skin rejuvenation. However, these treatments belong to cosmetic dermatology, not medical dermatology, so practical medicine does not consider skin "rejuvenation" a medical priority. The lack of reliable scientific data on the effectiveness of supplements creates opportunities for misleading marketing claims.

11.2. Acne

Acne, a condition that affects almost every girl or woman at some point, is not limited to the face but can also appear on the back, shoulders, or chest. While not all cases of breakouts are medically classified as acne, the term specifically refers to an inflammatory process in hair follicles involving sebaceous glands. An increased production of keratinocytes and excessive sebum secretion mark this condition.

Up to 85% of teenagers experience acne, and about 20% seek medical help due to significant emotional and physical discomfort. Since the skin naturally harbors many bacteria, microbial involvement in the inflammatory process can worsen the condition. Acne is commonly triggered by Propionibacterium acnes, a type of bacteria that thrives in sebaceous glands. Blackheads, widely referred to as comedones, are also considered a form of acne.

Acne most frequently appears between ages 15 and 19. While its exact cause remains unknown, elevated levels of male sex hormones (androgens) can trigger it. However, acne is not limited to adolescence — it also occurs in adult women and is often linked to stress, fatigue, fasting, sleep deprivation, and synthetic clothing.

Previously, acne was primarily attributed to hormonal imbalances (hyperandrogenism). Today, genetics is considered the most critical factor, meaning that acne has a strong hereditary component.

There are multiple types of acne, each with its causes. For instance, hormonal shifts, such as those during pregnancy, can lead to pregnancy-related acne. Other factors, such as medication or stress, can also trigger acne. The acne formation process involves several stages that often occur simultaneously, making it difficult to determine whether inflammation, follicular blockage, bacterial overgrowth, or excessive sebum production plays the primary role.

The skin is actively metabolizing sex hormones, progesterone, and thyroid hormones. Certain androgens, including dehydroepiandrosterone (DHEA), DHEA sulfate (DHEA-S), and androstenedione, are converted into testosterone within the skin through sebaceous gland activity. These hormones, particularly testosterone, play a significant role in acne formation. Additionally, hair follicles, sweat glands, the epidermis, and the dermis contribute to converting androgen precursors into dihydrotestosterone (DHT) and testosterone. Notably, DHT is 5 to 10 times more active than testosterone.

Various enzymes regulate androgen metabolism in the skin, and genetic factors influence enzyme production and the ability to neutralize excess hormones, which explains individual differences in acne severity.

Autoimmune thyroiditis is associated with the production of antibodies that can stimulate sebaceous gland activity, leading to excess sebum production. The relationship between thyroid disorders and acne is currently an active area of research.

Previous chapters on adrenal hormones and stress discussed the role of corticotropin-releasing hormone (CRH), corticotropin (ACTH), and cortisol. These stress-related hormones influence sebaceous gland function, which explains why stress-related flare-ups are common.

Despite acne being extremely prevalent among teenagers and adults over 20, clinical research on the condition remains limited. This is because acne often resolves naturally with age without requiring medical treatment. Acne improves in girls once the menstrual cycle becomes regular, and skincare habits develop. Stress, particularly emotional stress, remains a key factor in flare-ups. Simply educating young women about the temporary nature of acne and emphasizing a healthy lifestyle and proper skin care can significantly reduce anxiety and improve skin condition.

Acne does not require extensive diagnostic testing, as the clinical picture is usually sufficient for diagnosis. Medical evaluation may be warranted in severe cases or when standard treatments fail.

The first step in managing acne is proper skincare. Many women mistakenly believe that aggressive cleansing and multiple skincare products will quickly eliminate acne. However, since acne is a chronic condition influenced by hormonal fluctuations, lifestyle, and stress, excessive cosmetic treatments are not only ineffective but may worsen the condition.

A common misconception is that removing excess oil through frequent cleansing, scrubs, or peels will help. However, excessive drying of the skin triggers increased sebum production, further exacerbating acne. Often, washing with lukewarm water and mild soap every other day is sufficient for maintaining skin hygiene. Additionally, frequent hair washing with shampoos and conditioners that come into contact with facial skin may worsen acne, so rinsing the face with clean water after washing the hair is advisable.

Women rarely pay attention to temperature fluctuations and their effect on the skin. Cold, heat, and abrupt temperature changes (such as moving indoors to outdoors) significantly influence sebum production as a protective response. Over-cleansing the skin disrupts this natural process, making it more sensitive and prone to inflammation.

Psychological support is a crucial component in treating acne. Emotional distress about acne can create a vicious cycle, preventing other treatments from working effectively. Consultation with a psychotherapist or psychologist is often overlooked but can be more beneficial than medication in some cases, providing reassurance and reducing anxiety.

Many medications and alternative acne treatments are available, most of which can be purchased without a prescription in pharmacies, beauty salons, supermarkets, and online stores. The sale of acne treatments has become highly profitable, generating significant revenue for manufacturers and retailers.

Medications used to treat acne include:

- Vitamins (such as synthetic vitamin A derivatives)
- Antibiotics
- Steroids and hormonal treatments
- Anti-androgen drugs

Topical treatments are generally preferred, as they are more effective and have fewer side effects than systemic treatments. In many cases, combination therapy is recommended.

Hormonal contraceptives, particularly new-generation synthetic progestins, have shown positive effects on skin health and can help reduce acne. However, modern guidelines do not consider this an optimal treatment, particularly for adolescents. Hormones should only be prescribed when there are underlying hormonal disorders or when contraception is required. Hormonal contraceptives do not offer superior effectiveness compared to other acne treatments and should not be used without strict medical indications.

Numerous alternative treatments for acne exist, including laser, light, and photodynamic therapy, but their effectiveness remains debatable. Additionally, there is ongoing debate regarding the duration of treatment, bacterial resistance to antibiotics, and the rational use of antibiotics in acne therapy. Since acne treatment may involve dermatologists, cosmetologists, and other specialists, the combined effect of different interventions may sometimes be counterproductive.

For this reason, it is crucial not to overcomplicate the diagnosis and treatment of acne—primarily through self-treatment—but rather to seek guidance from a qualified specialist.

11.3. Hair and Hormones

Hormonal levels play a significant role in determining the condition of hair. While genes control hair quantity, natural color, and structure, hormonal imbalances can lead to noticeable changes in hair quality.

The health of your hair is strongly influenced by several glands in your body, including the thyroid and parathyroid glands, adrenal glands, pancreas (insulin), and gonads.

Two common conditions influenced by hormones that affect hair are hair loss (alopecia) and hirsutism, which is excessive hair growth.

The causes of alopecia in men and women are different. In men, male sex hormones play a key role, whereas in women, the leading causes are sharp fluctuations in sex hormones and stress. This is why hair loss is often observed during adolescence, after stopping hormonal contraceptives, and in the postpartum period. Stress-related alopecia is the most common type of hair loss in women of reproductive age. Fortunately, this type of alopecia is usually reversible, meaning hair often returns to normal.

Having too little hair is undesirable, but excess hair is also a problem for many women.

11.3.1. Hirsutism

Hair growth in adolescent girls and young women who follow modern beauty standards of "smooth skin" often leads to tears, disappointment, and a desperate search for the cause of such hairiness. Society's perception of female (and male) body hair has changed radically over the past 50 years. Interestingly, in old photographs of the still-popular movie and music stars (from their younger years) and films produced up to the late 1970s, one can see hairy legs, underarm hair, and pubic hair (in nude scenes). Even today, in many regions of the world, body hair is considered a normal part of human life, except in rare cases.

The trend of removing body hair and artificially shaped eyebrows and eyelashes is now dominant in most parts of the world. It is prevalent among women of reproductive age living in cities.

The amount of hair on the skin primarily depends on hereditary factors, as the development of the hair follicle apparatus occurs in the embryonic period. Other factors that influence hair growth include the levels and metabolism of male sex hormones, the concentration of sex hormone-binding proteins in the blood, and the sensitivity of hair follicles to androgens. In the presence of skin infections (such as acne), the sensitivity of hair to androgens increases.

Androgens do not affect the growth of fine, vellus hair, meaning these hairs are androgen-independent. Long hair grows under the influence of various hormones. Therefore, when a woman complains about the appearance of fine hairs on her chin or cheeks, this is not a sign of disease.

Hirsutism is excessive hair growth in a male pattern triggered by increased levels of male sex hormones. Hair appears on the tip of the nose (inside the nostrils), above the upper lip, on the chin, cheeks (sideburns), ear lobes, back, chest, around the nipples, in the armpits, on the lower abdomen, in the pubic area, and on the front surface of the thighs. Again, hair in these areas can be completely normal, so its evaluation must be realistic.

A much more concerning condition is virilization, which requires urgent diagnosis. Virilization includes hirsutism as well as other signs of masculinization, such as a deepened voice, muscle development in a male pattern, clitoral enlargement, changes in hair growth and distribution, receding hairline at the temples, and acne. Virilization most often occurs when androgen levels are significantly elevated, usually due to hormone-producing ovarian or adrenal tumors. In such women, menstruation frequently stops.

Another condition associated with increased hair growth is hypertrichosis, a general increase in body hair without elevated levels of male sex hormones. Hypertrichosis is often constitutional, may be observed in families (hereditary), and can be either a normal variation or a sign of disease.

Sudden onset or progressive hirsutism is a sign of hormonal imbalances in the female body, primarily indicating increased androgen levels. This is often observed in various endocrine-metabolic disorders such as polycystic ovary syndrome, Cushing's syndrome, congenital adrenal hyperplasia, and hormone-producing ovarian tumors. In some cases, hirsutism develops due to disruptions in the production and metabolism of male sex hormones, even without a detected disease or tumor. However, in most cases, hirsutism is constitutional (familial), meaning it has a hereditary basis. It can also occur due to certain medications that increase androgen levels.

A comprehensive medical history and physical examination are crucial steps in identifying the cause of hirsutism. Many doctors recommend photographing the most affected areas to track treatment progress. Specific scales and scoring systems are used to assess the severity of hirsutism, and laboratory tests should be performed to rule out ovarian tumors that produce androgens.

The choice of treatment depends on the severity of hirsutism. It is essential to remember that hirsutism is not a disease but a possible sign of hormonal imbalance. Treatment of hirsutism can be medical and/or cosmetic. In cases of familial hirsutism, temporary or permanent hair removal methods are often used. The choice of treatment is the doctor's responsibility.

11.4. Cosmetics with Hormones

Almost all hormonal drugs (and there are several hundred of them, if not more) require a prescription in many countries. They are also banned in cosmetics and skincare products in developed countries. Therefore, if any hormonal substances are present in such products, they are most likely plant-based hormone precursors (phytosterols), which I have already mentioned, or hormone metabolites that do not have hormonal activity.

In countries where cosmetic product composition is not strictly regulated, some products may contain hormones, most commonly steroids, anabolic agents, or growth hormone.

Some cosmetic and skin care manufacturers bypass ingredient regulations by using plant—and animal-derived extracts, infusions, and broths, such as placenta extract and parabens and their derivatives.

Among all hormones, progesterone is most frequently used outside of medicine without supervision. Today, many cosmetic and hygiene products, anti-aging treatments, and dietary supplements containing micronized progesterone are sold online and in various "health stores."

These products are often advertised with persuasive claims about their ability to enhance libido and potency, reduce "estrogen dominance," support the prostate, and improve and rejuvenate the skin. However, the exact percentage and quantity of progesterone used in these products are rarely disclosed because their production is mainly unregulated worldwide. Even if a product is banned in one country, it can still be purchased online and shipped globally for "personal use."

Parabens are not hormonal substances, despite being marketed as such in advertisements and some publications. Their direct impact on the human body remains poorly studied (refer to the section on phytoestrogens), and neither their effectiveness nor safety has been proven.

If we are honest and not swayed by marketing or the warnings of some doctors, we do not know how beneficial or harmful cosmetics and other skincare and haircare products are. However, since these are purely commercial products, their popularity grows each year, leaving the final choice up to the consumer.

Final Thoughts

I want to express my heartfelt gratitude to every one of you who has read this book to the last lines. Your interest and engagement have been a source of inspiration and motivation. Yes, the time has come to put a final period, though the role of hormones in human life remains an open question.

Writing books has always been a pleasure for me. I work on them with inspiration, a smile, and a sense of fulfillment, knowing that I can share fascinating and important information with others. However, the more you know, the harder it becomes to select only the most essential pieces — and, most importantly, to know when to stop writing.

On the one hand, I am leaving many topics open-ended for future books. On the other hand, I hope that even the volume of knowledge presented here has enriched your understanding of your own body and hormones.

You can find more health information on my official website and social media pages, especially on women's health. I strive to share the most up-to-date, accurate, and accessible scientific and medical data.

Thank you to all my readers who, when asked in a poll on my social media about which book they would like me to write first, almost unanimously chose this one on hormones. Your wish has come true — just as mine has! Your input and interest are the driving force behind my work, and I am deeply grateful for your support.

I want to give a special thanks to my beloved family and friends for their unwavering support throughout the creation of this massive and unique work.

I am not saying goodbye because I have many more publications, including books, lectures, seminars, and videos, ahead. If new readers have discovered me through this book, I am delighted, and I hope it won't be the last book of mine that interests you.

Stay healthy!

Yours truly,

Olena Berezovska

References

1. Adlercreutz H, Mazur W (1997) Phyto-oestrogens and Western diseases Ann Med 29(2):95–120.
2. Ahmed A M (2005) Historical landmarks in thyroid disorder understanding including Graves' disease, thyroidectomy, and thyroxine definition EMHJ 11(3):459–469.
3. Albers EM, et al (2024) Sex-steroid hormones and risk of postmenopausal breast cancer Cancer Causes Control 35(4):395–407.
4. Albrecht ED, Pepe GJ (1990) Placental steroid hormone biosynthesis in primate pregnancy Endocr Rev 11(1):124–150.
5. Alexander E. K., et al. (2017). 2017 Guidelines of the American Thyroid Association for the diagnosis and management of thyroid disease during pregnancy and the postpartum. Thyroid, 27(3):315–389.
6. Allen M. J., Kumar P., Cho J. (2023). Physiology, Adrenocorticotropic Hormone (ACTH). StatPearls Publishing.
7. Allen N. E., et al (2002). Dietary fat, fiber, and ovarian function. Cancer Epidemiology, Biomarkers & Prevention, 11(11):1148–1151.
8. American Diabetes Association. (2025). Classification and diagnosis of diabetes: Standards of Medical Care in Diabetes. Diabetes Care, 48(Suppl 1):S17–S42.
9. American Society for Reproductive Medicine (2020) Practice Committee opinion: testing and interpreting measures of ovarian reserve Fertility and Sterility 114(6):1151–1156.
10. American Thyroid Association (2007) High-risk pregnant women should have TSH measured at first prenatal visit or by nine weeks gestation Journal of Clinical Endocrinology & Metabolism 92(1):203–207.
11. American Thyroid Association and American Association of Clinical Endocrinologists (2000) Recommendations for screening thyroid function starting at age 35 every five years Fertility and Sterility 74(5):829–838.
12. Anderson TJ, Haynes NB (1969) Plasma testosterone in pregnant women. J Endocrinol 45(1):69–78.
13. Apter D (1980) Serum steroids and pituitary hormones in female puberty: a longitudinal study Clinical Endocrinology 12(2):107–120.
14. Arey B. J. (1999). Identification and classification of FSH receptor antagonists. Journal of Reproductive Immunology, 44(1–2):41–52.
15. Argiolas A., Melis M. R. (2004). The neuropharmacology of dopamine and sexual behavior. Neuroscience & Biobehavioral Reviews, 28(6): 671–684.

16. Asa S. L., Ezzat S. (2009). The pathogenesis of pituitary tumors. Annual Review of Pathology: Mechanisms of Disease, 4:97–126.
17. ASRM Practice Committee (2021) Diagnosis and treatment of luteal phase deficiency: a committee opinion Fertility and Sterility.
18. Astwood E B (1943) The use of thiourea and thiouracil in the treatment of hyperthyroidism Journal of Clinical Endocrinology 3(5):487–492.
19. Azziz R, et al (2006) Diagnosis of polycystic ovary syndrome: which criteria to use? J Clin Endocrinol Metab 91(3):781–785.
20. Azziz R, et al (2016) Polycystic ovary syndrome Nat Rev Dis Primers 2:16057.
21. Babu P. S., Sairam M. R. (2004). Hormonal regulation, expression, cloning and immunological detection of follicle stimulating hormone receptor in extragonadal tissues. Molecular and Cellular Endocrinology, 224(1–2):85–96.
22. Baird D T (1983) Factors regulating the growth of the dominant follicle in the human ovary J Reprod Fertil 69(1):343–352.
23. Baird DD, et al (2003) High cumulative incidence of uterine leiomyoma in black and white women: ultrasound evidence Am J Obstet Gynecol 188(1):100–107.
24. Baird DT (1978) The secretion of progesterone and the oestrogens by the ovary in relation to follicular development and luteal function. Biochem Soc Trans 6(6):1129–1133.
25. Balen A. H., et al (2016). The management of anovulatory infertility in women with polycystic ovary syndrome: an analysis of the evidence to support the development of global WHO guidance. Human Reproduction Update, 22(6):687–708.
26. Banting F. G., Best C. H. (1922). The Internal Secretion of the Pancreas. Journal of Laboratory and Clinical Medicine, 7(5):251–266.
27. Basedow K A (1840) Exophthalmus durch Hypertrophie des Zellgewebes in der Augenhöhle Wochenschrift für die gesammte Heilkunde 6:197–204.
28. Basson R (2001) Human sex-response cycles J Sex Marital Ther 27(1):33–43.
29. Bayhan G, et al (2015) Luteoma of pregnancy: clinical, radiologic and pathologic findings. Case Rep Obstet Gynecol 2015:613029.
30. Bayliss W. M., Starling E. H. (1902). The Mechanism of Pancreatic Secretion. Journal of Physiology, 28(5):325–353.
31. Begbie J (1852) Description of exophthalmic goiter Edinburgh Medical and Surgical Journal 77:33–46.

32. Bellamy L, et al (2009) Type 2 diabetes mellitus after gestational diabetes: A systematic review and meta-analysis Lancet 373(9677):1773–1779

33. Ben-Jonathan N., et al. (2008). What can we learn from rodents about prolactin in humans? Endocrine Reviews, 29(1):1–41.

34. Berent-Spillson A, et al (2015) Distinct cognitive effects of estrogen and progesterone during verbal processing: an fMRI study Horm Behav 70:1–9.

35. Bernichtein S., et al (2010). New concepts in prolactin biology. Journal of Endocrinology, 206(1):1–11.

36. Bikle D. D. (2021). The free hormone hypothesis: When, why, and how to measure free hormone levels. Journal of Bone and Mineral Research, 36(1):112–118.

37. Biller B.M., et al (1999). Guidelines for the diagnosis and treatment of hyperprolactinemia. Journal of Reproductive Medicine, 44(12 Suppl):1075–1084.

38. Bingham SA, et al (1998) Phyto-oestrogens: Where are we now? Br J Nutr 79(5):393–406.

39. Biondi B., Cooper D. S. (2008). The clinical significance of subclinical thyroid dysfunction. Endocrine Reviews, 29(1):76–131.

40. Blackmore PF (1999) Extragenomic actions of progesterone in human sperm Comp Biochem Physiol A Mol Integr Physiol 122(3):481–485

41. Blümel J E (2014) Climacteric and menopause as distinct concepts Climacteric 17(5):504–510.

42. Boguszewski C. L. S., Boguszewski M. C. S. (2019). Growth hormone, IGFs, and cancer: potential tumorigenic pathways. Endocrine Reviews, 40(2):558–578.

43. Bole-Feysot C., et al (1998). Prolactin (PRL) and its receptor: actions, signal transduction pathways and phenotypes observed in PRL receptor knockout mice. Endocrine Reviews, 19(3):225–268.

44. Brandon DD, et al (1993) Progesterone receptor messenger ribonucleic acid and protein are overexpressed in human uterine leiomyomas Am J Obstet Gynecol 169(1):78–85.

45. Braunstein GD, et al (1976) Serum human chorionic gonadotropin levels throughout normal pregnancy Am J Obstet Gynecol 126(6):678–681.

46. Brent G. A. (2012). Mechanisms of thyroid hormone action. Journal of Clinical Investigation, 122(9):3035–3043.

47. Broekmans F J M, et al (2006) Anti-Müllerian hormone: ovarian reserve testing and clinical implications Human Reproduction Update 12(6):685–702.

48. Broekmans F J, et al (2007) Female reproductive ageing: current knowledge and future trends Trends in Endocrinology & Metabolism 18(2):58–65

49. Broekmans F. J., et al (2009). Ovarian aging: mechanisms and clinical consequences. Endocrine Reviews, 30(5):465–493.

50. Brownstein M. J., et al. (1980). Synthesis, transport, and release of posterior pituitary hormones. Science, 207(4429):373–378.

51. Buchanan TA, Xiang AH (2005) A clinical update on gestational diabetes mellitus Endocr Rev 26(5):697–738.

52. Bulun SE (2009) Endometriosis N Engl J Med 360(3):268–279.

53. Bulun SE (2013) Uterine fibroids N Engl J Med 369(14):1344–1355.

54. Bulun SE, et al (2010) Estrogen receptor-β, estrogen receptor-α, and progesterone resistance in endometriosis Semin Reprod Med 28(1):36–43.

55. Burchardt NA, et al. (2020) Oral contraceptive use and endometrial cancer risk — hazard ratio 0.43 for >10 years of use Eur J Epidemiol 35(11):1037–1045.

56. Burger H. G., et al (2007). A review of hormonal changes during the menopausal transition: focus on findings from the Melbourne Women's Midlife Health Project. Human Reproduction Update, 13(6):559–565.

57. Burney RO, Giudice LC (2012) Pathogenesis and pathophysiology of endometriosis Fertil Steril 98(3):511–519.

58. Cable J. K. (2023). Physiology, Progesterone. StatPearls Publishing.

59. Calderon R A, et al (2001) Increased incidence of thyroid cancer among children in Cumbria post-Chernobyl Radiation Research 156(2):131–136.

60. Carmichael MS, et al (1987) Plasma oxytocin increases in the human sexual response J Clin Endocrinol Metab 64(1):27–31.

61. Carmina E. (2017). Non-classic CAH due to 21-hydroxylase deficiency: Diagnosis via 17-OHP. Human Reproduction Update, 23(5):580–592.

62. Carter C. S. (1998). Neuroendocrine perspectives on social attachment and love. Psychoneuroendocrinology, 23(8):779–818.

63. Carter C. S., Altemus M. (2004). Integrative functions of lactational hormones in social behavior and stress management. Annals of the New York Academy of Sciences, 1032(1):289–301.

64. Catalano PM (2014) Trying to understand gestational diabetes Diabet Med 31(3):273–281.

65. Catenaccio E, et al (2016) Estrogen- and progesterone-mediated structural neuroplasticity in the female human limbic system Neuroimage 134:327–336.

451

66. Centers for Disease Control and Prevention (2024) U.S. Medical Eligibility Criteria and Selected Practice Recommendations for Contraceptive Use MMWR Recomm Rep 73(RR-3):1–128.

67. Cervantes A., et al (2018) Profile of gut hormones, pancreatic hormones and pro-inflammatory cytokines Gastroenterology Research 11(4):280–289.

68. Cetera GE, et al. (2023) Non-response to first-line hormonal treatments in endometriosis: role of progesterone resistance BMC Womens Health 23:449.

69. Chang S, et al (2021) Diagnosis of polycystic ovarian syndrome: the Rotterdam criteria and beyond J Clin Endocrinol Metab 106(6):1682–1691.

70. Chatuphonprasert W., et al. (2018). Physiology and pathophysiology of steroid biosynthesis in the human placenta. Frontiers in Pharmacology, 9:1021.

71. Cheung L P, et al (2017) Dietary fat intake and ovarian hormone secretion in premenopausal women The British Journal of Nutrition 117(9):1328–1334.

72. Christin-Maitre S (2013) History of oral contraceptive drugs and their use worldwide Best Pract Res Clin Endocrinol Metab 27(1):3–12.

73. Cianfarani S. (2019). GH therapy during childhood and cancer risk: A critical review. Annals of Pediatric Endocrinology & Metabolism, 24(2):92–101.

74. Clayton AH, Dennerstein L (2019) The role of sex hormones in female sexual dysfunction Endocrinol Metab Clin North Am 48(3):467–484.

75. Clayton AH, Kingsberg SA, Goldstein I (2018) Evaluation and management of hypoactive sexual desire disorder Sex Med 6(2):59–74.

76. Cole LA (2010) Biological functions of hCG and hCG-related molecules Reprod Biol Endocrinol 8:102.

77. Cole LA (2012) hCG, the wonder of today's science Reprod Biol Endocrinol 10:24.

78. Collaborative Group on Epidemiological Studies of Ovarian Cancer (2017) Combined oral contraceptives and ovarian and endometrial cancer risk — reduction persists for decades Lancet Oncol 18(9):1371–1381.

79. Collaborative Group on Hormonal Factors in Breast Cancer (1997) Breast cancer and hormone replacement therapy: Collaborative reanalysis of data from 51 epidemiological studies of 52,705 women with breast cancer and 108,411 women without breast cancer Lancet 350(9084):1047–1059.

80. Cooke P. S. (2017). Estrogens in male physiology. Physiological Reviews, 97(1).
81. Coomarasamy A, et al (2011) Progesterone for prevention of miscarriage: a randomized placebo-controlled trial N Engl J Med 364(19):1879–1887.
82. Coomarasamy A, et al (2015) A randomized trial of progesterone in women with recurrent miscarriages N Engl J Med 373(22):2141–2148.
83. Cooper DB, Mahdy H, Shah K (2024) Oral contraceptive pills initiation methods StatPearls Publishing.
84. Cooper W (1975) No Change: The Biological Revolution for Women. Arlington Books, London, 224 p.
85. Corner G W, Allen W M (1929) Physiology of the corpus luteum, its development and function Am J Anat 44(1):169–223.
86. Cornwell T, Cohick W, Raskin I (2004) Dietary phytoestrogens and health Phytochemistry 65(8):995–1016.
87. Costea D M (2000) Delayed luteo–placental shift of progesterone production Steroids 68(2):123–129.
88. Coustan DR (2013) Gestational diabetes mellitus Clin Chem 59(9):1310–1321.
89. Crowley W. F., Pitteloud N. (2005). Gonadotropin-releasing hormone deficiency. New England Journal of Medicine, 352(12):1228–1236.
90. Csapo A I (1956) Function, regulation and regression of the corpus luteum of pregnancy in mammals Physiol Rev 36(4):640–690.
91. Csapo AI (1981) Progesterone "block". Am J Anat 162(3):237–256.
92. Csapo AI, et al (1972) Effects of luteectomy and progesterone replacement therapy in early pregnant patients Am J Obstet Gynecol 112(7):1061–1067.
93. Csapo AI, Pulkkinen MO (1978) Indispensability of the human corpus luteum in the maintenance of early pregnancy. Lancet 312(8086):1061–1063.
94. Cushing H. (1912). The Pituitary Body and Its Disorders: Clinical States Produced by Disorders of the Hypophysis Cerebri. Philadelphia: J.B. Lippincott.
95. Cussen L (2022) Approach to androgen excess in women: clinical presentations Clinical Endocrinology 97(4):445–457.
96. D'Agostino G., et al. (2010). Alpha-Melanocyte-Stimulating Hormone: Production and processing. Peptides, 31(2).
97. Dale H. H. (1950). Reflections on the Term 'Hormone'. British Medical Bulletin, 6(4):323–326.
98. D'Angelo E, Prat J (2010) Uterine sarcomas: a review Gynecol Oncol 116(1):131–139.

99. Danilovich N., et al (2002). Estrogen deficiency, obesity and skeletal abnormalities in follicle-stimulating hormone receptor knockout (FORKO) female mice. Endocrinology, 143(2):471–486.

100. Davis S, et al (2004) Thyroid cancer risk related to radiation dose after Chernobyl Radiation Research 162(3):231–240.

101. Davison S. L. (2005). Androgen levels decline steeply from early reproductive years; minimal variation post-menopause. Journal of Clinical Endocrinology & Metabolism, 90(7).

102. de Angelis C, et al (2020) Smoke alcohol and drug addiction and female fertility Reproductive Biology and Endocrinology 18:21.

103. de Gardanne C P L (1816) Introduction of the term "ménopause" referring to the cessation of menstruation On Menopause, or the Critical Age of Women: A Medical Essay,

104. Dhage V D, et al (2024) A narrative review on the impact of smoking on female reproductive health Journal of Reproductive Health Research 12(1):34–41.

105. Dhont M (2010) History of oral contraception Eur J Contracept Reprod Health Care 15(3):164–170.

106. Donnez J (2021) PR deficiency and progesterone resistance in endometriosis: therapeutic consequences J Clin Med 10(5):1085.

107. Donnez J, Dolmans MM (2013) Endometriosis and medical therapy: from progestogens to progesterone resistance to GnRH antagonists: a review J Endocrinol Invest 36(7):603–611.

108. Dorn L D and Biro F M (2011) Puberty and its measurement: a decade in review Journal of Research on Adolescence 21(1):180–195

109. Douxfils J, et al. (2025) COC-related VTE in European region — 2- to 6-fold risk, tens of thousands of cases annually Front Endocrinol 16:1559162.

110. Dunselman GA, et al (2014) ESHRE guideline: management of women with endometriosis Hum Reprod 29(3):400–412.

111. Eaton L. (2005). College Looks Back to Discovery of Hormones. British Medical Journal, 331(7510):126.

112. Ehrmann D. A. (1992). Detection of functional ovarian hyperandrogenism. New England Journal of Medicine, 327(3):226–230.

113. Eisenberg DL, et al (2012) Distinguishing typical and perfect-use contraceptive failure rates Ann Intern Med 157(11):824–825.

114. Eisinger M, Li WH (2018) Hormones and skin aging Dermatoendocrinol 10(1):e1442169.

115. El Sayed S.A., Collins J. (2023). Physiology, Pancreas. StatPearls Publishing.

116. Elhassan Y. S. (2018). Causes, patterns, and severity of androgen excess in 1,205 women. Journal of Clinical Endocrinology & Metabolism, 103(3).
117. Emanuele M A, et al (2002) Alcohol's effects on female reproductive function Alcohol Research & Health 26(4):274–281.
118. Enriori P. J., Sinnayah P., Cowley M. A. (2016). α-MSH modulates glucose homeostasis via skeletal muscle. PLoS ONE, 11(10).
119. Epplein M, et al (2008) Risk of complex and atypical endometrial hyperplasia in relation to anthropometric measures and reproductive history Am J Epidemiol 168(6):563–570.
120. Erdheim J (1914) Parathyroid hyperplasia in osteomalacia and rickets Wiener Klinische Wochenschrift 27:279–281.
121. ESHRE/ASRM (2004) Revised 2003 consensus on diagnostic criteria and long-term health risks related to polycystic ovary syndrome Hum Reprod 19(5):41–48
122. Eyth E.M., Basit H. (2023). Glucose Tolerance Test. StatPearls Publishing.
123. Ezziz R (2005) Diagnostic criteria for polycystic ovary syndrome— Rotterdam versus NIH definitions Fertil Steril 83(6):1365–1369.
124. Fabbrocini G et al (2018) Acne scars: pathogenesis, classification and treatment Dermatol Res Pract 2010:893080.
125. Falck B (1959) Site of production of oestrogen in rat ovary as studied in microtransplants Acta Physiol Scand 47:1–101.
126. Fan D, et al (2017) Female alcohol consumption and fecundability Scientific Reports 7:13815.
127. Farquhar M. G., Rinehart J. F. (1954). A cytological study of prolactin secretion by the rat anterior pituitary gland. American Journal of Anatomy, 94(1):83–107.
128. Fauser B. C., et al. (1999). Minimal ovarian stimulation for IVF: appraisal of potential benefits and drawbacks. Human Reproduction, 14(11):2681–2686.
129. Filicori M., et al. (2003). The use of LH activity to drive folliculogenesis: exploring uncharted territories in ovulation induction. Human Reproduction Update, 9(5):483–497.
130. Flores VA, et al. (2018) Progesterone receptor status predicts response to progestin therapy in endometriosis J Clin Endocrinol Metab 103(12):4561–4570.
131. Forest MG, et al (1980) Hypothalamic-pituitary-gonadal relationships in man from birth to puberty. Clin Endocrinol (Oxf) 13(6):567–588.
132. Fortner RT, et al (2013) Premenopausal endogenous steroid hormones and breast cancer risk Cancer Epidemiol Biomarkers Prev 22(1):14–24.

133. Fraser H M, Lunn S F (2000) Regulation and manipulation of angiogenesis in the primate corpus luteum Reproduction 121(3):355–362.
134. Freeman M. E., et al (2000). Prolactin: structure, function, and regulation of secretion. Physiological Reviews, 80(4):1523–1631.
135. Freud S (1905) Three Essays on the Theory of Sexuality. Deuticke, Leipzig and Vienna, 239 p.
136. Frisch R E and McArthur J W (1974) Menstrual cycles: fatness as a determinant of minimum weight for height necessary for their maintenance or onset Science 185(4155):949–951.
137. Frye CA (2025) Progestogens promote anti-anxiety and anti-depressive behavior via allopregnanolone in hippocampus/amygdala Int J Mol Sci 26(3):1173.
138. Funder J W (2010) From 1953 until 1990: some pivotal discoveries regarding aldosterone biology and epithelial sodium retention Endocrinology 151(11):5098–5104.
139. Gallo-Payet N. (2016). 60 years of POMC: Adrenal and extra-adrenal functions. Journal of Molecular Endocrinology, 56(4).
140. Gallos ID, Shehmar M, Thangaratinam S, Papadopoulou A, Coomarasamy A, Gupta JK (2010) Oral progestogens vs levonorgestrel-releasing intrauterine system for endometrial hyperplasia: a systematic review and meta-analysis Am J Obstet Gynecol 203(6):547.e1–547.e10.
141. Gaskill P J (2022) Catecholamines and neuroimmune communication Neuroscience Review.
142. Gaskins A. J., Chavarro J. E. (2018). Diet and fertility: Carbohydrates and hormones. Fertility and Sterility, 109(3):384–392.
143. Geist SH, Spielman AJ (1932) The use of estrogens in the treatment of climacteric syndrome Am J Obstet Gynecol 24:76–82.
144. Giudice LC, Kao LC (2004) Endometriosis Lancet 364(9447):1789–1799.
145. Gley E (1891) Demonstration that removal of parathyroid glands causes tetany Comptes Rendus de l'Académie des Sciences (Paris) 113:688–691.
146. Glinoer D. (1997). The regulation of thyroid function in pregnancy: pathways of endocrine adaptation from physiology to pathology. Endocrine Reviews, 18(3):404–433.
147. Goffin V., et al (2002). Prolactin: the new biology of an old hormone. Annual Review of Physiology, 64:47–67.
148. Gold E B (2011) Median age at menopause and variation across populations Menopause 18(2):126–127.

149. Goldman A. L. (2017). Reappraisal of testosterone's binding in circulation. Endocrine Reviews, 38(4):302–328.
150. Goldstein SR (2010) Modern evaluation of the endometrium Obstet Gynecol 116(1):168–176.
151. Goldstuck N D (2011) Progestin potency – assessment and relevance to choice of oral contraceptives Eur J Contracept Reprod Health Care 16(4):281–290.
152. Golos T G, Strauss J F (1996) Progesterone regulation of endometrium and contraception Endocr Rev 17(3):331–355.
153. Grady D, et al (2002) Cardiovascular disease outcomes during 6.8 years of hormone therapy: Heart and Estrogen/progestin Replacement Study follow-up (HERS II) JAMA 288(1):49–57.
154. Grattan D. R. (2002). Behavioural significance of prolactin signalling in the central nervous system during pregnancy and lactation. Reproduction, 123(4):497–506.
155. Graves R J (1835) Newly observed affection of the thyroid gland in females London Medical and Surgical Journal 7(2):516–520.
156. Grumbach M M (2002) The neuroendocrinology of human puberty revisited Hormone Research 57(Suppl 2):2–14.
157. Guevara-Aguirre J., et al (2023). Cancer in growth hormone excess and deficit: current evidence and controversies. Endocrine-Related Cancer, 30(10).
158. Guo SW (2009) Recurrence of endometriosis and its control Hum Reprod Update 15(4):441–461.
159. Gurgan T., et al (1997). A prospective randomized study comparing recombinant FSH (Gonal-F) and urinary FSH (Metrodin) in ovulation induction. Human Reproduction, 12(10):2143–2148.
160. Guttmacher Institute (2020) Contraceptive effectiveness in the United States Guttmacher Fact Sheet.
161. Haas DM, et al (2009) Progestogen for preventing miscarriage Cochrane Database Syst Rev 2:CD003511.
162. Hammond G. L. (2011). Diverse roles for sex hormone-binding globulin in reproduction. Endocrine Reviews.
163. Hammond G. L. (2016). Plasma steroid-binding proteins: primary gatekeepers of steroid action. Journal of Endocrinology, 230(1):R43–R55.
164. Han SJ, et al (2015) Progesterone receptor signaling in the uterus and ovary Front Endocrinol 6:157.
165. Handwerger S, Freemark M (2000) The roles of placental growth hormone and placental lactogen in the regulation of human fetal growth and development J Pediatr Endocrinol Metab 13(4):343–356
166. Harris B S (2022) Diminished ovarian reserve is not associated with reduced future reproductive capacity Reproduction 164(1).

167. Havelock J C, et al (2004) Adrenarche — physiology, biochemistry and human disease Clinical Endocrinology 60(3):288–296.
168. Henderson J. (2005). Ernest Starling and 'Hormones': An Historical Commentary. Journal of Endocrinology, 184(1):7–10.
169. Herman-Giddens M E et al. (1997) Secondary sexual characteristics and menses in young girls seen in office practice: a study from the Pediatric Research in Office Settings network Pediatrics 99(4):505–512.
170. Hertz S and Roberts A (1943) Radioactive iodine as therapy for Graves' disease Journal of Clinical Investigation 22(5):729–740.
171. Hillier. S. G. (2001). Gonadotropic control of ovarian follicular growth and development. Molecular and Cellular Endocrinology, 179(1–2):39–46.
172. Hirschberg A. L. (2023). Hirsutism as a measure of hyperandrogenism. Journal of Clinical Endocrinology & Metabolism, 108(5):1243–1256.
173. Hod M, et al (2015) The International Federation of Gynecology and Obstetrics (FIGO) initiative on gestational diabetes mellitus: A pragmatic guide for diagnosis, management, and care Int J Gynaecol Obstet 131 Suppl 3:S173–S211.
174. Hod M, et al (2020) Evidence in support of the International Association of Diabetes and Pregnancy Study Groups' criteria for diagnosing gestational diabetes: A systematic review Diabetes Care 43(10):2390–2397.
175. Horseman N. D., Yu-Lee L. Y. (1994). Prolactin in man and other mammals: actions and regulation. Trends in Endocrinology and Metabolism, 5(8):277–282.
176. IARC Working Group on the Evaluation of Carcinogenic Risks to Humans (1999) Combined oral contraceptives, progestogens only, and post-menopausal oestrogen therapy IARC Monographs No. 72.
177. IARC Working Group on the Evaluation of Carcinogenic Risks to Humans (2007) Combined estrogen–progestogen contraceptives and combined estrogen–progestogen menopausal therapy IARC Monographs No. 91
178. Ikoma D. M., et al (2017). Threshold progesterone level of 25 ng/ml to sustain pregnancy in first trimester in women with history of infertility or miscarriage. Clin Obstet Gynecol Reprod Med.
179. Ishimoto H and Jaffe R B (2010) Development and function of the human fetal adrenal Endocrine Reviews 31(5).
180. Iwasaki Y. (2024). Biological roles of growth hormone/prolactin from an evolutionary standpoint. Endocrine Journal, 71(9).
181. Jabbour HN, et al (2006) Endocrine regulation of menstruation Endocr Rev 27(1):17–46.

182. Jacob P, et al (1999) Chernobyl accident and thyroid cancer in children: excess risk assessment Nature 388(6643):810–811.

183. Jarvis G (2017) Early embryo mortality in natural human reproduction: What the data say F1000Res 5:9616.

184. Jensen T K, et al (1998) Does moderate alcohol consumption affect fertility BMJ 317(7155):505.

185. Johnson NP, et al (2017) World Endometriosis Society consensus on the classification of endometriosis Hum Reprod 32(2):315–324.

186. Johnson WS, Bartlett WR (1971) Total synthesis of progesterone J Am Chem Soc 93(13):4329–4331.

187. Johnston Z C et al (2018) Human fetal adrenal produces cortisol but no aldosterone in the second trimester BMC Medicine 16:23.

188. Junod SW, Marks L (2002) Women's trials: the approval of the first oral contraceptive pill in the United States J Hist Med Allied Sci 57(2):117–160.

189. Kao A (2000) History of oral contraception AMA J Ethics 2(6):171–177.

190. Kao LC, et al (2003) Expression profiling of endometrium from women with endometriosis reveals candidate genes for disease-based implantation failure and infertility Endocrinology 144(7):2870–2881,

191. Kaufman KD (2002) Androgens and alopecia Mol Cell Endocrinol 198(1-2):89–95.

192. Kaunitz A M (2007) Injectable and implantable contraception Obstet Gynecol Clin North Am 34(1):73–91.

193. Kelly P. A., et al. (2001). Prolactin: from physiology to pathology. Journal of Clinical Endocrinology & Metabolism, 86(10):4589–4596.

194. Kendall E C (1914) The isolation of thyroxine from the thyroid gland Journal of Biological Chemistry 19(1):1–16.

195. Kendall E. C. (1915). The Isolation in Crystalline Form of the Thyroid Hormone. Journal of Biological Chemistry, 23:287–293.

196. Kerr J. B., et al (2006). Quantification of healthy follicles in the neonatal and adult mouse ovary: evidence for maintenance of primordial follicle supply. Reproduction, 132(1):95–109.

197. Kim B. (2008). Peroxisome proliferator-activated receptors and thyroid hormone signaling. PPAR Research, 2008:1–12.

198. Kim J (2025) Estrogens and breast cancer: progestin signaling amplification Cancer Lett 530:215–223.

199. Kingsberg SA, Clayton AH (2020) The women's sexual health continuum: merging clinical medicine with science Fertil Steril 114(1):70–77.

200. Kiriyama Y., Nochi H., Ichinose S. (2018). Role and cytotoxicity of amylin and protection. Cells, 7(8).

201. Kocher T (1910) Jod-Basedow: hyperthyroidism induced by iodine exposure Deutsche Medizinische Wochenschrift 36(19):835–837.

202. Koniares K., et al. (2023). Macroprolactinemia: a mini-review and update on clinical significance. Hormones (Athens), 22(2): 183–188.

203. Kopp P. (2001). Human thyroglobulin: From gene structure to defects in thyroid function. Endocrine Reviews, 22(4):485–501.

204. Ku C.W., et al. (2021). Gestational age-specific normative serum progesterone values and the luteal–placental shift. Scientific Reports, 11(1).

205. Kühl H (2005) Pharmacology of progestogens Maturitas 52(1):1–13.

206. Kurman RJ, et al (1985) Endometrial hyperplasia and carcinoma: clinical and pathologic correlations Am J Obstet Gynecol 152(4):505–512.

207. Kurman RJ, et al (1985) The behavior of endometrial hyperplasia: a long-term study of "untreated" hyperplasia in 170 patients Cancer 56(2):403–412.

208. La Marca A., et al (2009). Anti-Müllerian hormone (AMH): what do we still need to know? Human Reproduction, 24(9):2264–2275.

209. Lacey JV Jr, et al (2008) Endometrial carcinoma risk among women diagnosed with endometrial hyperplasia: the 34-year experience in a large health plan Br J Cancer 98(1):45–53.

210. Larsen P. R., et al. (1998). Thyroid physiology and diagnostic evaluation of patients with thyroid disorders. In: Williams Textbook of Endocrinology, 9th ed.

211. Lee JR, Hopkins V (1996) What Your Doctor May Not Tell You About Menopause: The Breakthrough Book on Natural Progesterone. Warner Books, New York, 368 p.

212. Lee JR, Hopkins V (2001) What Your Doctor May Not Tell You About Premenopause: Balance Your Hormones and Your Life from Thirty to Fifty. Warner Books, New York, 464 p.

213. Leeners B, et al (2017) Lack of associations between female hormone levels and attention, working memory, and cognitive bias across the menstrual cycle Front Behav Neurosci 11:120.

214. Legro RS, et al (2013) Diagnosis and treatment of polycystic ovary syndrome Fertil Steril 100(1):13–15.

215. Lesnewski R, Prine L (2021) Initiating hormonal contraception: evidence-based flexibility Am Fam Physician 104(3):187–194.

216. Lethaby A, Vollenhoven B (2015) Fibroids (uterine myomatosis, leiomyomas) BMJ Clin Evid 2015:0814.

217. Levine S., et al (2018). Stress-induced hyperprolactinemia: pathophysiology and diagnostic implications. Journal of Clinical Endocrinology and Metabolism, 103(5):1876–1881.
218. Levitz M, Young BK (1977) Estrogens in pregnancy Vitam Horm 35:109–147.
219. Levothyroxine efficacy (2024) Pre-conceptional LT4 does not significantly reduce miscarriage or improve fertility Thyroid 34(2):207–215.
220. Levothyroxine in subclinical hypothyroidism (2023) Improved pregnancy outcomes in women with TPO antibodies and SCH Obstetrics & Gynecology 142(5):948–957.
221. Li Z., et al (2016). Growth hormone replacement therapy reduces risk of cancer in adults with GH deficiency: A meta-analysis. European Journal of Endocrinology, 175(4).
222. Liao P V (2012) Half a century of the oral contraceptive pill Postgrad Med J 88(1041):234–238.
223. Lightman S. L. (2008). The neuroendocrinology of stress: A never ending story. Journal of Neuroendocrinology, 20(6):880–884.
224. Liu H, Lang JH (2017) Is abnormal eutopic endometrium the cause of endometriosis? The role of eutopic endometrium in pathogenesis of endometriosis Med Sci Monit 23:635–643.
225. Liu J, et al (2018) Diagnostic accuracy of single progesterone test to predict early pregnancy outcome in women with pain or bleeding: meta-analysis of cohort studies BMJ 337:a1391.
226. Liu PY, et al (2009) Clinical review: The rationale, efficacy and safety of androgen therapy in women J Clin Endocrinol Metab 94(10): 3811–3821.
227. Lizneva D, et al (2016) Prevalence, diagnostic criteria, and phenotypes of polycystic ovary syndrome: a systematic review and meta-analysis Hum Reprod Update 22(6):789–805.
228. Lobo RA, et al (2016) Back to the future: Hormone replacement therapy as part of a prevention strategy for women at the onset of menopause Atherosclerosis 254:282–290.
229. Loewi O. (1921). Über humorale Übertragbarkeit der Herznervenwirkung. Pflügers Archiv für die gesamte Physiologie, 189(1):239–242.
230. Loriaux DL, Lipsett MB (1971) The role of human placental lactogen in pregnancy N Engl J Med 285(13):711–714.
231. MacCallum W G (1908) Role of parathyroid glands in calcium metabolism and tetany Journal of Experimental Medicine 11(4):133–148.

232. Mahoney M C, et al (2004) Rising thyroid cancer incidence in Ukraine after Chernobyl International Journal of Epidemiology 33(5):1025–1031.
233. Makinen N, et al (2011) MED12, the mediator complex subunit 12 gene, is mutated at high frequency in uterine leiomyomas Science 334(6053):252–255.
234. Makrantonaki E, Zouboulis CC (2007) Androgens and ageing of the skin Curr Opin Endocrinol Diabetes Obes 14(3):240–245.
235. Mandl F (1925) First successful parathyroidectomy for osteitis fibrosa in humans Wiener Medizinische Wochenschrift 75:1451–1453.
236. Manson JE, et al (2013) Menopausal hormone therapy and health outcomes during the intervention and extended poststopping phases of the Women's Health Initiative randomized trials JAMA 310(13):1353–1368.
237. March W A, et al (2010) The prevalence of polycystic ovary syndrome in a community sample under the Rotterdam criteria Hum Reprod 25(2):544–549.
238. Marker RE (1940) Sterols. CXIII. Steroidal sapogenins. XLI. The preparation of steroidal hormones from sarsasapogenin and diosgenin J Am Chem Soc 62(9):2543–2555.
239. Marks L (2001) Sexual chemistry: a history of the contraceptive pill Yale University Press.
240. Marks L (2010) Public health and the pill Am J Public Health 100(11):2020–2028.
241. Marshall W A and Tanner J M (1969) Variations in the pattern of pubertal changes in girls Archives of Disease in Childhood 44(235):291–303.
242. Martin K. A. (2018). Evaluation and treatment of hirsutism in premenopausal women. Journal of Clinical Endocrinology & Metabolism, 103(4):1233–1250.
243. Martin KA, et al (2008) Evaluation and treatment of hirsutism in premenopausal women: an Endocrine Society Clinical Practice Guideline J Clin Endocrinol Metab 93(4):1105–1120.
244. Martinerie L (2013) Aldosterone discovered and purified in 1953; its importance in sodium metabolism highlighted Steroids 68(2).
245. Matheson E., Bain J. (2019). Hirsutism in women. American Family Physician, 100(3):168–175.
246. Matthews SC, et al. (2024) Long-term oral contraceptive use and endometrial cancer risk — up to 69% reduction with extended use Acta Obstet Gynecol Scand 103(8):810–818.
247. Mauvais-Jarvis F. (2013). The role of estrogens in control of energy balance and glucose homeostasis. Molecular Metabolism, 2(3).

248. Mayo C H (1907) Clinical notes on hyperthyroidism American Journal of Medical Sciences 134(2):187–193

249. Mayo Clinic Staff. (2024). Glucose tolerance test. Mayo Clinic Proceedings.

250. McCarthy O. J., et al. (2022). The endocrine pancreas during exercise in people with impaired metabolic function. Frontiers in Endocrinology.

251. McGowan P O et al (2018) Prenatal stress glucocorticoids and developmental programming Endocrinology 159(1):69–82.

252. McKenzie L. J. (2002). Progesterone in early pregnancy: measuring it, giving it. Contemporary OB/GYN.

253. Melmed S. (2011). Medical progress: Pathogenesis and diagnosis of pituitary tumors. New England Journal of Medicine, 324(10):705–715.

254. Melmed S. (2011). Pathogenesis and diagnosis of pituitary tumors. Nature Reviews Endocrinology, 7(5):257–266.

255. Mesen T. B. (2015). Progesterone and the luteal phase: A requisite to reproductive success. Reproductive Sciences.

256. Mesiano S (2019) Roles of estrogen and progesterone in human pregnancy J Steroid Biochem Mol Biol 189:142–150.

257. Messinis I. E. (2003). Excessive exercise and menstrual disturbances. Journal of Reproductive Medicine, 48(7):563–569.

258. Metzger BE, Coustan DR (1998) Summary and recommendations of the Fourth International Workshop-Conference on Gestational Diabetes Mellitus Diabetes Care 21 Suppl 2:B161–B167.

259. Metzger BE, et al (2010) International association of diabetes and pregnancy study groups recommendations on the diagnosis and classification of hyperglycemia in pregnancy Diabetes Care 33(3):676–682.

260. Michaud D. S., et al. (1998). Fat intake and hormone levels in women: Prospective study. Journal of the National Cancer Institute, 90(10):738–741.

261. Michels KB, et al. (2018) Duration of oral contraceptive use and ovarian cancer risk — long-term use consistently protective JAMA Oncol 4(6):881–888.

262. Mikkelsen E M, et al (2016) Alcohol consumption and fecundability: prospective Danish cohort study BMJ 354:i4262.

263. Miller J, et al (2016) Epidemiology of uterine fibroids with race, age, and smoking status Am J Obstet Gynecol 214(1):76.e1–76.e9.

264. Miller W L (2022) History of adrenal research from ancient anatomy to modern endocrinology Endocrine Reviews 43(1).

265. Miller W. L. (2010). The molecular biology, biochemistry, and physiology of steroidogenesis. Physiological Reviews, 90(2):777–795.

266. Miller W. L. (2011). Early steps in steroidogenesis: intracellular cholesterol transport and conversion. Endocrine Reviews, 32(4):Omitted pagination.

267. Million Women Study Collaborators (2003) Breast cancer and hormone-replacement therapy in the Million Women Study Lancet 362(9382):419–427.

268. Missmer SA, et al (2004) Endogenous estrogen, androgen, and progesterone levels and breast cancer risk JNCI 96(24):1856–1865.

269. Mokrysheva N G and Krupinova J A (2019) History of the discovery of parathyroid glands and their role in the body Vestnik Rossiiskoi Akademii Meditsinskikh Nauk 74(1):35–43.

270. Molitch M.E. (2005). Medication-induced hyperprolactinemia. Mayo Clinic Proceedings, 80(8):1050–1057.

271. Moll A (1897) Untersuchungen über die Libido sexualis, Leipzig: F.C.W. Vogel 379 p.

272. Momodu I. I. (2023). Congenital adrenal hyperplasia: Diagnostic approach. StatPearls Publishing.

273. Monaco C F (2023) Angioregression of the corpus luteum: vascular dynamics and functional implications Front Physiol 14:1254943.

274. Moore A M (2018) The rise of the term la ménopause and its shift from age-critical notions Feminist History of Medicine 32(2):226–244.

275. Morimont L, et al. (2021) History and reduction of VTE risk in combined oral contraceptives Hum Reprod Update 27(1):21–33.

276. Mukherjee S (2010) The Emperor of All Maladies: A Biography of Cancer. Scribner, New York, 592 p.

277. Mulders P., et al (2018). POMC: The physiological power of hormone processing. Physiological Reviews, 98(3).

278. Muniyappa R., et al. (2021). Assessing insulin sensitivity and resistance in humans. NCBI Bookshelf.

279. Murphy PA, et al (1999) Isoflavones in retail and institutional soy foods J Agric Food Chem 47(7):2697–2704.

280. Nagy B (2021) Progesterone production by the corpus luteum and its luteal phase dynamics Frontiers in Reproductive Health 12(8):101–113.

281. Nagy B. (2021). Physiological role and clinical implications of progesterone. International Journal of Molecular Sciences, 22(20):11039.

282. National recommendation (2022) Screening women with infertility for TSH and anti-TPO due to elevated risk of miscarriage Frontiers in Endocrinology 13:768363.

283. Neill JD (2006) Prolactin and reproductive hormones in human pregnancy Reproduction 131(4):583–592.

284. Nelson A L (2007) Transdermal and vaginal hormonal contraception Am J Obstet Gynecol 197(2):134.e1–134.e11.

285. NICE Guideline (2021) Ectopic pregnancy and miscarriage: diagnosis and initial management NICE Clinical Guideline NG126

286. Niswender G D, et al (2000) Mechanisms controlling the function and life span of the corpus luteum Physiol Rev 80(1):1–29.

287. North American Menopause Society (2011) The role of soy isoflavones in menopausal health: Report of The North American Menopause Society Menopause 18(7):732–753.

288. North American Menopause Society (2017) The 2017 hormone therapy position statement of The North American Menopause Society Menopause 24(7):728–753.

289. O'Shea J D, et al (1989) Cellular composition and morphological changes in the corpus luteum during luteolysis and early pregnancy in the cow J Reprod Fertil 85(2):483–496.

290. Odent M. (2013). The function of orgasms: The highways to transcendence. Pinter & Martin.

291. Ogasawara M, et al (1996) Prognostic significance of serum progesterone and estradiol in early pregnancy Hum Reprod 11(10):2300–2303.

292. Oliver G., Schäfer E. A. (1895). The Physiological Effects of Extracts of the Suprarenal Capsules. Journal of Physiology, 18(3):230–276.

293. Oliver R. (2023). Anatomy, Abdomen and Pelvis, Ovary Corpus Luteum. NCBI Bookshelf.

294. Owen R (1852) Description of parathyroid gland in Indian rhinoceros Transactions of the Zoological Society of London 4:189–190.

295. Panicker V., et al. (2008). A common variation in the phosphodiesterase 8B gene is associated with TSH levels and thyroid function. American Journal of Human Genetics, 82(6):1270–1280.

296. Papadopoulou-Marketou N (2023) Adrenal androgens and adrenopause Endotext NCBI Bookshelf.

297. Papanikolaou EG, et al (2005) hCG as a luteotropic agent in early pregnancy Reprod Biomed Online 11(4):427–433

298. Paravati S (2022) Catecholamines include dopamine, norepinephrine, and epinephrine StatPearls Publishing.

299. Parent A S, et al (2003) The timing of normal puberty and the age limits of sexual precocity: variations around the world, secular trends, and changes after migration Endocrine Reviews 24(5):668–693.

300. Parker WH (2007) Etiology, symptomatology, and diagnosis of uterine myomas Fertil Steril 87(4):725–736.

301. Parry C H (1825) Cases of exophthalmic goiter preceding Graves' disease Collections from the Unpublished Writings of Caleb Hillier Parry II:111–120.

302. Patisaul HB, Jefferson W (2010) The pros and cons of phytoestrogens Front Neuroendocrinol 31(4):400–419.

303. Peluso J J (2006) Multiplicity of progesterone's actions and receptors in the mammalian ovary Biol Reprod 75(1):2–8.

304. Pepe GJ, Albrecht ED (1995) Actions of placental and fetal adrenal steroid hormones in primate pregnancy Endocr Rev 16(5):608–648.

305. Petersen M. C., et al. (2018). Mechanisms of insulin action and insulin resistance. Physiological Reviews, 98(3).

306. Peterson C. M., et al. (2015). Impact of weight loss and exercise on reproductive hormones in women. The Journal of Clinical Endocrinology & Metabolism, 100(1).

307. Pierce J. G., Parsons T. F. (1981). Glycoprotein hormones: structure and function. Annual Review of Biochemistry, 50:465–495.

308. Piltonen TT, et al (2023) AMH as part of the diagnostic PCOS workup in large population-based study Hum Reprod 38(9):1655–1679

309. Piltonen TT, et al (2024) Validation of an AMH cutoff for PCOM diagnosis in PCOS JMIR Res Protoc 13(1):e48854.

310. Plant T M (1988) Neuroendocrine control of the onset of puberty in the rhesus monkey: regulation by GABA Journal of Endocrinology 119(2):175–184.

311. Pletzer B, Kronbichler M, Aichhorn M, et al (2019) The cycling brain: Menstrual cycle-dependent changes in brain activation and connectivity Neuropsychopharmacology 44(3):431–439.

312. Podolskyi V V, et al (2025) The effect of alcohol on sex hormone levels in fertile aged women Reproductive Endocrinology 55(2):145–152.

313. Poromaa I-S, Gingnell M (2014) Menstrual cycle influence on cognitive function and emotion recognition Front Psychol 5:386.

314. Prapas Y, et al (1998) Vaginal progesterone supplementation during early pregnancy in patients with unexplained recurrent miscarriage Hum Reprod 13(12):3484–3487.

315. Prevalence (1996) Hypothyroidism affects about 1.4–2% of women; Hashimoto's prevalent in 30–50 age group Lancet 348(9045):274–278.

316. Priedkalns J, Weber AF (1968) Functional morphology of the bovine corpus luteum. Biol Reprod 1(2):77–106.

317. Rabe T, Oettel M (2006) Clinical pharmacology of estradiol, estrone, estriol and progesterone in skin aging Horm Mol Biol Clin Investig 2(1):5–20.

318. Reed SD, et al (2009) Incidence of endometrial hyperplasia Am J Obstet Gynecol 200(6):678.e1–678.e6.

319. Reichrath J (2011) Hormones and skin: An endless story Dermatoendocrinol 3(3):111–112.

320. Reifenstein EC (1941) The relation of osteoporosis to the menopause Endocrinology 28(1):33–38.

321. Röder P.V., et al (2016). Pancreatic regulation of glucose homeostasis. Experimental & Molecular Medicine, 48(3): e219.

322. Rosenfield R L and Cooke D W (2019) The ovary and puberty in girls Endocrine Reviews 40(4):895–936.

323. Rosenfield R. L., Ehrmann D. A. (2016). The pathogenesis of polycystic ovary syndrome (PCOS): the hypothesis of PCOS as functional ovarian hyperandrogenism revisited. Endocrine Reviews, 37(5):467–520.

324. Rosner W. & Laurent M. R. (2016). SHBG regulation of androgen and estrogen action. Scientific Reports.

325. Rosner W. (2015). Free estradiol and sex hormone-binding globulin. Steroids.

326. Rousseau-Merck M. F., et al. (1991). The prolactin gene: structure, evolution and transcriptional regulation. Molecular and Cellular Endocrinology, 76(1–3):175–179.

327. Ruffaner-Hanson C et al (2022) Fetal HPA-axis adaptations to prenatal stress Frontiers in Neuroscience.

328. Russell J. M., Grossman A. B. (2010). The hypothalamus and pituitary gland: From anatomy to pathology. Clinical Medicine, 10(3):235–238.

329. Sadovsky R. (2001). Androgen deficiency in women: testosterone potency relative to DHEA and DHEA-S. American Family Physician.

330. Samaras K. (2006). Insulin levels in insulin resistance: phantom metabolic opera. Medical Journal of Australia, 185(3).

331. Sampson JA (1927) Peritoneal endometriosis due to the menstrual dissemination of endometrial tissue into the peritoneal cavity Am J Obstet Gynecol 14(4):422–469.

332. Sandström I V (1880) On a new gland in man and several animals ("glandulæ parathyroideæ") Upsala Läkareförenings Förhandlingar 17:385–416.

333. Santen RJ, et al (2010) Postmenopausal hormone therapy: An Endocrine Society scientific statement J Clin Endocrinol Metab 95(7 Suppl 1):s1–s66.

334. Santoro N., et al (1996). FSH and estradiol secretion in the perimenopause: changes in the hypothalamic–pituitary–ovarian axis. Menopause, 3(2):84–94.

335. Saper C. B., et al (2002). The need to feed: homeostatic and hedonic control of eating. Neuron, 36(2):199–211.

336. Saso S, et al (2011) Endometrial hyperplasia BMJ 343:d2650.

337. Sato F, et al (2002) Progesterone receptor expression in uterine leiomyoma and myometrium Steroids 67(8-9):741–751.

338. Sawchenko P. E., Swanson L. W. (1982). The organization of noradrenergic pathways from the brainstem to the paraventricular and supraoptic nuclei in the rat. Brain Research Reviews, 4(3):275–325.

339. Scherwitzl R, et al (2017) Contraceptive failure rates based on cycle analysis Contraception 95(5):420–426.

340. Schloffer H. (1907). Zur Frage der Operationen an der Hypophyse. Wiener Klinische Wochenschrift, 20:621–624.

341. Schumacher M. (2012). Progesterone synthesis in the nervous system. Frontiers in Neuroscience, 6:10.

342. Selye H (1956) The Stress of Life. McGraw-Hill, New York.

343. Serón-Ferré M, et al (1978) Role of hCG in regulation of the corpus luteum during early pregnancy in the rhesus monkey. Nature 272(5655):759–761.

344. Setchell KD, Cassidy A (1999) Dietary isoflavones: Biological effects and relevance to human health J Nutr 129(3):758S–767S.

345. Sharma R, et al (2021) Progesterone and estradiol modulate emotion processing during working memory tasks: an fMRI study Cogn Affect Behav Neurosci 21(6):1197–1211.

346. Sherman ME (2000) Theories of endometrial carcinogenesis: a multidisciplinary approach Mod Pathol 13(3):295–308.

347. Shifren JL, Davis SR (2017) Androgens in postmenopausal women: a review Menopause 24(8):970–979.

348. Short RV (1969) Implantation and the maternal recognition of pregnancy. Ciba Found Symp 2:2–26.

349. Simoni M., et al (1997). The follicle-stimulating hormone receptor: biochemistry, molecular biology, physiology, and pathophysiology. Endocrine Reviews, 18(6):739–773.

350. Simpson ER, MacDonald PC (1981) Endocrine physiology of the placenta. Annu Rev Physiol 43:163–188.

351. Sirtori CR (2001) Risks and benefits of soy phytoestrogens in cardiovascular diseases, cancer, climacteric symptoms and osteoporosis Drug Saf 24(9):665–682.

352. Sitruk-Ware R (2006) New progestagens for contraceptive use Hum Reprod Update 12(2):169–178.

353. Smith JF, et al (2013) Progesterone activates the principal Ca^{2+} channel of human sperm Proc Natl Acad Sci U S A 110(5):E288–E297.

354. Smith M F (1986) Recent advances in corpus luteum physiology J Anim Sci 63(1):1–10.

355. Solymoss S (2011) Combined oral contraceptives increase VTE risk three- to five-fold Thromb Res 128(6):636–639.

356. Somers S (2006) Ageless: The Naked Truth About Bioidentical Hormones. Crown Publishers, New York, 464 p.

357. Spencer C. A., et al (2007). National Health and Nutrition Examination Survey III: Thyroid-stimulating hormone levels in the US population (1988 to 1994). Journal of Clinical Endocrinology & Metabolism, 92(2):457–464.

358. Speroff L, Darney P D (2010) A clinical guide for contraception 5th ed. Lippincott Williams & Wilkins.

359. Speroff L., Glass R. H., Kase N. G. (1999). Clinical Gynecologic Endocrinology and Infertility. 6th ed. Baltimore: Lippincott Williams & Wilkins.

360. Steiner A Z (2011) Antimüllerian hormone as a predictor of natural fecundability Obstetrics & Gynecology 117(1):57–63.

361. Steiner A Z (2017) Biomarkers of ovarian reserve and fertility in older women JAMA 318(20):1986–1991.

362. Steiner A Z, et al (2017) Ovarian reserve tests and natural fertility in women aged 30–44 without infertility history JAMA 318(20):1986–1991.

363. Stenman UH, Tiitinen A, Alfthan H, Valmu L (2006) The classification, functions and clinical use of different isoforms of HCG Hum Reprod Update 12(6):769–784.

364. Stewart EA (2015) Uterine fibroids Lancet 379(9822):293–299.

365. Stocco C, et al (2007) The molecular control of corpus luteum formation, function, and regression Endocr Rev 28(1):117–149.

366. Stouffer RL (2006) The function and regulation of corpus luteum in the primate ovary Annu Rev Physiol 68:329–351.

367. Stuckey BG (2008) Female sexual function and dysfunction: impact of endocrinological, gynecological and psychological factors Int J Impot Res 20(1):35–44.

368. Stuenkel CA, et al (2015) Treatment of symptoms of the menopause: An Endocrine Society Clinical Practice Guideline J Clin Endocrinol Metab 100(11):3975–4011.
369. Stute P, et al (2018) The impact of micronized progesterone on breast cancer risk Climacteric 21(2):117–124.
370. Sumigama S, et al (2015) Progesterone triggers massive calcium influx into human sperm through activation of the sperm-specific calcium channel CatSper Mol Hum Reprod 21(7):563–571.
371. Sun S S et al. (2002) National estimates of the timing of sexual maturation and racial differences Pediatrics 110(5):911–919.
372. Sun X, et al (2017) The CatSper channel and its roles in male fertility: a systematic review Reprod Biol Endocrinol 15(1):1–14
373. Sundström-Poromaa I (2020) Progesterone, emotional memory, and limbic system modulation Neuroendocrinology 110(1):54–62.
374. Suzuki H., et al. (1965). Antithyroid antibodies in thyroid diseases. Journal of Clinical Endocrinology & Metabolism, 25(7):827–835.
375. Swaab D. F. (2004). The human hypothalamus: Basic and clinical aspects. Part I: Nuclei and anatomy. Handbook of Clinical Neurology, 79:1–54.
376. Swanson L. W. (2000). Cerebral hemisphere regulation of motivated behavior. Brain Research, 886(1–2):113–164.
377. Takahashi Y. (2018). Minimum values for midluteal plasma progesterone. Reproductive Biology and Endocrinology.
378. Takamine J. (1901). The Blood-Pressure Raising Principle of the Suprarenal Gland. American Journal of Physiology, 6(3):203–210.
379. Tamburrino L, et al (2020) Progesterone, spermatozoa and reproduction Rev Reprod (Review)
380. Tanbek K., et al (2024). Neurohormonal actions of glucagon in the central nervous system. European Review for Medical and Pharmacological Sciences, 28(1).
381. Tang HC (2024) Progesterone resistance in endometriosis—clinical implications J Clin Reprod Biol.
382. Taraborrelli S. (2015). Physiology, production and action of progesterone. Acta Obstetricia et Gynecologica Scandinavica, 94(12):1378–1386.
383. Tata J. R. (2005). One Hundred Years of Hormones. Journal of Endocrinology, 184(1):5–6.
384. te Velde E R and Pearson P L (2002) The variability of female reproductive ageing Human Reproduction Update 8(2):141–154.
385. Teal S (2021) Typical effectiveness of hormonal contraceptives JAMA 325(4):341–342.
386. Téblick A., et al (2021). The role of proopiomelanocortin in the ACTH–cortisol dissociation of sepsis. Critical Care, 25.

387. Teede HJ, et al (2023) International evidence-based guideline for the assessment and management of polycystic ovary syndrome Fertil Steril 120(4):767–793.

388. Thiboutot D, et al (2000) Activity of the type 1 5α-reductase exhibits regional differences in isolated sebaceous glands and whole skin J Invest Dermatol 114(6):1001–1006.

389. Tomaszewski JJ, et al (2010) Theca-lutein cysts associated with high hCG states: review and case report. Obstet Gynecol Int 2010:847041.

390. Trabert B, et al (2020) Progesterone and breast cancer risk in menopausal hormone therapy Endocr Rev 41(2):320–339.

391. Treloar A E, et al (1967) Variation of the human menstrual cycle through reproductive life International Journal of Fertility 12(1 Pt 2):77–126.

392. Trimble Cl, et al(2006) Concurrent endometrial carcinoma in women with a biopsy diagnosis of atypical endometrial hyperplasia: a Gynecologic Oncology Group study Cancer 106(4):812–819

393. Trompoukis C (2016) Bartolomeo Eustachio and early adrenal anatomy Hormones 15(2).

394. TSH and antibodies (2023) High anti-TPO levels correlate with recurrent pregnancy loss in women Reproductive Endocrinology 49(3):112–118.

395. Tsigos C., Chrousos G. P. (2002). Hypothalamic–pituitary–adrenal axis, neuroendocrine factors and stress. Journal of Psychosomatic Research, 53(4):865–871.

396. Tuckerman E, et al (2014) Progesterone and recurrent miscarriage Reprod Biomed Online 28(5):614–624.

397. Tulchinsky D, et al (1972) Plasma estriol in human pregnancy: I. Daily levels measured by radioimmunoassay during late gestation J Clin Endocrinol Metab 34(2):242–248.

398. Tulchinsky D, et al (1972) Plasma estrone, estradiol, estriol, progesterone, and 17-hydroxyprogesterone in human pregnancy Am J Obstet Gynecol 112(8):1095–1100.

399. U.S. Preventive Services Task Force (2015) Screening tests—TSH as primary test with follow-up free T4 for abnormal results Annals of Internal Medicine 162(14):158–165.

400. UCSF Health. (2023). Serum progesterone reference ranges during luteal phase and early pregnancy. UCSF Health Clinical Guidelines.

401. Ulrich N D (2019) Ovarian reserve testing: review of options and limitations Reproductive Biology and Endocrinology 17(1):35.

402. Ulrich-Lai Y. M., Herman J. P. (2009). Neural regulation of endocrine and autonomic stress responses. Nature Reviews Neuroscience, 10(6):397–409.

403. US Institute of Medicine (2000) Dietary Reference Intakes for iodine: RDA and UL values National Academies Press (US).

404. US National Toxicology Program (2021) Progesterone is reasonably anticipated to be a human carcinogen Report on Carcinogens, 15th Edition.

405. Uvnäs-Moberg K. (1998). Oxytocin may mediate the benefits of positive social interaction and emotions. Psychoneuroendocrinology, 23(8):819–835.

406. Vale W., et al (1981). Characterization of a 41-residue ovine hypothalamic peptide that stimulates secretion of corticotropin and β-endorphin. Science, 213(4514):1394–1397.

407. Valente R., et al. (2024). Interactions between the exocrine and the endocrine pancreas. Journal of Clinical Medicine, 13(4).

408. van Anders SM, Goldey KL, Bell SN (2014) Measurement of testosterone in human sexuality research: Methodological considerations Arch Sex Behav 43(2):231–250.

409. van der Linden M, et al (2011) Luteal phase support for assisted reproduction cycles Cochrane Database Syst Rev 10:CD009154.

410. van Hooff M H et al. (1998) Predictors of first menstruation and the relationship with body composition in adolescent Dutch girls European Journal of Endocrinology 139(1):75–83.

411. van Wingen G, et al (2007) A single dose of progesterone impairs memory for faces by reducing neural response in the amygdala Proc Natl Acad Sci U S A 104(39):16388–16393.

412. Vercellini P, et al (2009) Surgery for endometriosis-associated infertility: a pragmatic approach Hum Reprod 24(2):254–269.

413. Vercellini P, et al (2014) Endometriosis: pathogenesis and treatment Nat Rev Endocrinol 10(5):261–275.

414. Vermeulen A (2000) Age-related decline in adrenal androgen secretion Journal of Endocrinological Investigation 23(8):515–520.

415. VeryWell Health Editorial Team. (2017). Understanding estrogen's effects on the body. General Health Publication.

416. Wallace W H B and Kelsey T W (2010) Human ovarian reserve from conception to the menopause PLoS ONE 5(1):e8772.

417. Wang R., et al. (2014). High dietary fiber intake and reproductive hormone levels in women. American Journal of Clinical Nutrition, 99(4):930–938.

418. Wang X, et al (2003) Conception, early pregnancy loss and time to clinical pregnancy: A population-based prospective study Fertil Steril 79(3):577–584.

419. Warde K M (2023) Age-related changes in the adrenal cortex Journal of Endocrinological Science 7(9).

420. Watkins ES (1998) On the pill: a social history of oral contraceptives, 1950–1970 Johns Hopkins University Press.
421. Whitcomb B W, et al (2010) Ovarian function and cigarette smoking in the BioCycle Study Environment International 36(8):932–938.
422. Wierman ME, et al, Endocrine Society (2014) Androgen therapy in women: an Endocrine Society Clinical Practice Guideline J Clin Endocrinol Metab 99(10):3489–3510.
423. Wilson RA (1966) Feminine Forever. M. Evans & Company, New York, 198 p.
424. Wong F. C. K. (2019). Hyperandrogenism, elevated 17-hydroxyprogesterone. [Journal Title Placeholder].
425. World Health Organization / United Nations Scientific Committee (2006) Increased incidence of childhood thyroid cancer in Belarus, Russia, and Ukraine Bulletin of the WHO 84(12):919–924.
426. Writing Group for the Women's Health Initiative Investigators (2002) Risks and benefits of estrogen plus progestin in healthy postmenopausal women: Principal results from the Women's Health Initiative randomized controlled trial JAMA 288(3):321–333.
427. Yiallouris A et al (2019) Adrenal aging and implications on stress responses Frontiers in Endocrinology 10.
428. Young J M, McNeilly A S (2010) Theca: the forgotten cell of the ovarian follicle Reproduction 140(4):489–504.
429. Zhang M, et al (2023) The reference value of anti-Müllerian hormone to diagnose PCOS — impact of BMI Reprod Biol Endocrinol 21(1):15
430. Zhang P, Wang G (2023) Progesterone resistance in endometriosis: current evidence and mechanisms Int J Mol Sci 24(8):6992.
431. Zhang Q, et al (2010) Growth factors and uterine fibroids Endocrinol Metab Clin North Am 39(2):331–342.
432. Zhou J., et al (1997). Insulin-like growth factor I regulates gonadotropin responsiveness in the murine ovary. Molecular Endocrinology, 11(14):1924–1933.
433. Zondervan KT, et al (2020) Endometriosis N Engl J Med 382(13):1244–1256.
434. Zouboulis CC (2009) Endocrinology and skin: Lessons learned from acne Horm Res 71(2):75–81.

List of Olena Berezovska's books

1. Мій шлях до істини. Березовська О.А. — 90 стор. Самовидав. Івано-Франківськ, Україна, 1986.

2. Интернет: Мифы и реальность заработка. Березовская Е.П. — 110 стр. Несколько онлайн-публикаций. Украина-Россия-Беларусь, 2000. (ISBN 978-0-9867786-5-0)

3. Тысячиии... вопросов и ответов по гинекологии. Березовская Е.П. — 360 стр. Пресс-экспресс. Львов, Україна, 2008. (ISBN 966-8360-08-7)

4. Ангел. Березовская Е.П. — 94 стр. Электронная версия. Торонто, Канада, 2008. (ISBN 978-0-9867786-2-9)

5. День серебристого дождя. Березовская Е.П. — 107 стр. Электронная версия. Торонто, Канада, 2008. (ISBN 978-0-9867786-3-6)

6. Настольное пособие для беременных женщин. Березовская Е.П. — 400 стр. Канада-Украина, 2010. (ISBN 978-0-9867786-1-2)

7. Подготовка к беременности. Березовская Е.П. — 200 стр. International Academy of Healthy Life. Канада-Украина, 2011. (ISBN 978-0-9867786-0-5)

8. Гормонотерапия в акушерстве и гинекологии: иллюзии и реальность. Березовская Е.П. — 600 стр. International Academy of Healthy Life. Канада, 2013. (ISBN 978-0-9867786-6-7)

9. 9 месяцев счастья. Настольное пособие для беременных женщин. Березовская Е.П. — 596 стр. ЭКСМО. Москва, Россия, 2015. (ISBN 978-5-699-80102-2)

10. Настільний посібник для вагітних. Березовська О.П. — 400 стор. Электронна версія. International Academy of Healthy Life. Торонто, Канада, 2016. (ISBN 978-0-9867786-1-2)

11. Підготовка до вагітності. Березовська О.П. — 205 стор. Электронна версія. International Academy of Healthy Life. Торонто, Канада, 2016. (ISBN 978-0-9867786-0-5)

12. Посібник для вагітних. Березовська О.П. — 392 стор. Манускрипт. Львів, Україна, 2016. (ISBN 978-966-2400-55-7)

13. 1000 вопросов и ответов по гинекологии. Березовская Е.П. — 432 стр. ЭКСМО. Москва, Россия, 2017. (ISBN 978-5-699-80101-5)

14. Дочки-матери: Все, о чем вам не рассказывала ваша мама и чему стоит научить свою дочь. Березовская Е.П. — 288 стр. ЭКСМО. Москва, Россия, 2018. (ISBN 978-5-04-090021-3)

15. 9 місяців щастя. Березовська О.П. — 576 стор. BookChef. Київ, Україна, 2018. (ISBN 978-617-7559-18-3)

16. 9 месяцев счастья (второе издание). Настольное пособие для беременных женщин. Березовская Е.П. — 596 стр. ЭКСМО. Москва, Россия, 2019. (ISBN 978-5-04-098981-2)

17. Это все гормоны! Березовская Е.П. — 410 стр. ЭКСМО. Москва, Россия, 2019. (ISBN 978-5-04-101870-2)

18. Малыш, ты скоро? Березовская Е.П. — 384 стр. ЭКСМО. Москва, Россия, 2019. (ISBN 978-5-04-103359-0)

19. Когда ты будешь готова. Березовская Е.П. — 348 стр. ЭКСМО. Москва, Россия, 2020. (ISBN 978-5-04-116932-9)

20. Здравствуй, малыш. Березовская Е.П. — 320 стр. ЭКСМО. Москва, Россия, 2021. (ISBN 978-5-04-121120-2)

21. Педіатрія: у 3-х т. Т. 3: підручник для студ. вищих мед. навч. закладів IV рівня акред. Катілов О., Варзарь А., Валіуліс А., Дмитрієв Д., та ін. — 656 стор. Нова Книга. Вінниця, Україна, 2022. (ISBN 978-966-382-931-9)

22. 9 місяців щастя. Посібник для вагітних (оновлене й доповнене видання). Березовська О.П. — 624 стор. BookChef. Київ, Україна, 2023. (ISBN 978-617-548-122-6)

23. Коли тобі 35+. Як завагітніти й народити дитину. Березовська О.П. — 256 стор. BookChef. Київ, Україна, 2023. (ISBN 978-617-548-124-0)

24. Когда тебе 35+. Как забеременеть и родить ребенка. Березовская Е.П. — 290 стр. International Academy of Healthy Life. Торонто, Канада, 2024. (ISBN 978-0-9867786-7-4)

25. Angel. Olena Berezovska. — 256 p. International Academy of Healthy Life. Toronto, Canada, 2024. (ISBN 978-0-9867786-8-1)

26. Ангел. Березовська О.П. — 270 стор. International Academy of Healthy Life. Торонто, Канада, 2024. (ISBN 978-0-9867786-9-8)

27. Grandma Lena's Bedtime Stories. Olena Berezovska. — 154 p. International Academy of Healthy Life. Toronto, Canada, 2024. (ISBN 978-1-0691603-0-0)

28. Привіт, малюк! Як пройти четвертий триместр без турбот і хвилювань. Березовська О.П. — 290 стор. International Academy of Healthy Life. Торонто, Канада, 2024. (ISBN 978-1-0691603-3-1)

29. Growing Up Strong: A Guide to Girls' Health and Well-Being. Olena Berezovska. — 422 p. International Academy of Healthy Life. Toronto, Canada, 2025. (ISBN 978-1-0691603-4-8)

30. Вечірні казочки бабусі Олени. Березовська О.П. 180 стор. International Academy of Healthy Life. Toronto, Canada, 2025 (ISBN: 978-1-0691603-1-7)

31. Вечерние сказки бабушки Лены. Березовская Е.П. 172 стр. International Academy of Healthy Life. Toronto, Canada, 2025 (ISBN: 978-1-0691603-2-4).

32. The Curious Escapades of a Corpse Named Jack. Book 1. Olena Berezovska. 148 p. International Academy of Healthy Life. Toronto, Canada, 2025 (ISBN: 978-1-0691603-5-5)

33. Основи здоров'я дівчаток: Практичний путівник для батьків. Березовська О..570 стор. International Academy of Healthy Life. Toronto, Canada, 2025 (ISBN: 978-1-0691603-6-2)

34. The Curious Escapades of a Corpse Named Jack. Book 2. Olena Berezovska. 112 p. International Academy of Healthy Life. Toronto, Canada, 2025 (ISBN: 978-1-0691603-7-9)

35. Hormonal Intelligence: How Hormones Shape Health and Well-being. Olena Berezovska. 475 p. International Academy of Healthy Life. Toronto, Canada, 2025 (ISBN 978-1-0691603-8-6)

36. Все про гормони: Таємна мова вашого тіла. Олена Березовська. 460 с. International Academy of Healthy Life. Торонто, Канада, 2025 (ISBN 978-1-0691603-9-3)

37. Дивовижні пригоди трупа на ім'я Джек: Книга 1. Олена Березовська. 180 с. International Academy of Healthy Life. Торонто, Канада, 2025 (ISBN 978-1-0694544-0-9)

38. Підготовка до вагітності: Посібник з усвідомленого батьківства. Олена Березовська. 468 с. International Academy of Healthy Life. Торонто, Канада, 25 травня 2025 (ISBN 978-1-0694544-41-6)

39. DIY Bestseller: How to Write, Publish, and Market Your Book in the AI Era. Olena Berezovska. 432 p. International Academy of Healthy Life. Toronto, Canada, 2025. (ISBN 978-1-0694544-2-3)

40. Mind Over Muscle: A Journal for Teen Athletes. Olena Berezovska. 56 p. International Academy of Healthy Life. Toronto, Canada, 2025. (ISBN 978-1-0694544-3-0)

www.ingramcontent.com/pod-product-compliance
Lightning Source LLC
Chambersburg PA
CBHW052118270326
41930CB00012B/2668